CORONARY PRESSURE

Coronary Pressure

Second Edition

by

Nico H. J. Pijls
Catharina Hospital, Eindhoven,
The Netherlands

and

Bernard De Bruyne
Cardiovascular Center, Aalst,
Belgium

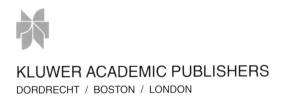

KLUWER ACADEMIC PUBLISHERS
DORDRECHT / BOSTON / LONDON

Library of Congress Cataloging-in-Publication Data

Pijls, Nico H. J., 1952-
      Coronary pressure / by Nico H.J. Pijls and Bernard de Bruyne.-- 2nd ed.
         p. ; cm. -- (Developments in cardiovascular medicine ; v. 227)
      Includes bibliographical references and index.
      ISBN 0-7923-6170-9 (HB : alk. paper)
         1. Coronary artery stenosis--Diagnosis. 2. Blood pressure--Measurement. 3. Coronary
      circulation. I. Bruyne, Bernard de. II. Title. III. Series.
         [DNLM: 1. Coronary Vessels--physiology. 2. Blood Flow Velocity. 3. Blood Pressure.
      4. Coronary Circulation. 5. Coronary Vessels--physiopathology. WG 300 P634c 2000]
      RC685.C58 P54 2000
      616.1'23--dc21

                                                                    99-089548
      ISBN 0-7923-6170-9

Published by Kluwer Academic Publishers,
P.O. Box 17, 3300 AA Dordrecht, The Netherlands.

Sold and distributed in North, Central and South America
by Kluwer Academic Publishers,
101 Philip Drive, Norwell, MA 02061, U.S.A.

In all other countries, sold and distributed
by Kluwer Academic Publishers,
P.O. Box 322, 3300 AH Dordrecht, The Netherlands.

Printed on acid-free paper

Printed in the Netherlands.

This book is dedicated to our wives and children,

Francine
Marjolijn, Reinier, and Margot

Françoise
Géraldine, Aurélie, Martin, and Ségolène

Preface

A little bit more than two years after the first edition, we are pleased to publish the second edition of this book. More than half of the chapters have been remodeled and completed as the result of technical improvements and recently acquired clinical data. During these two years, the number of coronary pressure measurements performed worldwide both during diagnostic and interventional procedures has increased almost exponentially. Most of the initial problems associated with this new approach have been overcome. Many colleagues have explored new research avenues and in many catheterization laboratories the method has matured from a research toy to a clinical tool. Classical indications such as the intermediate stenosis and guidance of PTCA or stent implantation, have been largely extended and coronary pressure measurement has proven to be useful in multivessel disease, diffuse disease, long and serial stenosis, after myocardial infarction, and in many other diagnostic and interventional situations encountered in the catheterization laboratory. Quite unexpectedly, this approach has also enforced the ties with our surgical colleagues in the selection of patients suitable for minimal invasive surgery or hybride revascularization. Also in mild and intermediate left main disease, there is a role for coronary pressure measurement in the process of decision making.

We would like to express our gratitude to all those many colleagues who trusted and applied this new approach for the benefit of their patients.

Aalst,   Eindhoven,
Bernard De Bruyne.   Nico H.J.Pijls.

March, 2000.

Table of Contents (overview)

Table of Contents

List of Abbreviations

CFR	: (absolute) coronary flow reserve
CFVR	: coronary flow velocity reserve
ΔP	: transstenotic pressure gradient
ΔP_{rest}	: transstenotic pressure gradient at rest
ΔP_{max}	: transstenotic pressure gradient after administration of a maximum vasodilatory (hyperemic) stimulus
FFR	: fractional flow reserve
FFR_{cor}	: coronary fractional flow reserve
FFR_{myo}	: myocardial fractional flow reserve
IHDVPS	: instantaneous hyperemic diastolic velocity pressure slope
IVUS	: intravascular ultrasound
LAD	: left anterior descending coronary artery
LM	: left main coronary artery
LCX	: left circumflex coronary artery
MLD	: minimal luminal diameter
P_a	: aortic pressure
P_d	: distal coronary pressure or transstenotic coronary pressure
P_v	: central venous pressure
P_w	: coronary occlusion (wedge) pressure
P_{fem}	: femoral artery pressure
PET	: positron emission tomography
QCA	: quantitative coronary angiography
Q_c	: collateral blood flow at maximum vasodilation
Q_s	: coronary blood flow at maximum vasodilation
Q	: myocardial blood flow at maximum vasodilation
Q^N	: normal maximum myocardial blood flow
Q_s^N	: normal maximum coronary artery blood flow
Q_c/Q^N	: fractional collateral blood flow
$(Q_c/Q^N)_{max}$	: maximum recruitable fractional collateral blood flow, at coronary artery occlusion
RFR	: relative flow reserve
R	: minimal resistance of the myocardial vascular bed
R_c	: minimal resistance of the collateral vascular bed
R_s	: minimal resistance of the epicardial coronary artery

Chapter 1

INTRODUCTION

When evaluating and treating patients with a coronary artery stenosis, cardiologists must answer three important questions. As a physiologist: "What is the effect of this stenosis on coronary blood flow and myocardial function?"; as a clinician: " Is this lesion responsible for the patient's symptoms?"; and finally as an interventionalist: "Will revascularization of this artery improve the patient?"

Fundamentally, the answer to these questions can be given to a large extent by measuring coronary pressure. That is the rationale of writing this book.

1.1   Historical overview.

Andreas Gruentzig and most interventional cardiologists in the early days of PTCA, had the intuitive feeling that pressure measurement could help to establish the severity of a coronary stenosis and to monitor the progress and result of a coronary intervention. At that time, measuring coronary pressure by the balloon catheter was part of a standard procedure. A residual transstenotic gradient of less than 15 mmHg was generally considered as a good result. Later, however, it turned out that measuring these (resting) gradients with balloon catheters was inaccurate an only had a limited prognostic value. Moreover, because there was no consistent theory to correlate pressure measurements to blood flow, the interest in measuring coronary pressure faded and disappeared almost completely with the introduction of new balloon catheters not intended for pressure measurement.

Following the rapid progress in quantitative coronary angiography (QCA) in the mid- and late 1980's, many cardiologists and cardiac surgeons hoped that anatomic information alone, enhanced by the new digital imaging techniques, would become so comprehensive that there would be no further need for physiologic assessment of stenosis severity and physiologic confirmation of angioplasty results. Fifteen years later, however, the opposite is true and it has turned out that QCA could not fulfill its promise to predict the functional significance of a coronary stenosis. Clinicians have realized that direct physiologic information about pressure and flow is necessary for complete evaluation and understanding of coronary artery disease. Guide wire based physiologic techniques for the assessment of coronary blood flow velocity and distal coronary pressure have become widely available now and can be routinely implemented in both diagnostic and interventional procedures. A consistent theory about the meaning and interpretation of coronary pressure has become available with a sound scientific background, which has overcome the limitations of pressure measurements in the early days and which has been thoroughly validated step by step, both in animals and humans.

At the same time, major technical progress has been made with respect to pressure monitoring guide wires. Presently, several reliable 0.014-in pressure guide wires are available which can be used as first line guide wires and enable continuous coronary pressure recording throughout the procedure. At present, the additional value of these physiologic measurements above anatomic assessment alone, is beyond any doubt. Based upon the valuable insights obtained, its prognostic relevance, and the rapid technical progress, an increasing number of catheterization laboratories uses coronary pressure as an integral part of their diagnostic and therapeutic armamentarium.

The purpose of this book is to give a practical, but comprehensive overview of the rapidly developing and exciting field of coronary pressure measurements.

1.2   How to use this book.

Once having performed coronary pressure measurement in 10 or 20 patients, its performance and interpretation becomes extremely easy and the measurements can be implemented in routine diagnostic and interventional procedures with minimal disturbance of the daily routine, minimal extra time, and minimal costs.

Therefore, one of the background considerations in writing this book, is to provide a practical manual for the cardiologist, who likes to get started quickly with coronary pressure measurements without spending too much time on the theory. By just reading paragraph 4.1 to 4.4, chapter 5, chapter 6, and chapter 17, a first quick acquaintance with coronary pressure and fractional flow reserve is made.

For a more extensive physiologic background of coronary pressure interpretation and fractional flow reserve, reading of chapter 2 and paragraph 4.5 and 4.6, is advised.

The place of coronary pressure measurements among other anatomic and physiologic invasive techniques, is outlined in chapter 3.

For a better understanding of the cut-off points used for clinical decision-making and to monitor interventions, as well as for applications in a variety of pathologic conditions chapter 11 to 15 should be read.

The interventionalist, interested in the in-depth validation of the different and unique features of fractional flow reserve, should read chapter 7 to 10.

Finally, to understand the potential of fractional flow reserve to distinguish separately the contribution of coronary and collateral blood flow to maximum myocardial flow, the last part of chapter 4 and chapter 16 can be studied.

In several chapters some sections have been printed with a smaller font. These sections contain issues which may be important but can be skipped without affecting the general understanding of this book.

At last, a few good examples often better clarify an issue than a lot of theory. Therefore, a number of selected case studies have been compiled at the end of this book (chapter 17). Reading of these examples is strongly recommended for the cardiologist just starting coronary pressure measurements.

1.3   Acknowledgements.

The principles described in this book would not have been developed and the book would never have been written without the continuous support of a number of people.

In the first place we are much indebted to some colleagues, older and wiser than we are, who inspired and stimulated us in developing the theory and translating basic physiologic principles into the everyday practice of cardiology: K. Lance Gould and Richard L. Kirkeeide (Houston, TX), Patrick W. Serruys (Rotterdam, NL), Paul Yock (Stanford, CA), Morton Kern (St.Louis, MO), Mamdouh I.H. El Gamal (Eindhoven, NL), and Guy R. Heyndrickx and William Wijns (Aalst, BE).

We owe a lot to our friends and colleagues at the Catharina Hospital, Eindhoven, NL and the Cardiovascular Center Aalst, BE, for their never fading support, stimulation, and sympathy. These people created the indispensable atmosphere in which the development and maturation of the principles and practice of coronary pressure measurements could take place. We like to mention Erik Andries, Hans Bonnier, Cees Joost Botman, Frank Bracke, Pedro Brugada, Jan Melle van Dantzig, Marc Goethals, Jacques Koolen, Albert Meijer, Rolf Michels, Paul Nellens, Walter Paulus, Kathinka Peels, and Dorus Relik, who were actively involved in the many studies and gave us the room and time necessary for further developments.

We also like to give special thanks to the technicians and nurses working in our catheterization laboratories. We clearly realize how much the quality of patient care and research depends on their everlasting enthusiasm and assistance.

A special word of thank should be given to Jozef Bartunek, Jan Willem Bech, and Clara Hanekamp for their help in collecting and analyzing patients data and their great contribution to several of the studies described in this book. We are sincerely grateful to Neal G. Uren (Edinburgh, UK) for correcting the manuscript.

The round-the-clock availability of Guy Van Dael, medical photographer, and Jan Kalter, clinical engineer, is particularly appreciated, as is the unequaled help of our fabulous secretaries, Anne Hol and Jozefa Cano, who prepared the manuscript of this book.

Last, but not least, we owe an immeasurable debt to our wives and children to whom this book is dedicated and whose unwavering love and affection keep our hearts beating.

Chapter 2

THE CORONARY CIRCULATION

As this book deals with the relationship between coronary pressure and myocardial blood flow, some basic anatomic and physiologic concepts should be well understood. This chapter does not claim to be an extensive review of the physiology of the coronary circulation but aims at providing the reader with the anatomic and physiologic background required to understand the principles, advantages, and limitations of the concept of pressure-derived fractional flow reserve.

For more detailed considerations of this subject, the reader is referred to recent comprehensive reviews[1-6].

2.1 The coronary tree.

2.1.1 The arterial system.

The inlet of the coronary arterial system consists of two major vessels which are the first to branch from the aorta. In the dog, the right ventricle is perfused by the right coronary artery while the left coronary artery perfuses the interventricular septum and the free wall of the left ventricle. Yet, in humans, the inferior part of the septum and the left ventricular free wall are perfused by the right coronary artery in approximately 80% of cases (right dominance). The arterial tree consists of large arteries ranging from several mm to 400 μm and branching like a tree into small arteries and arterioles (with a diameter < 400 μm). The arterioles are the smallest arterial conduits surrounded by smooth muscle cells. Although the distinction between large and smaller arteries is somewhat arbitrary, it corresponds to physiological and clinical differences.

Large arteries include the left main stem, the right coronary artery, the left anterior descending artery, the left circumflex artery, and their diagonal, marginal, and septal branches. The latter penetrate straight into the septum and are completely surrounded by myocardial tissue. All other large arteries run over the epicardial surface of the heart. Therefore, in this book these large arteries will be referred to as *epicardial arteries*. Epicardial arteries follow a regular, dichotomous branching system. The edges of the vascular lumen of these vessels are sharply delineated at coronary angiography. These epicardial vessels can be the site of atherosclerotic narrowings which are the main cause of exercise-induced myocardial ischemia and may lead to thrombotic occlusion and myocardial infarction. The large coronary arteries are the only part of the coronary circulation amenable to mechanical revascularization.

Normal epicardial coronary arteries do not create any significant resistance to blood flow. Even at high flow rates induced by intravenous infusion of adenosine, only a negligible pressure difference exists between central aorta and the most distal part of angiographically smooth epicardial coronary arteries in humans[7]. This corroborates data obtained in beating cat hearts (figure 2.1) showing that resistance to coronary blood flow is negligible in arteries larger than 400 μm[8]. The epicardial coronary arteries, therefore, are also called *conduit* or *conductance vessels*. As will be discussed in the next chapters, the absence of a pressure drop along a normal epicardial coronary artery during maximal vasodilation is an essential prerequisite for the concept of pressure-derived fractional flow reserve.

The arteries of less than 400 μm will be referred to in this book as *resistive vessels*. At coronary angiography they are not clearly delineated but appear as a myocardial *blush* of contrast medium. Resistive vessels are able to vasodilate under physiological and pharmacological stress. This modulation of resistance is paramount for matching myocardial blood flow to variable energy requirements. The ability of coronary resistive vessels to vasodilate may be impaired before the development of angiographically visible atherosclerosis [9-11]. Often, the vasodilatory reserve is also abnormal in angiographically normal arteries in patients with remote coronary artery disease[12]. This latter point will be further discussed in chapter 10.

The classical two-compartments model of the coronary circulation (*conduit* and *resistive* vessels) does not account for the heterogeneity in the distribution of coronary resistance with respect to regulation of coronary blood flow[13]. Based on sequential differences in the response to shear stress and adenosine, resistive vessels in the human coronary circulation have been divided into two groups:

The proximal compartment consists of the pre-arteriolar vessels with a diameter ranging from 100-400 μm. Their tone is controlled by coronary

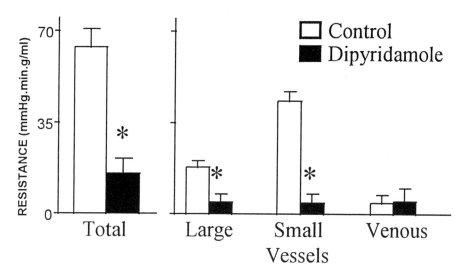

Figure 2.1 *Resistance distribution in the cat coronary arterial tree as established by Chilian. The data are grouped in ranges of diameters. Each group forms a compartment. In this study, the arterial compartment contains the arteries with diameters above 170 μm, and the venous compartment, the venules and veins with diameters larger than 150 μm. The small vessel compartment contains arteries smaller than 170 μm, and the capillaries and venules smaller than 150 μm. The resistance was calculated in control conditions with intact vasomotor tone (white bars) and after administration of dipyridamole (black bars). Most of the resistance during autoregulation is within the microvessels. The resistance of the "large compartment" was mainly provided by small arteries with diameters up to 400 μm. During infusion of dipyridamole, the contribution of the small vessels to total resistance decreased to the level of the resistance of the venous system. The resistance distribution during the dilated state is fairly even over the compartments. (From Chilian et al[8], with permission of the author and the American Physiological Society)*

flow, distending pressure and myogenic tone, and modulated by the autonomic nervous system and endothelial function.

The distal compartment consists of arterioles with a diameter of less than 100 μm. They are influenced primarily by the perfusion pressure at the origin of the vessel and by myocardial metabolism.

2.1.2   Capillaries.

The capillary bed does not have a branching structure but consists of a network of interconnected vessels of similar diameter. The myocytes are organized within the capillary network and are connected to the capillary wall by collagen struts[14]. The diameter of the capillaries is approximately 5 μm[15-17]. However, the capillary bed is distensible and will be influenced by its inner pressure and by the contractile state of the adjacent myocytes[17]. The capillary density reported in the human heart approximates 3500/mm², and appears to be lower in the subendocardium than in the subepicardium[17-20]. The distance between two capillaries averages 17 μm. The normal diameter of a myocyte is 18 μm and increases up to 30 μm with hypertrophy. Each myocyte is lined by at least one capillary. This close anatomic structure suggests an intense functional link.

2.1.3   Collaterals.

Collaterals are vessels structured as a connecting network between different coronary arteries. Their function is to bypass obstructions in arterial branches and, thus, to protect myocardial tissue that otherwise would become ischemic. Unlike a generally accepted impression that collaterals were the privilege of only a happy few, it is now well recognized that rudimentary connecting vessels are always present at birth. They are probably remnants of the embryonal arterial network and may develop progressively under the influence of various stimuli.

Collaterals growth.
Because the presence of well developed collaterals correlates strongly with recurrent myocardial ischemia, it has been postulated that the ischemic myocardial cells produce angiogenic growth factors. However, collateral growth, expansion, and maturation take one month whereas ischemia is only transient. In addition, at least in the canine heart, collateral growth takes place in the subepicardium while ischemia has a subendocardial predilection. Finally, it is well known that the collateral "stem" which connects the collateral network with the normal arteries is surrounded by normal tissue that does not belong to the region of the occluded artery. For these reasons, collateral growth does not seem to be determined by the myocardium in its direct vicinity[21]. The role of the pressure gradient between the normal and the

stenotic vascular regions appears to be more important than initially believed. The pressure difference induces an increase in blood flow velocity in the rudimentary anastomoses and connections. The increased shear stress in turn activates the endothelium, leading to the expression of adhesive molecules, subsequent monocyte attachment, and production of growth factors.

The combination of heparin and ischemia has been demonstrated in animal models to enhance collateral growth and function[22-25]. Similarly, pharmacologic enhancement of collateral growth has been achieved in dogs by the heparin-binding vascular endothelial growth factor[26]. Recent data suggest that exercise and low molecular weight heparin therapy may also enhance collateral function in humans[27].

A variety of growth factors is in the stage of clinical testing now and although clear increase in myocardial perfusion by these factors could not be convincingly demonstrated so far in humans, it is generally believed that different growth factors and gene-transfer techniques will constitute a new, exciting, and promising way to treat coronary artery disease in the first decade of the new millennium.

Structure and localization of collaterals.
Unlike the canine heart where collaterals are restricted to the subepicardial zone, a predominant localization in the human heart is also the subendocardium where a dense plexus develops. The histological structure of these vessels is that of abnormally thin-walled arteries. Macroscopically identifiable interconnecting larger vessels have a normal arterial wall structure but show often extensive subintimal proliferation[28].

Protective role of collaterals.
In the presence of an epicardial coronary narrowing, collateral channels develop, and the contribution of collateral flow to myocardial flow increases progressively. Hence, it is obvious that in the presence of coronary artery disease, myocardial blood flow represents the sum of coronary and collateral flow, and that myocardial blood flow can be strikingly different from coronary flow. At the extreme, in case of total coronary occlusion, myocardial flow is provided only via collaterals. Even though the cardiologist is prone to focus on the coronary artery, from the point of view of the patient, myocardial blood flow is the most important parameter, whether it is provided by the epicardial vessel or by collaterals. It is now well accepted that collateral circulation has a protective effect with respect to left ventricular damage, attenuation of myocardial ischemia during stress, and patient survival. In patients with a totally occluded but fully collateralized artery, myocardial function is often

normal at rest. Moreover, in some of these patients myocardial flow reserve as determined by positron emission tomography, can be even close to normal[29]. Our own data on the protective role of collaterals against left ventricular dysfunction and symptoms of ischemia in patients with coronary artery disease will be discussed in chapter 16.

2.2   Coronary flow mechanics.

In contrast to all other organs, coronary arterial blood flow occurs predominantly during diastole. As shown in figure 2.2 coronary arterial blood flow at rest is low during systole, while it is high during diastole. At maximum vasodilation, diastolic flow further increases and also some increase in systolic flow occurs. Generally, the systolic component at hyperemia is less than 25% of total flow. The reverse occurs with coronary venous blood flow which is high during systole and low during diastole[30,31]. Therefore, although coronary perfusion is needed to sustain myocardial contraction, the latter seems to be an impeding factor for coronary perfusion. This impeding effect has been ascribed to ventricular pressure or to varying myocardial elastance.

Effects of ventricular pressure.
The difference in right and left coronary flow signals has provided evidence that the mechanisms of systolic inhibition was related to the pressure in the ventricles. In a small right coronary artery, blood flow is equally distributed over the heart cycle. In a large right coronary artery with large branches to the left ventricle, a flow pattern is seen which is more alike the left coronary artery with only little systolic and predominantly diastolic blood flow at rest. The concept of systolic inhibition of blood flow by intraventricular pressure was also supported by the observation that systolic flow was interrupted in the right coronary artery in case of pulmonary hypertension[32]. The inverse relationship between transmural myocardial flow distribution and tissue pressure also reinforces this concept[33].

Time varying elastance.
Incidental observations that coronary flow was also pulsatile when the heart was beating but empty as occurs during bypass surgery, were ascribed to tissue pressure generated by the large deformation of the ventricle in this condition[34]. Confirming previous experiments, it has been recently evidenced that the pulsatility of coronary arterial blood flow is related more to the contractility of the ventricular wall than to the left ventricular pressure generated in it[35-37]. This is illustrated in figure 2.2. Accordingly, the impediment to coronary blood flow during systole was ascribed to a direct interaction between myocyte contraction and myocardial microvessels. This theory is supported by the finding that flow in atrial arteries is interrupted during atrial contraction although this inhibition is unlikely to be caused by the atrial pressure[38]. Yet, this theory is at odds with the different flow velocity patterns in the right and left coronary arteries as well as with the fact that myocardial flow in the subendocardium is inhibited by cardiac contraction in contrast to the perfusion of the subepicardium.

2.3   Regulation of myocardial blood flow.

Mechanical and electrical activity of the heart are supported by myocardial perfusion which represents approximately 5% of cardiac output under baseline conditions. In case of normal epicardial coronary arteries, coronary flow equals myocardial flow or "nutritive flow". Even under resting conditions the myocardial oxygen demand is high (8-10 ml/min/100g of tissue) as compared to that of skeletal muscles (0.5 ml/min/100g)[39]. The high density of coronary capillaries is optimally suited to meet high oxygen consumption. Nevertheless, extraction of oxygen by the myocardium is close to its maximum, much higher than in any other organ, and oxygen saturation of the coronary sinus venous blood is low (close to 20%) . Hence, since oxygen extraction cannot increase much further, the coronary circulation can only meet increasing oxygen demand by increasing blood flow. A close linear relation, therefore, exists between metabolic demand and myocardial blood flow[40]. Myocardial blood

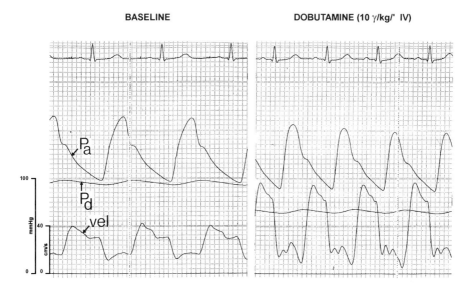

Figure 2.2 *Simultaneous aortic pressure* (P_a), *distal coronary pressure* (P_d), *and coronary flow velocity (Vel) recordings in a stenotic left anterior descending coronary artery. Coronary blood flow occurs predominantly during diastole. During administration of dobutamine an increase in flow velocity is observed during diastole, while almost no increase in systolic flow velocity occurs. Since aortic pressure remains almost unchanged, these pressure tracings suggest that the pulsatility of coronary artery blood flow is related more to the contractility of the left ventricular wall than to left ventricular pressure itself.*

flow is regulated by a changing balance of interacting, cumulative, and non-linear control mechanisms. These include an intrinsic autoregulation, external compressive forces, neural regulation, metabolic demand, and endothelial factors.

2.3.1 Autoregulation.

Autoregulation refers to the intrinsic mechanisms which maintain blood flow constant when the perfusion pressure varies[2]. Myocardial perfusion is maintained relatively constant when perfusion pressure varies from 70 to 130 mmHg in anesthetized dogs[41]. In conscious, chronically instrumented dogs, however, the lower limit of autoregulation is 40 mmHg[42]. When coronary perfusion pressure falls below this limit, small additional reductions in pressure are associated with marked reduction in both myocardial flow and wall thickening. Recently, we studied a series of 26 patients with an isolated lesion in the proximal left anterior descending coronary artery, a normal resting electrocardiogram and normal left ventricular function as assessed by left ventricular angiography[43]. Distal coronary perfusion pressure was measured with a pressure guide wire and myocardial perfusion was assessed by positron emission tomography and oxygen labeled water. The main results are given in figure 2.3. Myocardial perfusion remains relatively constant over a wide range of perfusion pressure. The lower limit, i.e. the lowest distal coronary pressure recorded in a patient with normal left ventricular function, was 46 mmHg. These data demonstrate that the autoregulatory range in humans is as large as that reported in conscious dogs and ranges from 45 to 130 mmHg approximately. Several mechanisms to explain autoregulation have been proposed.

Myogenic mechanism. This theory supposes that the increase of vasomotor tone opposing a transient vascular stretch is secondary to an increase in perfusion pressure. Although, it has been observed in other organs, no clear evidence of myogenic responses in the control of coronary blood flow has been provided. In the coronary circulation, evidence for myogenic mechanisms in the control of coronary blood flow is extremely difficult to obtain since even short-lasting changes in coronary blood flow alter myocardial metabolism. Thus, it is almost impossible to distinguish myogenic from metabolic control of coronary blood flow.

Local metabolic regulation. This theory is, at present, the most favored one. Even when the heart is cut-off from external control mechanisms (nerves, hormonal, and humoral factors) its ability to adjust blood flow to its metabolic requirements remains almost unaffected. This is due to a number of factors including metabolites released from the working myocardium which act to provide an appropriate arteriolar tone. Several metabolic mediators have been studied and include oxygen, carbon dioxide, hyperosmolarity, changes in H^+, K^+, and Ca^{++} concentration, and adenosine. The latter has been studied extensively. It is one of the most potent coronary dilators [44], and diffuses rapidly from the cardiomyocyte cytosol into the interstitial space [45]. A good correlation was found between myocardial oxygen consumption, the release of adenosine, and coronary flow in vitro[46]. However, neither reactive hyperemia following complete coronary occlusion nor resting coronary flow are altered by adenosine deaminase[47-49]. Likewise, the administration of the adenosine antagonist aminophylline does not change the flow increment induced by atrial pacing in humans[50]. Therefore it is generally thought that adenosine is not the only factor for coronary flow autoregulation. The role of nitric oxyde (NO) is discussed in paragraph 2.3.4.

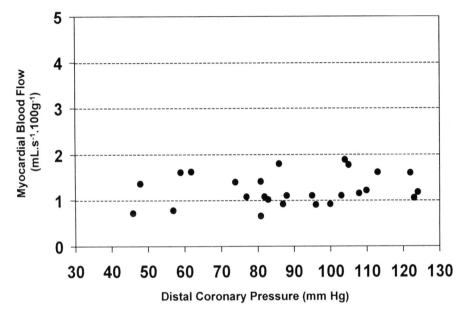

Figure 2.3 *Scatter plot of distal coronary pressure and myocardial blood flow as assessed by positron emission tomography and oxygen-labeled water at rest in 26 patients with an isolated proximal stenosis of the left anterior descending coronary artery and normal left ventricular wall motion at rest.*

2.3.2 Extravascular coronary compression.

Rises in peak left ventricular pressure, end-diastolic pressure, heart rate, and contractility can all independently enhance extravascular coronary resistance. This extravascular compression is of functional importance in the presence of coronary stenoses and decreased post-stenotic pressure[51,52].
Moreover, since extravascular compression is higher in the subendocardium than in the subepicardium, the influence of extravascular compression on transmural myocardial blood flow distribution becomes fully apparent in the

presence of a coronary stenosis when the autoregulatory reserve is partially consumed. Any increase in heart rate, left ventricular pressure, or aortic pressure will then predominantly compromise the perfusion of the subendocardial layers[53,54]. The beneficial effect of nitroglycerin on myocardial blood flow can be largely attributed to a decrease in extravascular compression.

2.3.3   Neural regulation.

The effects of both the parasympathetic and sympathetic systems on transmural myocardial perfusion are summarized in table 2.1 They are difficult to evaluate because stimulation or blockade of cardiac nerves usually has profound effects on many of the mechanical and metabolic determinants of regional myocardial perfusion. Thus, although primary neural control of blood flow is most often surpassed by mechanical and metabolic factors, neural mechanisms may still influence coronary flow response to metabolic needs. Moreover, the density of different receptor types is not uniformly distributed throughout the left ventricular wall. Finally, sympathetic and vagal stimulation might have different effects at the level of the epicardial coronary artery, on the resistive vessels, and on the collateral circulation.

2.3.4   Coronary endothelium.

The coronary endothelium has been recognized to play a major role in the regulation of vasomotor tone of large arteries[55]. Under normal conditions, several vasoactive substances are constantly released by the endothelial cells, among which nitric oxyde (NO) has received the greatest attention. Under the influence of various stimuli such as low oxygen tension, thrombin, platelet products, and increased shear stress, synthesis and release of these vasoactive substances increase above baseline. This release is both luminal and abluminal and induces relaxation of subendothelial smooth muscle cells, leading to decrease of vacular tone. In addition, it has become evident that NO can influence coronary resistance vessels and recent data suggest that NO contributes to the maintenance of myocardial perfusion distal to a flow limiting coronary artery stenosis during exercise[56-62]. Blunted NO-dependent vasodilation of coronary resistance vessels in patients with endothelial dysfunction can render these patients more vulnerable to hypoperfusion distal to an epicardial stenosis.

Table 2.1: *Neural control of transmural myocardial perfusion*			
	Primary Effects	**Secondary Effects**	**Net Effect on myocardial flow**
Parasympathetic system	- Vasodilation of large coronary arteries →↑Flow - ↓Heart rate - ↓Blood pressure	↓ metabolic demand →vasoconstriction of coronary arterioles	↓
Sympathetic system β₁ receptors	- ↑ Contractility - ↑Heart rate - ↑ Sinus node and AV conduction	↑ metabolic demand → coronary vasodilation	↑
β₂ receptors	- vasodilation of coronary conductance and resistance vessels - (vasodilation of peripheral arteries)		↑
α receptors	- vasoconstriction of coronary conductance and resistance arteries - (vasoconstriction of peripheral arteries)		↓

2.4   The concept of flow reserve.

2.4.1   Reactive hyperemia.

When a coronary artery is occluded for more than a few seconds, the heart is deprived of oxygen and the smooth muscle cells in the smaller coronary arteries relax. When the occlusion is released, coronary flow increases far above the control values. Typically, the post-occlusion hyperemia, or reactive hyperemia, consists of about three to five times the volume deficit during the temporary occlusion (figure 2.4). The peak value of flow following an occlusion of about 20 seconds is the maximum flow that can be obtained for an ischemic stimulus, and varies linearly with coronary arterial pressure[63].

During this hyperemic flow, arterio-venous difference in oxygen decreases, indicating that the relative extraction of O_2 is smaller than under resting flow conditions before hyperemia. In contrast, after brief perfusion with an anoxic solution, the repayment of the oxygen debt is much less pronounced[64]. This suggests that factors other than the mere lack of O_2 stimulate coronary flow disproportionately. Adenosine release was initially thought to be the principle mediator of hyperemic blood flow[65]. More recent work has de-emphasized the role of adenosine as a mediator of increased coronary blood flow following temporary occlusion, hypoxemia, or increased metabolic demand[50,66-69]. High shear stress on the arterial wall after sudden restoration of flow can stimulate NO release which, in turn, will prolong the vasodilation. A direct relaxant effect of oxygen tension on vascular smooth muscle is another potential mechanism[70,71]. In conclusion, the precise mechanism of post-occlusion reactive hyperemia, is not yet completely understood.

2.4.2   Minimal coronary resistance.

It was initially believed that short-lasting myocardial ischemia is the most potent stimulus to achieve minimal myocardial resistance and hence maximal myocardial flow. Yet, in animals it seems that even during low flow ischemia the resistance vessels retain some degree of vasomotor tone and can respond to vasodilating stimuli[72-82]. Similarly, during demand ischemia produced by the combination of rapid atrial pacing and coronary artery stenosis, infusion of adenosine resulted in significant increases in transmural flow[83]. In humans also, some residual reserve has been described even in the presence of ischemia[84]. Apparently, a distinction should be made between physiologic and pharmacologic minimal coronary resistance, the former sometimes seeming to exceed the latter. In contrast to these results, Canty and Smith recently showed

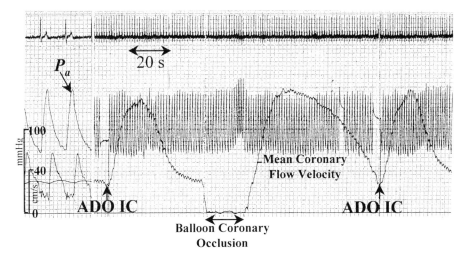

Figure 2.4 *Mean coronary flow velocity recorded in the mid left anterior descending coronary artery (LAD) after stent implantation. A balloon coronary occlusion of approximately 20 s is accompanied by a disappearance of antegrade flow in the LAD. After release of occlusion, flow velocity reaches approximately three times the pre-occlusional level of flow velocity (reactive hyperemia). After administration of intra-coronary adenosine (ADO IC) a similar level of flow velocity is reached. P_a: aortic pressure.*

that in unanesthetized dogs, adenosine-recruitable flow reserve is absent during ischemia[85]. In patients studied after successful angioplasty, Serruys et al found a similar increase in flow velocity during post-occlusion hyperemia and during intracoronary administration of papaverine[86]. This suggests that intrinsic autoregulatory mechanisms are actually able to match local vasodilator reserve to the pharmacologically recruitable reserve. From here onwards, we will refer to *hyperemia* as the maximum coronary or myocardial flow induced by adenosine or papaverine.

Several conditions can produce such a maximum flow or minimal coronary and myocardial resistance. The conditions which can be used in clinical practice to induce maximum hyperemia are summarized below:

Physical exercise. This is far out the most "physiological" stress, but has the disadvantage of being difficult to apply in the catheterization laboratory, where flow and/or pressure measurements are performed. In animal experiments, maximal physical exercise does not seem to exhaust myocardial flow reserve completely. To date, there are no data in humans comparing myocardial flow during maximal exercise and after pharmacologic stimuli.

Pacing tachycardia. The increase in flow achieved by atrial pacing is only modest (2 to 2.5 fold increase) and is far below maximum hyperemic flow induced by pharmacologic agents[87].

Brief coronary occlusion. In man, brief coronary occlusions can only be performed in the setting of coronary angioplasty (figure 2.4), and therefore can not be proposed for diagnostic purposes.

Pharmacological agents. The characteristics of various pharmacological agents used to produce hyperemia, have been well documented. In clinical practice, resistive vessel vasodilation is easily obtained by administration of pharmacological agents. The choice of the coronary vasodilator depends mainly on the imaging modality which is used (echocardiography, perfusion scintigraphy, intracoronary flow velocity or pressure measurements). Their respective dosage, hemodynamic effects, and mode of administration is discussed in detail in chapter 5.

2.4.3 Coronary flow reserve.

Absolute flow reserve.
The extent to which coronary (or myocardial) flow can increase is generally referred to as absolute coronary (or myocardial) flow reserve. The concept of absolute coronary flow reserve is defined as the ratio of hyperemic to resting coronary (or myocardial) blood flow and was initially proposed by Gould[6]. The normal four to six-fold increase in flow after a maximum vasodilatory stimulus identifies a normal coronary flow reserve. In the presence of a stenosis, the resting flow does not change until a tight narrowing of at least 80 to 85% in diameter is reached. However, hyperemic coronary flow begins to decline when a short 50% diameter stenosis is present. Several factors such as heart rate, blood pressure, and left ventricular hypertrophy will affect the level of resting flow and therefore also absolute flow reserve, and need to be accounted for.

Relative flow reserve.
Relative flow reserve is defined as the maximum blood flow in a stenotic artery (or myocardial territory) divided by maximum blood flow in an adjacent normal artery (or myocardial territory). The concept of relative flow reserve is referred to when performing perfusion scintigraphy. Relative flow reserve does not account for baseline blood flow and is therefore less dependant on changes in cardiac workload[88]. Yet, relative flow reserve requires the presence

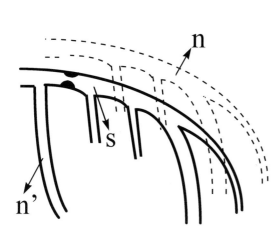

Absolute flow reserve

$$= \frac{Q^s_{max}}{Q^s_{rest}}$$

Relative flow reserve

$$= \frac{Q^s_{max}}{Q^{n'}_{max}}$$

Fractional flow reserve

$$= \frac{Q^s_{max}}{Q^n_{max}}$$

Fig 2.5 *Schematic illustration of the concepts of absolute, relative, and fractional flow reserve.*

of a territory perfused by a normal epicardial vessel and cannot be applied in case of balanced 3-vessel disease. As already noted, even in case of 1- or 2-vessel disease, one cannot be sure that flow reserve is normal in the remote control artery (cf. figure 10.4).

Fractional flow reserve.
Fractional flow reserve is defined as the ratio of the hyperemic flow in the stenotic coronary artery (or myocardial territory) to the hyperemic flow in that same artery (or territory) in the hypothetical case the epicardial vessel were completely normal[89]. Stated another way, the fractional flow reserve expresses maximum hyperemic blood flow as a fraction of its normal value. Fractional flow reserve can be calculated from intracoronary pressure measurements obtained during maximum hyperemia. The theory, experimental basis, and clinical applications of pressure-derived fractional flow reserve, constitute the body of this book.

The definitions of absolute, relative and fractional flow reserve are illustrated in figure 2.5 and some of their characteristics are summarized in table 2.2. A diagram clarifying some specific features of and differences between coronary and fractional flow reserve, is presented in figure 9.6.

Table 2.2: *Characteristics of absolute, relative, and fractional flow reserve (CFR, RFR, FFR respectively)*			
	Absolute Flow Reserve	Relative Flow Reserve	Fractional Flow Reserve
Definition	Ratio of hyperemic to resting blood flow	Ratio of hyperemic flow in the stenotic region to hyperemic flow in a contralateral normal region	Ratio of hyperemic flow in the stenotic region to hyperemic flow in that same region if no lesion were present
Independent of driving pressure	NO	YES	YES
Easily applicable in humans	YES (flow velocity measurements, positron emission tomography)	YES (flow velocity measurements, perfusion scintigraphy, positron emission, tomography)	YES (coronary pressure measurements)
Applicable to 3 vessel disease	YES	NO	YES
Assessment of collateral flow	NO	perfusion: YES velocity: NO	YES
Unequivocal reference value	NO (=3 to 6)	YES (=1)	YES (=1)

References.

1.   Bassenge E, Heusch G. Endothelial and neuro-humoral control of coronary blood flow in health and disease. *Rev Physiol Biochem Pharmacol.* 1990;116:77-165.
2.   Dole WP. Autoregulation of the coronary circulation. *Prog Cardiovasc Dis* 1987;29:293-323.
3.   Hoffman JIE. Transmural myocardial perfusion. *Prog Cardiovasc Dis* 1987;29:429-464.
4.   Hoffman JIE, Spaan JAE. Pressure-flow relations in coronary circulation. *Physiol Rev* 1990;70:331-390.
5.   Spaan JAE Coronary blood flow. *Kluwer Academic Publishers* 1991.
6.   Gould KL. Coronary artery stenosis. *Elsevier Science Publishing Co, Inc* 1991.

7. Pijls NHJ, Van Gelder B, van der Voort P, Peels K, Bracke FALE, Bonnier HJRM, El Gamal MIH. Fractional flow reserve. A useful index to evaluate the influence of an epicardial coronary stenosis on myocardial blood flow. *Circulation*, 1995;92:3183-3193.

8. Chilian WM, Layne SM, Klausner EC, Eastham CL, Marcus ML. Redistribution of coronary microvascular resistance produced by dipyridamole. *Am J Physiol* 1989;256: H383-H390.

9. Lopez JAG, Amstrong ML, Piegors DJ, Heistad DD. Effect of early and advanced atherosclerosis on vascular response to serotonine, thromboxane A2, and ADP. *Circulation* 1989;79:698-705

10. Yokoyama I, Ohtake T, Momommura S, Nishikawa J, Sasaki Y, Omata M. Reduced coronary flow reserve in hypercholesterolemic patients without overt coronary stenosis. *Circulation* 1996;94:3232-3238.

11. Pitkänen O-P, Raitakari OT, Niinikoski H, Nuutila P, Iida H, Voipio-Pulkki LM, Härkönen R, Wegelius U, Rönnemaa T, Viikari J, Knuuti J. Coronary flow reserve is impaired in young men with familial hypercholesterolemia. *J Am Coll Cardiol* 1996; 28:1705-1711.

12. Kern MJ, Bach RG, Mechem CJ, Caracciolo EA, Aguirre FV, Miller LW, Donohue TJ. Variations in normal coronary vasodilatory reserve stratified by artery, gender, heart transplantation and coronary artery disease. *J Am Coll Cardiol* 1996;28:1154-1160.

13. Uren NG, Crake T. Resistive vessel function in coronary artery disease. *Heart* 1996; 76:299-304.

14. Borg TK, Caulfied JB. The collagen matrix of the heart. *Fed Proc* 1981;40:2037-2041.

15. Henquell L, Odoroff CL, Honig CR. Coronary intercapillary distance during growth: relation to P0$_2$ and aerobic capacity. *Am J Physiol* 1978;231:1852-1859.

16. Potter RF, Groom AC. Capillary diameter and geometry in cardiac and skeletal muscle studied by means of corrosion casts. *Microvasc Res* 1983;25:68-84.

17. Fung YC, Zweifach BW, Intaglietta M. Elastic environment of the capillary bed. *Circ Res* 1966; 19: 441-461.

18. Levy BI, Samuel JL, Tedgui A, Kotelianski V, Marotte F, Poitevin P, Chadwick RS. Intramyocardial blood volume measurement in the left ventricle of rat arrested hearts. In: *Cardiovascular Dynamics and Models 1988.* Eds. Brun P, Chadwick RS, Levy BI, INSERM, Paris: 65-76.

19. Roberts JT, Wearn JT. Quantitative changes in the capillary-muscle relationship in human hearts during normal growth and hypertrophy. *Am Heart J* 1941;21: 617-633.

20. Gerdes AM, Kasten FH. Morphometric study of endomyocardium and epimyocardium of the left ventricle in adult dogs. *Am J Anat* 1980; 159:389-394.

21. Schaper W, Ito WD. Molecular mechanisms of coronary collateral vessel growth. *Circ Res* 1996;79:911-919.

22. Thornton SC, Mueller SN, Levine EM. Human endothelial cells: use of heparine in cloning and longterm serial cultivation. *Science* 1983;222:623-625.

23. Folkman J, Klassbrun M. Angiogenic factors. *Science* 1987;235:442-447.

24. Unger SF, Sheffield CD, Epstein SE. Heparine promotes the formation of extracardiac to coronary anastomoses in a canine model. *Am J Physiol* 1991;260:H1625-H1634.

25. Caroll SM, White FC, Roth DM, Bloor CM. Heparine accelerates coronary collateral development in a porcine model of coronary artery occlusion. *Circulation* 1993; 88:198-207.

26. Banai S, Jaklitsch MT, Shou M, Lazarous DF, Scheinowitz M, Biro S, Epstein SE, Unger E. Angiogenic-induced enhancement of collateral blood flow to ischemic myocardium by vascular endothelial growth factor in dogs. *Circulation* 1994;89:2183-2189.

27. Quyumi AA, Diodati JG, Lakatos E, Bonow RO, Epstein SE. Angiogenic effects of low molecular weight heparine in patients with stable coronary artery disease : a pilot study. *J Am Coll Cardiol* 1993;22:635-641.

28. Schaper W, Görge G, Winckler B, Schaper J. The collateral circulation in the heart. *Prog Cardiovasc Diseases* 1988; 31:57-77.
29. Vanoverschelde JL, Wijns W, Depre C, Essamri B, Heyndrickx GR, Borgers M, Bol A, Melin JA. Mechanisms of chronic regional post-ischemic dysfunction in humans. New insights from the study of non-infarcted collateral-dependent myocardium. *Circulation* 1993; 87:1513-1523.
30. Sabiston DC Jr, Gregg DE. Effect of cardiac contraction on coronary blood flow. *Circulation* 1957;15: 14-20.
31. Katz SA, Feigl EO. Systole has little effect on diastolic coronary blood flow. *Circ Res* 1988; 62: 443-451.
32. Lowensohn HS, Khouri EM, Gregg DE, Pyle RL, Patterson RE. Phasic right coronary artery flow in conscious dogs with normal and elevated right ventricular pressures. *Circ Res* 1976;39:760-766.
33. Bruinsma P, Arts T, Dankelman J, Spaan JAE. Model of the coronary circulation based on pressure dependence of coronary resistance and compliance. *Basic Res Cardiol* 1988;83:510-524.
34. Reneman RS. Cited by Spaan, in Spaan JAE. Coronary blood flow. *Kluwer Academic Publishers* 1991.
35. Marzilli M, Goldstein S, Sabbah HN, Lee T, Stein PD. Modulating effect of regional myocardial performance on local myocardial perfusion in the dog. *Circ Res* 1979; 45:634-640.
36. Krams R, Sipkema P, Zegers J, Westerhof N. Contractility is the main determinant of coronary systolic flow impediment. *Am J Physiol* 1989;257:H1936-H1944.
37. Krams R, Sipkema P, Westerhof N. Varying elastance concept may explain coronary systolic flow impediment. *Am J Physiol* 1989; 257:1471-H1479.
38. Kajiya F, Tsujioka K, Ogasaware Y, Hiramatsu O, Wada Y, Goto M, Yanaka M. Analysis of the characteristics of the flow velocity waveforms in the left atrial small arteries and veins in the dog. *Circ Res* 1989;65:1172-1181.
39. Camici P, Ferranni E, Opie LH. Myocardial metabolism in ischemic heart disease: Basic principles and application to imaging by positron emission tomography. *Prog Cardiovasc Dis Disease* 1989; 32:217-238.
40. Eckenhoff JE, Hafkenschiel JH, Landmesser CM, Harmel M. Cardiac oxygen metabolism and control of the coronary circulation. *Am J Physiol* 1947; 149:634-639.
41. Mosher P, Ross Jr J, McFate PA, Shaw RF. Control of coronary blood flow by an autoregulatory mechanism. *Circ Res* 1964;14:250-259.
42. Canty JM. Coronary pressure-function and steady-state pressure-flow relations during autoregulation in the unanesthetized dog. *Circ Res* 1988;63:821-836.
43. De Bruyne B, Melin JA, Heyndrickx GR, Wijns W. Autoregulatory plateau in patients with coronary artery disease. *Circulation* 1994;90:I-113 (abstract).
44. Berne RM. Cardiac nucleotides in hypoxia: possible role in regulation of coronary blood flow. *Am J Physiol* 1963;204:317-322.
45. Olsson RA, Bünger R. Metabolic control of coronary blood flow. *Prog Cardiovasc Dis* 1987;29:369-387.
46. Katori M, Berne RM. Release of adenosine from anoxic hearts. Relationship to coronary flow. *Circ Res* 1966;19:420-425.
47. Dole WP, Yamada N, Bishop VS, Olsson RA. Role of adenosine in coronary blood flow regulations after reductions in perfusion pressure. *Circ Res* 1985;56:517-524.
48. Hanley FL, Messina LM, Baer RW, Uhlig PN, Hoffman JIE. Direct measurement of left ventricular interstitial adenosine. *Am J Physiol* 1983;245:H327-H335.
49. Kroll K, Feigl EO. Adenosine is unimportant in controlling coronary blood flow in unstressed dog hearts. *Am J Physiol* 1985;249:H1176-H1187.

50. Rossen JD, Oskarsson H, Minor RL Jr, Talman CL, Winniford MD. Effect of adenosine antagonism on metabolically mediated coronary vasodilation in humans. *J Am Coll Cardiol* 1994;23:1421-1426.

51. Heusch G, Yoshimoto N. Effects of heart rate and perfusion pressure on segmental coronary resistances and collateral perfusion. *Pfluegers Arch* 1983;397:284-289.

52. Heusch G, Yoshimoto N. Effects of cardiac contraction on segmental coronary resistances and collateral perfusion. *Int J Microcirc* 1983;2:131-141.

53. Bache RJ, Cobb FR. Effect of maximal coronary vasodilation on transmural myocardial perfusion during tachycardia in the awake dog. *Circ Res* 1977;41:648-653.

54. Ellis AK, Klocke FJ. Effects of preload on the transmural distribution of perfusion and pressure-flow relationships in the canine coronary vascular bed. *Circ Res* 1979;46:68-77.

55. Furchgott RF, Zawadzki JV. The obligatory role of endothelial cells in the relaxation of smooth muscle by acetylcholine. *Nature* 1980;288:373-376.

56. Myers PR, Banitt PF, Guerra R Jr, Harrison DG. Characteristics of canine coronary resistance arteries: importance of endothelium. *Am J Physiol* 1989;257:H603-H610.

57. Woodman OL, Dusting GJ. *N*-Nitro L-arginine causes coronary vasoconstriction and inhibits endothelium-dependent vasodilation in anaesthetized greyhounds. *Br J Pharmacol* 1991;103:1407-1410.

58. Ishizaka H, Okumura K, Yamabe H, Tsuchiya T, Yasue H. Endothelium-derived nitric oxide as a mediator of acetylcholine-induced coronary vasodilation in dogs. *J Cardiovasc Pharmacol* 1991;18:665-669.

59. Komaru T, Lamping KG, Eastham CL, Harrison DG, Marcus ML, Dellsperger KC. Effect of an arginine analogue on acetylcholine-induced dilatation of isolated coronary arterioles. *Am J Phsyiol* 1990;259:H1063-H1070.

60. Parent R, Paré R, Lavallée M. Contribution of nitric oxide to dilatation of resistance coronary vessels in conscious dogs. *Am J Physiol* 1992;262:H10-H16.

61. Kuo L, Chilian WM, Davis MJ. Interaction of pressure- and flow-induced responses in porcine coronary resistance vessels. *Am J Physiol* 1991;261:H1706-H1715.

62. Duncker DJ, Bache RJ. Inhibition of nitric oxide production aggravates myocardial hypoperfusion during exercise in the presence of a coronary artery stenosis. *Circ Res* 1994;74:629-640.

63. Dole WP, Montville WJ, Bishop VS. Dependency of myocardial reactive hyperemia on coronary artery pressure in the dog. *Am J Physiol* 1981;240: H709-H715.

64. Kelly KO, Gould KL. Coronary reactive hyperemia after brief occlusion and after deoxygenated perfusion. *Cardiov Res* 1981;15:615-622.

65. Berne RM. Regulation of coronary blood flow. *Prog Cardiovasc Dis* 1975;18:105-21.

66. Downing SE, Chen V. Dissociation of adenosine from meabolic regulation of coronary flow in the lamb. *Am J Physiol* 1986;251:H40-H46.

67. Gewirtz H, Olsson RA, Most AS. Role of adenosine in mediating the coronary vasodilative response to acute hypoxia. *Cardiov Res* 1987;21:81-89.

68. Dole WP, Yamada N, Bishop VS, Olsson RA. Role of adenosine in coronary blood flow regulation after reductions in perfusion pressure. *Cir Res* 1985;56:517-524.

69. Hanley FL, Grattan MT, Stevens MB, Hoffman JIE. Role of adenosine in coronary autoregulation. *Am J Physiol* 1986;250:H558-H566.

70. Dole WP, Nuno DW: Myocardial oxygen tension determines the degree and pressure range of coronary autoregulation. *Circ Res* 1986;59:202-215.

71. Downey HF, Crystal GJ, Bockman EL, Bashour FA. Nonischemic myocardial hypoxia: coronary dilatation without increased tissue adenosine. *Am J Physiol* 1982;243:H512-H516.

72. Gorman MW, Sparks HV. progressive coronary vasoconstriction during relative ischemia in canine myocardium. *Circ Res* 1982;51:411-420.

73. Pantely GA, Bristow JD, Swenson LJ, Ladley HD, Johnson WB, Anselone CG. Incomplete coronary vasodilation during myocardial ischemia in swine. *Am J Physiol* 1985;249:H638-H647.

74. Canty JM, Klocke F. Reduced regional myocardial perfusion in the presence of pharmacologic vasodilator reserve. *Circulation* 1985;71:370-377.

75. Aversano T, Becker LC. Persistence of coronary vasodilator reserve despite functionally significant flow reduction. *Am J Physiol* 1985;248:H403-H411.

76. Grattan MT, Hanley FL, Stevens MB, Hoffman JIE. Transmural coronary flow reserve patterns in dogs. *Am J Physiol* 1986;250:H276-H283.

77. Laxson DD, Dai XZ, Homans DC, Bache RJ. Coronary vasodilator reserve in ischemic myocardium of the exercising dog. *Circulation* 1992;85:313-322.

78. Heusch G, Deussen A. The effects of cardiac sympathetic nerve stimulation on the perfusion of stenotic coronary arteries in the dog. *Circ Res* 1983;53:8-15.

79. Seitelberger R, Guth BD, Heusch G, Lee JD, Katayama K, Ross J. Intracoronary α_2-adrenergic receptor blockade attenuates ischemia in conscious dogs during exercise. *Circ Res* 1988;62:436-442.

80. Laxson DD, Dai X-Z, Homans DC, Bache RJ. The role of α_1- and α_2-adrenergic receptors in mediation of coronary vasoconstriction in hypoperfused ischemic myocardium during exercise. *Circ Res* 1989;65:1688-1697.

81. Bache RJ, Dai X-Z. The thromboxane A2 mimetic, U46619, worsens myocardial hypoperfusion during exercise in the presence of a coronary artery stenosis. *Cardiovasc Res* 1992;26:351-356.

82. Laxson DD, Homans DC, Bache RJ. Inhibition of adenosine-mediated coronary vasodilation exacerbates myocardial ischemia during exercise. *Am J Physiol* 1993; 265:H1471-H1477.

83. Gorman MW, Sparks HV Jr. Progressive vasoconstriction during relative ischemia in canine myocardium. *Cir Res* 1982;51:411-420.

84. Parodi O, Sambucetti G, Roghi A, Testa R, Inglese E, Pirelli S, Spinelli F, Campolo L, L'Abbate A. Residual coronary reserve despite decreased resting blood flow in patients with critical coronary lesions. A study by technetium-99m human albumin microsphere myocardial scintigraphy. *Circulation* 1993;87:330-344.

85. Canty JM, Smith TP Jr. Adenosine-recruitable flow reserve in absent during myocardial ischemia in unanesthetized dogs studied in the basal state. *Circ Res* 1995; 76:1079-1087.

86. Serruys PW, Di Mario C, Meneveau N, de Jaegere P, Strikwerda S, de Feyter PJ, Emanuelsson H. Intracoronary pressure and flow velocity from sensor tip guide wires. A new methodological comprehensive approach for the assessment of coronary hemodynamics before and after interventions. *Am J Cardiol* 1993;71:41D-53D.

87. Sambucetti G, Marzullo P, Giorgetti A, Neglia D, Marzilli M, Salvadori P, L'Abbate A, Parodi O. Global alteration in perfusion response to increasing oxygen consumption in patients with single-vessel coronary artery disease. *Circulation* 1994;90:1696-1705.

88. Gould KL, Kirkeeide RL, Buchi M. Coronary flow reserve as a physiological measure of stenosis severity. *J Am Coll Cardiol* 1990;15:459:474.

89. Pijls NHJ, Van Son JAM, Kirkeeide RL, De Bruyne B, Gould KL. Experimental basis of determining maximum coronary myocardial, and collateral blood flow by pressure measurements for assessing functional stenosis severity before and after PTCA. *Circulation* 1993;87:1354-1367.

Chapter 3

INTRODUCTION TO INVASIVE ASSESSMENT OF THE CORONARY CIRCULATION

The problem of knowing whether a given epicardial stenosis can be held responsible for myocardial ischemia and, consequently, whether the patient will be improved by the revascularization of that stenosis, are among the most common and important questions in the catheterization laboratory. Traditionally, cardiologists base their clinical decisions about the adequacy or inadequacy of myocardial perfusion in any given patient on inferences or predictions deduced from patients' symptoms, non-invasive testing, and morphological data provided by the coronary angiogram. Direct information about myocardial perfusion is mostly not available. Boosted by the emergence of interventional cardiology, several catheter-based techniques have been developed to assist cardiologists in clinical decision-making with respect to the appropriateness of revascularization of a particular stenosis. These techniques are based on a morphological or a functional approach and are briefly reviewed in this chapter.

3.1 Morphological approaches.

3.1.1 Quantitative coronary angiography.

Since its introduction in the late fifties, coronary angiography has been used as the reference method of the diagnosis of coronary artery disease[1,2]. At present, the definitive diagnosis of coronary artery disease cannot reliably be made without angiographic confirmation. Coupled to left ventricular pressure recordings and to left ventricular angiography, selective coronary arteriography provides an unsurpassed amount of information and is paramount for therapeutic decision making in patients complaining of chest pain. The development of mechanical revascularization procedures has further given a pivotal role to coronary arteriography serving as a map for the surgeon or the interventionalist. Although considerable progress in non-invasive techniques for imaging of the coronary arteries has been made, such as MRI, non-invasive coronary angiography will remain for a while the Holy Grail for cardiologists.

Despite the pivotal role of coronary angiography, visual interpretation of coronary angiograms ("eye balling") is hampered by several limitations. Severe discrepancies have been reported between the angiographic degree of stenosis and post-mortem measurements[3-5]. Angiographers tend to underestimate mild stenoses and to overestimate tighter ones as if reasoning in terms of percent diameter narrowing in the lower range of stenosis severity and in terms of percent area narrowing in the highest range. Moreover, a large inter- and intraobserver variability has been reported in several studies especially after coronary angioplasty[6-9]. To overcome these limitations, quantitative analysis of the coronary arteriogram has been developed and validated[10-12]. As quantitative coronary angiography significantly limits the variability of the measurements, this technique is suitable for comparing the effects of different therapeutic strategies[13,14]. Thus, quantitative coronary angiography became an absolute methodological prerequisite for studying the efficacy of new interventional devices[15,16] or for evaluating the effects of drugs or diets on coronary atherosclerosis[17,18].

In daily practice, however, the most common problem is not knowing how a given lesion compares with the situation of some months or years before, but to determine whether a given epicardial coronary narrowing can be flow-limiting, and thus responsible for the complaints of the patient. The usefulness of quantitative coronary angiography for clinical decision making in lesions of intermediate severity remains controversial. Studies reporting close correlations between angiographic and functional assessment have been carried out in highly selected patients and are not really representative for the "all round" coronary lesion posing a problem for clinical decision-making in everyday practice[19,20]. In a large group of patients, it is not surprising to find a statistically significant correlation between quantitative angiographic stenosis severity and the physiological impact of the lesion. In the individual patient, however, the variability is too large to rely upon for clinical decision-making[21-23].

Figure 3.1 shows the relationship between angiographic indexes and pressure-derived myocardial fractional flow reserve. These data were obtained in 221 patients before angioplasty or during diagnostic coronary angiography. Although there is an overall correlation between anatomic and functional approaches, the very wide dispersion of the data precludes angiography-based prediction of the functional significance of the stenosis in individual patients.

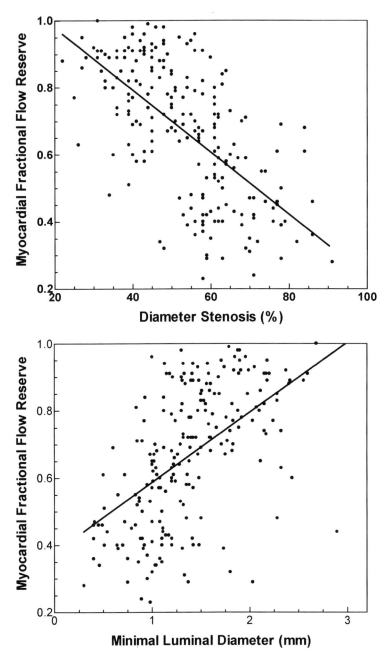

Figure 3.1 *Plot of the relationship between a functional index of coronary stenosis severity, namely pressure-derived myocardial fractional flow reserve (FFR$_{myo}$), and angiographic indexes of stenosis severity, namely percent diameter stenosis (*upper panel*) and minimal luminal diameter (lower panel).*

An example of quantitative coronary angiography of an intermediate lesion is given in figure 3.2.

There are several reasons why even the most precise QCA system will not closely reflect the impact of a given stenosis on myocardial flow:

(1) The edge detection, which is the most widely implemented technique in catheterization laboratories, consists of a projection of a lumenogram and is theoretically not ideal to assess irregular segments especially those obtained after balloon angioplasty. In those cases, quantitative coronary angiography obtained by edge detection will tend to overestimate the cross-sectional area of the vessel. Some studies have suggested that both pre- and post-angioplasty geometric assessments by edge detection yielded a better reproducibility between different views than QCA-techniques based on videodensitometry[24-26]. However, more recent work demonstrated a particularly good correlation between videodensitometry and IVUS, presumably because measurements of the luminal area is the basic quantification approach of both techniques[27].

(2) Intrinsic shortcomings of the radiographic methods may limit its applicability: overlapping side branches, the emergence of a side branch immediately before or after the stenosis, foreshortening of the stenotic segment, post-stenotic dilatation, and marked irregularities of the segment adjacent to the lesion are frequent so that optimal conditions to analyze a lesion are present only in a minority of cases[28].

(3) QCA assesses minimal luminal diameter, percent diameter stenosis, and lesion length which are the major determinants of the physiological impact of an epicardial lesion on translesional blood flow. However, other factors such as entrance and exit angles, blood viscosity, lesional roughness and eccentricity, and coronary flow pulsatility are rarely accounted for and may affect the value of flow reserve for a given degree of stenosis[29].

(4) Coronary angiography does not take into account collateral contribution to myocardial perfusion. The extreme example is that of a total coronary occlusion with well developed collaterals: angiography will consider the lesion as extremely severe, while it has been shown that myocardial blood flow in some of these cases might be close to normal even during stress[30].

(5) Small measurement inaccuracies are difficult to avoid even though the precision of most available algorithms goes down to one tenth of a mm. The fluid dynamic equation describes the factors responsible for the resistance of a given narrowing[31]. Minimal lesion dimensions, percent diameter stenosis and the length of the lesion all affect this resistance and thus the physiological significance of a stenosis. One could, therefore, expect that the larger the number of geometric parameters taken into account, the closer the relation would be with functional assessment of the narrowing. Actually, clinical studies contradict these theoretical considerations[23,32]. Myocardial fractional flow reserve and the results of the exercise ECG correlate better with minimal luminal diameter (which only takes into account one single measurement) than with percent diameter stenosis (taking into account two measurements : minimal diameter and "normal" reference diameter) and than with stenosis flow reserve (which in addition takes into account lesional length). This suggest that multiple measurements, by amplifying the effect of measuring errors, lead paradoxically to a weaker functional depiction of the stenosis.

In conclusion, notwithstanding the indisputable merits of QCA for follow-up of coronary lesions after mechanical or pharmacological interventions, its value for assessing the physiologic impact of a stenosis in the individual patient, remains poor. The advantages and limitations of QCA are summarized in table 3.1

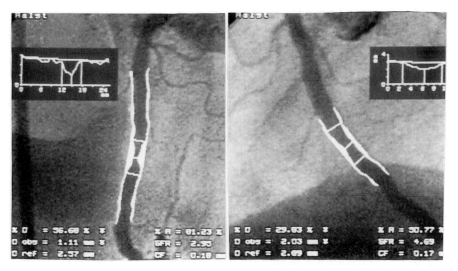

Figure 3.2 *Example of quantitative assessment of an intermediate stenosis in the right coronary artery.*

Table 3.1 *Advantages and limitations of quantitative coronary angiography.*
Advantages   ◆ reproducible   ◆ no additional material required   ◆ cheap   ◆ rapid and safe   *Limitations*   ◆ applicable in only a minority of stenoses   ◆ the reference segment is often not normal   ◆ not all dimensions are taken into account   ◆ physiologic parameters are not taken into account   ◆ collaterals are not taken into account

3.1.2   Intracoronary ultrasound.

The unique feature of intravascular ultrasound (IVUS) is its ability to study the vascular wall beneath the endothelial surface. Presently available ultrasound imaging devices are built in catheters which are advanced over an intracoronary guide wire. The morphology and pathology of the three layers of the wall (intima, media and adventitia) as well as intraluminal content (plaque, thrombus, intimal dissections) can be viewed on cross-sectional bidimensional images, perpendicular to the long axis of the vessel (figure 3.3).

From a technical point of view, two ultrasound catheter systems are currently available. The first is based on a mechanical rotation of a single crystal. It provides high resolution imaging without near-field artifact.

The second consists of multiple crystals mounted around the circumference of the catheter tip. The crystals are activated one after the other. Problems with near-field artifacts precluding the visualization of structures close to the catheter, have been largely resolved.

Studies on longitudinal and three-dimensional reconstruction of the arterial segment are also possible (figure 3.4). The principle is based on sequential cross-sectional image acquisition, digitalization, and reconstruction. Volumetric changes of lumen and wall can be displayed and analyzed[33].

At last, absolute quantitation of coronary blood flow by colour Doppler techniques combined with 2-D echo in one IVUS catheter, has become possible recently[34]. The value of this elegant technique remains to be determined because of the intrinsic limitations of absolute blood flow to represent the severity of disease if the mass of tissue to be perfused is unknown.

Intracoronary ultrasound has several potential advantages as compared to angiography:

(1) *Intravascular ultrasound is more sensitive than angiography in detecting coronary atherosclerosis.* Post-mortem and intraoperative data have shown that luminal changes do not occur in the early stages of coronary atherosclerosis. Compensatory enlargement in diseased segments occurs and results in a significant underestimation of atherosclerosis by luminal coronary angiography[36-41]. The most impressive observation in any center's initial experience with intravascular ultrasound is that extensive atherosclerotic involvement may be present in angiographically normal arterial segments[42-46]. An example is shown in figure 3.3.

(2) *Study of plaque composition.* The value of intravascular ultrasound to study the morphology of the native vessel wall and atherosclerotic lesions, is

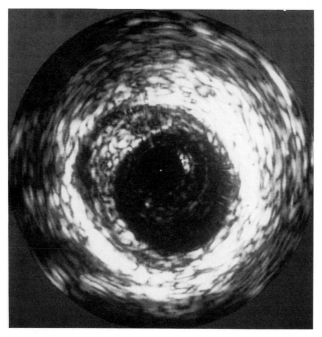

Figure 3.3 *Example of intravascular ultrasound image of an angiographically apparently normal segment. An atherosclerotic plaque occupies more than half of the circumference of the vessel. A significant compensatory enlargement of the vessel wall has prevented any decrease in luminal size.*

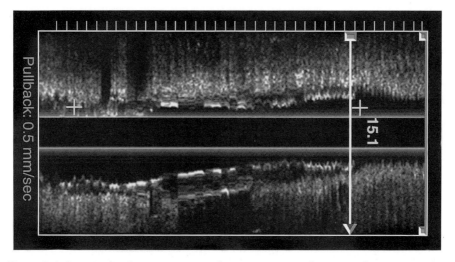

Figure 3.4 *Longitudinal reconstruction of a coronary vessel segment, by intravascular ultrasound.*

Table 3.2 *Advantages and limitations of intravascular ultrasound.*

Advantages
- ◆ accurate assessment of luminal borders and external elastic lamina
- ◆ assessment of the longitudinal extent of the lesion
- ◆ unsurpassed ability to study plaque composition and visualization of the vascular wall beneath the surface
- ◆ accurate assessment of optimal stent deployment

Limitations
- ◆ expensive
- ◆ interpretation of data is not trivial
- ◆ collaterals and physiologic parameters are not taken into account

unsurpassed. The potential to determine the risk of rupture of the atherosclerotic plaque by analysis of its composition represents one of the major challenges of modern cardiology[47]. Intravascular ultrasound is able to distinguish highly echogenic lesions ("hard" plaque) which are likely to be composed of dense fibrous tissue and calcified deposits, from less echogenic lesions ("soft" plaque) which are likely to be composed of thrombus, fibromuscular tissue, loose collagen, lipid deposition or intraplaque necrotic degeneration. This thin fibrous cap covering lipid deposits as well as the juxtaposition of hard and soft plaques might create an ideal substrate for plaque rupture leading to an acute coronary syndrome[48-51]. Therefore, the precise knowledge of plaque composition could bear prognostic information not provided by angiography nor by coronary flow assessment and could influence the therapeutic strategy[52]. While some authors have observed a high prevalence of soft plaques with fewer intralesional calcium deposits in unstable syndromes, others observed similar echographic characteristics of the plaque in stable and unstable syndromes[53,54].

(3) *New insights in the mechanisms of coronary interventions.* The structural changes associated with balloon angioplasty, atherectomy, and stent deployment, as well as the mechanisms of immediate complications of coronary interventions have been better understood by the use of intravascular ultrasound[55-66]. Despite a satisfactory angiogram after PTCA, IVUS sometimes shows just fissure of plaques without true luminal improvement (figure 14.5). Of direct clinical importance is the evaluation of stent deployment[67]. An increased risk for stent thrombosis is associated with incomplete expansion of the stent. This suboptimal apposition of the struts to the vessel wall can be observed by intravascular ultrasound in a large proportion of stent deployment

despite a satisfactory angiographic appearance. The importance of optimal apposition of the stent against the vessel wall has been demonstrated by intravascular ultrasound studies and has largely contributed to less aggressive anticoagulation therapy after stent implantation[68-71].

(4) *New insights in the mechanisms of restenosis.* Recent data, obtained immediately and 6 months after angioplasty, have changed our understanding of the mechanisms of restenosis. Until recently, neo-intimal cellular proliferation was considered as the main cause of restenosis after balloon angioplasty. In parallel to animal experimental data, IVUS data have shown that the increase in plaque area at 6 months follow-up, accounted for only 32% of the loss in luminal gain[72-78]. These studies suggest that a chronic recoil or adverse remodeling of the artery accounts for a significant part of the late luminal loss after balloon angioplasty, while in-stent restenosis is the result of neo-intimal proliferation[79,80].

(5) *Clinical outcome data.* The bottom line of any new diagnostic or therapeutic technique is patients' clinical outcome. So far, in spite of abundant literature on this issue, hard data proving that the use of IVUS during coronary intervention can improve the prognosis of the patient are scarce.

At present, the potential of intravascular ultrasound has created an increasing enthusiasm among interventional cardiologists[81,82]. However, this imaging technique remains an expensive and sometimes time-consuming diagnostic tool [83,84]. Moreover, the correct interpretation of IVUS images is not trivial and needs considerable experience. IVUS gives an anatomic assessment and does not provide true physiologic information. Although an absolute luminal area of less than 4mm^2 is used to distinguish hemodynamically significant lesions, it will be clear that such measure must also be dependent on the size of the vessel and the myocardial tissue mass to be supplied[85]. At last, it remains to be demonstrated that the knowledge of composition and structure of the atherosclerotic plaque provides additional prognostic information which cannot be obtained by competitive non-invasive techniques like magnetic resonance imaging[86]. The advantages and limitations of intracoronary ultrasound, are summarized in table 3.2.

3.1.3 Intracoronary angioscopy.

Direct visualization of the coronary lumen and the inner surface of the arterial wall has been made possible by miniaturization of angioscopes.

Coronary angioscopes consist of a central imaging bundle of optic fibers surrounded by fibers acting as light source.The angioscope is advanced over a guide wire into the segment to be examined. A compliant cuff is inflated to stop antegrade blood flow. To clear up the image field from blood, Ringer's lactate solution is infused (± 0.8cc/s). The tip of the angioscope can then be advanced to explore the segment under study.

In vitro and in vivo angioscopic studies have shown a higher sensitivity for detecting thrombi and superficial tears as compared to angiography and intravascular ultrasound[87]. A complex lumen shape (including spontaneous dissection and ulceration) and protruding thrombi were more often seen in unstable than in stable syndromes[88-94]. Some potential usefulness of coronary angioscopy has been suggested during coronary interventions[95]. The technique remains limited by the need for replacing blood by saline which creates myocardial hypoxemia, a condition often less well tolerated than regular balloon coronary occlusion[96]. It can be foreseen that further development of intravascular angioscopy will be limited due to its limited clinical benefit and poor cost-effectiveness.

The fundamental problem shared by quantitative coronary angiography, intravascular ultrasound, angioscopy, and other morphologic approaches is that the epicardial narrowing represents only one component of a system in which vasodilatory capacity of coronary resistive vessels, collateral circulation, the amount of myocardium to be supplied, heart rate, blood pressure, myocardial contractility, viscosity, and oxygen-carrying capacity of the blood also play a major role. Therefore, in individual patients it remains difficult to assess the physiologic importance of a coronary stenosis by a morphologic approach alone.

3.2   Functional approaches.

3.2.1   Myocardial videodensitometry.

After injection of contrast medium into the coronary arteries, temporal changes in contrast density of the myocardium can be studied to calculate the flow according to the indicator dilution theory[97-99]. The principle was first proposed by Rutishauser who measured transit time of a bolus of contrast agent in a well-delineated arterial segment. The use of digital methods and ECG-triggered subtraction imaging substantially improved the assessment of contrast agent passage through the myocardium[100-102]. According to indicator dilution theory, flow (F) can be calculated as:

$$F = \frac{V}{T_m}$$

where T_m is the mean transit time of the indicator, and V is the vascular volume between injection site and measuring site. Videodensitometry is a particularly elegant technique since, by a single diagnostic modality, namely the injection of contrast medium into the coronary arteries, both functional and morphologic information can be obtained. The conventional coronary angiogram (morphologic data) could thus be compared side-by-side with parametric images of myocardial perfusion (physiological data). Because of the technical difficulties in determining mean transit time of contrast passage through the myocardium, Vogel et al and several other investigators substituted mean transit time by other time parameters (T), derived from the ascending limb of the time-density curve; appearance time or time to maximum contrast intensity[100-107]. Furthermore, since calculation of vascular volume is impossible, contrast density (D) was used as a surrogate for vascular content. Coronary flow reserve (CFR) was then determined by performing studies at baseline (b) and after a hyperemic stimulus (h), and expressed as:

$$CFR = \frac{D_h}{D_b} \times \frac{T_b}{T_h}$$

In carefully selected patients, reasonable correlations were obtained between coronary flow reserve determined by videodensitometry and angiographic severity of the lesions[100-107]. However, in an unselected patient population videodensitometric measurements were not found to correlate with lesion severity[108]. The reason therefore lies in the three prerequisites for myocardial flow assessment by videodensitometry according to the indicator dilution theory [109]: (1) Images should be of such a quality that T_m can be determined reliably. This requires long and absolutely motionless cine runs. (2) Blood flow should be constant during image acquisition. (3) The vascular volume must remain constant between different states during which flow is compared. Since these conditions are rarely met, Pijls et al proposed to work merely under hyperemic conditions which implies that no information about resting flow has to be obtained and ensures constancy of blood flow and vascular volume[110,111]. Under those circumstances, hyperemic mean transit time was inversely proportional to hyperemic blood flow and could be used to assess functional improvement after a coronary intervention in selected patients[111,112]. Nevertheless, practical factors have limited the widespread application of videodensitometry. They include the long lasting post-processing of the data and the prerequisite for atrial pacing, for absolute patient immobility during the different image acquisitions, and especially for long-lasting held inspiration necessary to allow proper determination of the mean transit time of contrast medium. Moreover, only changes in maximum blood flow or coronary flow reserve can be reliably assessed whereas the use of videodensitometry for diagnostic purposes remains troublesome. The overlap between normal and abnormal values is too large to be useful in clinical decision making in individual patients[108,109]. Therefore, videodensitometry has been abandoned for clinical decision making and may be used occasionally when flow reserve is to be studied in the same patient under different conditions[112,113].

3.2.2 Coronary flow velocity measurements.

Although the first intracoronary Doppler catheters were developed approximately 15 years ago [114-118], the interest for coronary blood flow velocity measurements was greatly stimulated by the development of a 0.014-in steerable Doppler angioplasty guide wire with a flexible distal end (Endosonics Inc, Rancho Cordova, CA)[119-121]. The sample volume is positioned at 5.2 mm from the transducer and has an approximate width of 2.25 mm due to divergent ultrasound so that a large part of the flow velocity profile is included in the sample volume in case of eccentric position of the Doppler guide wire. A fast-Fourier transform algorithm increases the reliability of velocity measurements as compared to the classical zero-crossing detector analysis[122]. Flow velocity measurements obtained with this system have been validated in vitro and in an animal model[117,119].

The Doppler wire can be advanced into the distal part of the coronary tree without significantly impeding the flow. Furthermore the wire has handling characteristics that are similar to the majority of currently available PTCA guide wires so that it can be used to perform coronary angioplasty without the need for another guide wire. The handling characteristics of the Doppler wire allow to explore the human coronary circulation safely and without prolonging the procedure excessively. Doppler wire velocity measurements can be useful (1) to evaluate lesions of "intermediate" severity (i.e. lesions whose functional significance is not evident on the basis of contrast angiography) to decide at the time of diagnostic catheterization whether or not any revascularization procedure is warranted, (2) to monitor coronary flow during coronary interventions, and (3) to evaluate microvascular disease, the latter probably the most important application of the Doppler wire at present.

Several indexes of flow velocity have been proposed for assessing the physiological consequences of epicardial stenoses:

Coronary flow velocity reserve. Defined as the ratio of maximum to baseline flow velocity, coronary flow velocity reserve (CFVR) has been used as a surrogate for coronary flow reserve[123]. This approach is illustrated in figure 3.5. The advantages and limitations of this technique for evaluating lesion severity are summarized in table 3.3. In addition to the factors known to influence baseline flow and thus coronary flow reserve, i.e. blood pressure, heart rate, contractility, myocardial hypertrophy and microvascular disease [124-126], velocity reserve is influenced by changes in vessel cross-sectional area. Since absolute coronary flow (F) is given by the formula:

$$F = V \times CSA$$

where V is mean blood flow velocity and CSA is vessel cross-sectional area, it is evident that changes in absolute coronary flow can be mediated by changes in flow velocity, in vessel cross-sectional area, or both. Confounding effects of the interposition of side branches between the site of the measurement and the stenosis can further complicate the interpretation of velocity changes during hyperemia. Moreover, in a considerable number of patients, the Doppler signal is easily disturbed by positional changes, motion of the patient, or respiration. Finally, coronary flow velocity reserve does not take into account

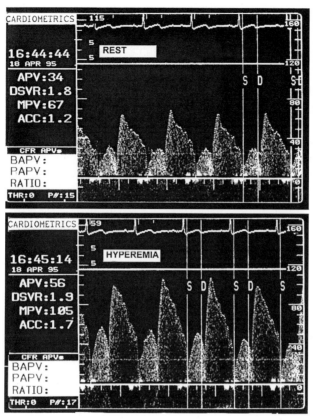

Figure 3.5 *Flow velocity recordings at rest and during hyperemia in a moderately stenotic left anterior descending artery.*

the collateral circulation which has been shown to play a major role in the functional status and prognosis of patients. Nevertheless, clinical studies have demonstrated that a coronary flow velocity reserve < 2 was most often associated with an abnormal perfusion scintigram[127]. Moreover, in patients with a coronary flow velocity reserve > 2 and in whom the planned angioplasty was deferred, a favorable medium-term prognosis was documented[128,129]. Therefore, from these studies it can be concluded that flow velocity measurements can be helpful in clinical decision-making in patients with stenosis of intermediate severity.

Several other velocity-derived indexes have been investigated to evaluate blood flow limitations by a coronary stenosis. Most of them do not have much clinical significance.

Table 3.3 *Advantages and limitations of Doppler flow velocity.*

Advantages
- ◆ all dimensions of the lesion are taken into account
- ◆ physiologic parameters are taken into account
- ◆ account for both epicardial resistance *and* myocardial resistance
- ◆ useful in the study of microvascular disease.

Limitations
- ◆ not stenosis-specific
- ◆ sensitive to hemodynamic conditions
- ◆ no clearly defined normal values
- ◆ no clearly defined cut-off values

Diastolic to systolic velocity ratio. Coronary blood flow occurs essentially during diastole while the systolic contribution to total coronary flow is markedly smaller. Distal to a coronary stenosis, there is a trend towards an equalization of systolic and diastolic contribution to total coronary flow[130-134]. A significant difference between distal diastolic to systolic velocity ratio was observed between normal arteries and arteries with significant stenosis. A cut-off value of 1.7 was proposed to distinguish between significant and non-significant lesion[134]. However, changes in the diastolic to systolic velocity ratio due to contractility (see figure 2.2) and the various patterns of diastolic to systolic ratio observed in the different coronary arteries, limit the use of this index to evaluate the physiology of the stenosis.

Proximal to distal velocity ratio. Along normal coronary arteries, a slight decrease in mean blood flow velocity is observed. This is due to the increase in total vascular cross-sectional area. In stenotic vessels, the ratio between proximal and distal mean velocity has been found significantly larger than in normal vessels (2.4 ± 0.7 vs 1.1 ± 0.2; $p < 0.001$)[134]. However, the large overlap of values in normal and diseased vessels as well as the prerequisite of important side-branches between the site of proximal measurement and the stenosis, limit the clinical usefulness of the proximal-to-distal velocity ratio.

Instantaneous hyperemic diastolic flow pressure slope index (IHDFPS). The IHDFPS index was proposed and validated by Mancini et al[135-138]. The relation between coronary flow and aortic pressure during mid and late diastole is a true index of stenosis conductance, and has been shown to be independent of heart rate, blood pressure, and contractility in animals. Preliminary studies in humans were conducted by Di Mario et al[139,140]. These authors have used a slightly modified index and found an excellent discriminatory power of the value of 0.8 cm/s/mmHg to separate lesions less from lesions greater than 30% diameter stenosis. Yet, this elegant approach of coronary physiology does not account for collateral circulation and requires a particularly stable flow velocity signal. Our experience with the IHDFPS index measurements is described in chapter 8.

During coronary interventions the Doppler guide wire is left in place distal to the lesion in order to record continuously the flow velocity during the different stages of the procedure. During balloon inflation, recruitment of collateral flow has been observed[141]. After the procedure, restoration of antegrade flow can be immediately detected, before the disappearance of electrocardiographic changes or of symptoms. The rapid flow velocity increase in the phase of post-occlusion hyperemia can be used to assess the adequacy of post-angioplasty lumen enlargement immediately after deflation of the balloon. Similarly, a normal diastolic to systolic flow velocity ratio pattern is restored immediately after the achievement of a satisfactory result. Also, the trend of the coronary flow velocity observed during the first minutes after PTCA has been reported to be able to predict subacute arterial closure[142]. Results of the Debate I and II trials and the Destiny and Frost trials suggest that the higher the coronary flow velocity reserve immediately after balloon angioplasty, the lower the cardiac event rate will be at 6 month, independently of the immediate post-angioplasty angiographic data[143-146]. Also, the combination of a CFVR > 2.5 and a residual diameter stenosis < 35% by QCA, should have a particularly low chance of restenosis within 6 months. This excellent prognosis in patients with the combination of an excellent angiographic and functional result after PTCA, was also confirmed by coronary pressure measurements as described in chapter 14 of this book[147].

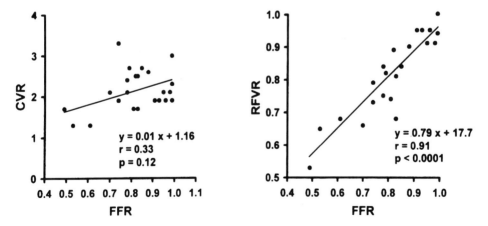

Figure 3.6 *Correlation between Doppler-derived absolute (left) and relative (right) coronary flow velocity reserve and pressure-derived fractional flow reserve in patients with a normal reference artery. (From Baumgart et al[148], with permission of the author and the American Heart Association, Inc).*

Even though the functional assessment of coronary stenosis by velocity measurements is hampered by some theoretical drawbacks, the latter are outweighed by the ease and the safety of obtaining the information. The Achilles' heel of Doppler velocity measurements remains the large overlap between normal and abnormal values inherent to every method using absolute coronary flow reserve as an endpoint, and the fact that there remains a subgroup of patients in whom only suboptimal signals can be obtained.

Some of the shortcomings of Doppler-derived coronary flow velocity reserve, can be overcome by calculating *relative flow velocity reserve (RFVR)* as recently shown in an elegant study by Baumgart et al[148]. Provided that microvascular disorders are equally distributed through the myocardium, RFVR is more stenosis-specific than absolute CFVR and less sensitive to hemodynamic variations. Reliable calculation of RFVR, however, is only possible if a truly normal reference artery is present. In those cases, RFVR correlates much better to fractional flow reserve than is the case for CFVR (figure 3.6). Besides the fact that RFVR measurement is not possible in all patients, a major disadvantage is that for obtaining this index 4 measurements should be performed: resting and hyperemic blood flow velocity in the stenotic vessel and resting and hyperemic blood flow velocity in the (normal) reference vessel whereas the same information can be obtained by a pressure wire by one measurement only. In addition, as shown in figure 10.4, the conductance of an apparently normal coronary artery in a patient with atherosclerotic heart disease, can be markedly abnormal even in the absence of a visible stenosis at angiography.

3.2.3   Coronary pressure measurements.

The body of this book is devoted to intracoronary pressure measurements and to the concept of pressure-derived fractional flow reserve, to be introduced in the next chapter. Chapter 5 and 6 describe the practical aspects of distal coronary pressure measurements with angioplasty guide wires in the catheterization laboratory. Chapter 7 to 10 validate the unique features of fractional flow reserve as an index for clinical decision making. The remaining chapters deal with clinical applications of coronary pressure measurements.

References.

1. Sones FM, Shirey EK. Cine coronary arteriography. *Med Concepts Cardiovasc Dis* 1962;31:735-738.
2. Judkins MP. Selective coronary arteriography. I. A percutaneous transfemoral approach. *Radiology* 1967;89:815-824.
3. Grondin CM, Dyrda I, Pasternac A, Campeau L, Bourassa MG, Lesperance J. Discrepancies between cine angiography and post-mortem findings in patients with coronary artery disease and recent revascularization. *Circulation* 1974;49:503-708.
4. Arnett EN, Isner JM, Redwood DR. Coronary artery narrowing in coronary heart disease: comparison of cine angiographic and necropsy findings. *Ann Intern Med* 1979; 91:350-356.
5. Isner JM, Kishel J, Kent KM. Accuracy of angiographic determination of left main coronary arterial narrowing. *Circulation* 1981;63:1056-1061.
6. Zir LM, Miller SW, Dinsmore RF, Gilbert JP, Harthorne JW. Interobserver variability in coronary arteriography. *Circulation* 1976;53:627-632.
7. De Rouen TA, Murray JA, Owen W. Variability in the analysis of the coronary angiograms. *Circulation* 1977;55:324-328.
8. Beauman GJ, Vogel RA. Accuracy of individual and panel visual interpretations of coronary arteriograms: implications for clinical decisions. *J Am Coll Cardiol* 1990; 16:108-113.
9. Meier B, Gruentzig AR, Goebel N, Pyle R, Van Gosslar W, Schlumf M. Assessment of stenoses in coronary angioplasty : inter-and intra observer variability. *Int J Cardiol* 1983;3:159-169.
10. Brown BG, Bolson E, Frimer M, Dodge HT. Quantitative coronary angiography: estimation of dimensions, hemodynamic resistance and atheroma mass of coronary artery lesions using the arteriogram and digital computation. *Circulation* 1977;53:329-337.
11. Gould KL, Kelly KO, Bolson EL. Experimental validation of quantitative coronary angiography for determining pressure flow characteristics of coronary stenosis. *Circulation* 1982;66:930-937.
12. Reiber JHC, Serruys PW, Kooijman CJ, Wijns W, Slager CJ, Gerbrands JJ, Schuurbiers JCH, den Boer A, Hugenholtz PG. Assessment of short-, medium-, and longterm variations in arterial dimension from computer assisted quantification of coronary cine angiograms. *Circulation* 1985;71:280-288.
13. de Feyter PJ, Serruys PW, Davies MJ, Richardson P, Lubsen J, Oliver MF. Quantitative coronary angiography to measure progression and regression of coronary atherosclerosis : value, limitations, and implications for clinical trials. *Circulation* 1991; 84:412-423.
14. Serruys PW, Foley DP, Kirkeeide RL, King SB. Restenosis revisited: Insights provided by quantitative coronary angiography. *Am Heart J* 1993;126:1243-1267.
15. Serruys PW, de Jaegere P, Kiemeneij F, Macaya C, Rutsch W, Heyndrickx GR, Emanuelsson H, Marco J, Legrand V, Materne P, Belardi J, Sigwart U, Colombo A, Goy JJ, Van Den Heuvel P, Delcan J, Morel M.A. A comparison of balloon-expandable-stent implantation with balloon angioplasty in patients with coronary artery disease. *New Engl J Med* 1994;331:489-495.
16. Topol EJ, Leya F, Pinkerton CA, Whitlow PL, Hofling B, Simonton CA, Masden RR, Serruys PW, Leon MB, Williams DO, King III SB, Mark DB, Isner JM, Holmes DR, Ellis SG, Lee KL, Keeler GP, Berdan LG, Hinohara T, Califf RM, for the Caveat study group. A comparison of directional atherectomy with coronary angioplasty in patients with coronary artery disease. *New Engl J Med* 1993;329:221-227.

17. Brown G, Albers JJ, Fischer LD. Regression of coronary artery disease as a result of intensive lipid-lowering therapy with high levels of apolipoprotein B. *New Engl J Med* 1990;323:1289-1298.

18. Scandinavian Simvastatin Survival Study Group. Randomized trial of cholesterol lowering in 4444 patients with coronary heart disease: the Scandinavian Simvastatin Survival Study (4S). *Lancet* 1994;344:1383-1389.

19. Wilson RF, Marcus ML, White CW. Prediction of the physiological significance of coronary arterial dimensions by quantitative lesion geometry in patients with limited coronary artery disease. *Circulation* 1987;75:723-732.

20. Zijlstra F, van Ommeren J, Reiber JHC, Serruys PW. Does quantitative assessment of coronary artery dimensions predict the physiological significance of a coronary stenosis? *Circulation* 1987;75:1154-1161.

21. White CW, Wright CB, Doty DB, Hiratza LF, Eastham CL, Harrison DG, Marcus ML. Does visual interpretation of the coronary arteriogram predict physiological importance of a coronary stenosis. *N Eng J Med* 1984;310:819-824.

22. Folland ED, Vogel RA, Hartigan P, Bates ER, Beauman GJ, Fortin T, Boucher C, Parisi AF, and the Veterans Affairs ACME Investigators. Relation between coronary artery stenosis assessed by visual, caliper and computer methods and exercise capacity in patients with single-vessel coronary artery disease. *Circulation* 1994;89:2005-2014.

23. Bartunek J, Sys SU, Heyndrickx GR, Pijls NHJ, De Bruyne B. Quantitative coronary angiography in predicting functional significance of stenoses in an unselected patient cohort. *J Am Coll Cardiol* 1995;26:328-334

24. Tobis J, Nalciogly O, Johnston WD, et al. Videodensitometric determination of minimum coronary artery luminal diameter before and after angioplasty. *Am J Cardiol* 1987;59:38-44.

25. Sans ML, Mancini GBJ, Lefree MT. Variability of quantitative digital subtraction coronary angiography before en after percutaneous transluminal coronary angioplasty. *Am J Cardiol* 1987;60:55-60.

26. Katritsis D, Lythall DA, Anderson MH, Looper IC, Webb-Peploe MM. Assessment of coronary angioplasty by an automated digital angiographic method. *Am Heart J* 1988; 116:1181-1187.

27. von Birgelen C, Kutryk MJ, Gil R, Ozaki Y, Di Mario C, Roelandt JR, De Feyter PJ, Serruys PW. Quantification of the minimal luminal cross-sectional area after coronary stenting by two- and three-dimensional intravascular ultrasound versus edge detection and videodensitometry. *Am J Cardiol* 1996;78:520-525.

28. Gurley JC, Nissen SE, Booth DC, DeMaria AN. Influence of operator- and patient-dependent variables on suitability of automated quantitative coronary arteriography for routine clinical use. *J Am Coll Cardiol* 1992;19:1237-1243.

29. Kalbfleisch SJ, McGillem MJ, Simon SB, DeBoe SF, Pinto IMF, Mancini GBJ. Automated quantitation of indexes of coronary lesion complexity. Comparison between patients with stable and unstable angina. *Circulation* 1990;82:439-447.

30. Vanoverschelde JL, Wijns W, Depre C, Essamri B, Heyndrickx GR, Borgers M, Bol A, Melin JA. Mechanisms of chronic regional post-ischemic dysfunction in humans. New insights from the study of non-infarcted collateral-dependent myocardium. *Circulation* 1993;87:1513-1523.

31. Gould KL, Lipscomb K, Hamilton GW. Physiological basis for assessing critical coronary stenosis: instantaneous flow response and regional distribution during coronary hyperemia as measures of coronary flow reserve *Am J Cardiol* 1974;33:87-94.

32. Rensing BJ, Hermans WR, Deckers JW, De Feyter PJ, Serruys PW. Which angiographic variable best describes functional status 6 months after successful single-vessel coronary balloon angioplasty ? *J Am Col Cardiol* 1993;21:317-324.

33. Roelandt JRTC, Di Mario C, Pandian NG, Wenguang L, Keane D, Slager CJ, de Feyter PJ, Serruys PW. Three dimensional reconstruction of intracoronary ultrasound images. Rationale, approaches, problems, and directions. *Circulation* 1994;90:1044-1055.

34. Li W. Image and signal processing in intravascular ultrasound. *Thesis, Rotterdam Thorax Center* 1997; ISBN 90-9010679-0.

35. Di Mario C. Intracoronary ultrasound. Introduction to catheter-based intracoronary diagnostic techniques; in *Intracoronary Ultrasound* 1993, Thesis, ICG Printing, Dordrecht, pp3-30.

36. Mc Pherson DD, Hiratzka LF, Lamberth WC, Brandt B, Hunt M, Kieso RA, Marcus ML, Kerber RE. Delineation of the extent of coronary atherosclerosis by high frequency epicardial echocardiography. *New Engl J Med* 1987;316:304-309.

37. Glagov S, Weisenberg E, Zarins CK, Stankunavicius R, Kolettis GJ. Compensatory enlargement of human atherosclerotic coronary arteries. *New Engl J Med* 1987; 316:1371-1375.

38. Stiel GM, Stiel LSG, Schofer MAJ, Donath K, Mathey DG. Impact of compensatory enlargement of atherosclerotic coronary arteries on angiographic assessment of coronary artery disease. *Circulation* 1989;80:1603-1609.

39. Mc Pherson DD, Sirna SJ, Hiratzka LF, Thorpe L, Armstrong ML, Marcus ML, Kerber RE. Coronary artery remodeling studies by high frequency epicardial echocardiography: An early compensatory mechanisms in patients with obstructive coronary atherosclerosis. *J Am Coll Cardiol* 1991;17:79-86.

40. Losordo DW, Rosenfield K, Kaufmann J, Pieczek A, Isner JM. Focal compensatory enlargement of human arteries in response to progressive atherosclerosis. In vivo documentation using intravascular ultrasound. *Circulation* 1994;89:2570-2577.

41. Hermiller JB, Tenaglia AN, Kisslo KB, Phillips HR, Bashore TM, Stack RS, Davidson GJ. In vivo validation of compensatory enlargement of atherosclerotic coronary arteries. *Am J Cardiol* 1993;71:665-668.

42. Nissen SE, Gurley JC, Grines CL, Booth DC, McClure R, Berk M, Fischer C, De Maria AN. Intravascular ultrasound assessment of lumen size and wall morphology in normal subjects and patients with coronary artery disease. *Circulation* 1991;84:1087-1099.

43. Alfonso F, Macaya C, Goicolea J, Inniguez 1, Hernandez R, Zamarano J, Perez-Viscaine MJ, Zarco P. Intraventricular ultrasound imaging of angiographically normal coronary segments in patients with coronary artery disease. *Am Heart J* 1994;127:536-544.

44. Gerber TC, Erbel R, Gorge G, Ge J, Rupprecht HJ, Meyer J. Extent of atherosclerosis and remodeling of the left main coronary artery determined by intravascular ultrasound. *Am J Cardiol* 1994;73:666-671.

45. Tuzcu EM, Hobbs RE, Rincon G, Bott-Silverman C, Defranco AC, Robinson K, McCarthy PM, Stewart RW, Guyer S, Nissen SE. Occult and frequent transmission of atherosclerotic coronary artery disease with cardiac transplantation. Insights from intravascular ultrasound. *Circulation* 1995;91:1706-1713.

46. Mintz GS, Painter JA, Pichard AD, Kent KM, Satler LF, Popma JJ, Chuang YC, Bucher TA, Sokolowicz LE, Leon MB. Atherosclerosis in angiographically "normal" coronary artery reference segments: an intravascular ultrasound study with clinical correlations. *J Am Coll Cardiol* 1995;25:1479-1485.

47. Fuster V. Mechanisms leading to myocardial infarction: insights from studies of vascular biology. *Circulation* 1994;90:2127-2146.

48. Davies MJ, Thomas AC. Plaque fissuring: the cause of acute myocardial infarction, sudden ischemic death and crescendo angina. *Br Heart J* 1985;53:363-373.

49. Falk E. Unstable angina with fatal outcome:dynamic coronary thrombosis leading to infarction and/or sudden death; autopsy evidence of recurrent mural thrombus with peripheral embolization culminating in total vascular occlusion. *Circulation* 1985; 71:699-708.

50. Fuster V, Badimon L, Badimon JJ, Chesebro JH. The pathogenesis of coronary artery disease and the acute coronary syndromes. *New Engl J Med* 1992;326:242-250.

51. Libby P. Lesion versus lumen. *Nature Med* 1995;1:17-18.

52. Little WC, Constantinescu M, Appelgate RJ, Kutcher MA, Burrows MT, Kahl FR, Santamore WP. Can coronary angiography predict the site of a subsequent myocardial infarction in patients with mild-to-moderate coronary artery disease ? *Circulation* 1988;78:1157-1166.

53. McHodgson JB, Reddy KG, Suneja R, Nair RN, Lesnefsky EJ, Sheehan HM. Intra coronary ultrasound imaging: correlation of plaque morphology with angiography, clinical syndrome and procedural results in patients undergoing coronary angioplasty. *J Am Coll Cardiol* 1993;21:35-44.

54. de Feyter PJ, Escaned J, Di Mario C. Combined intracoronary ultrasound and angioscopic imaging in patients with unstable angina. Target lesion characteristics (abstr). *Eur Heart J* 1993;14:25.

55. Tenaglia AN, Buller CE, Kisslo KB, Stack RS, Davidson CJ. Mechanisms of balloon angioplasty and directional coronary atherectomy as assessed by intracoronary ultrasound. *J Am Coll Cardiol* 1992;20:685-691.

56. The SHK, Gussenhoven EJ, Zhong Y, Li W, van Egmond F, Pieterman H, van Urk H, Gerritsen P, Borst C, Wilson RA, Bom N. Effect of balloon angioplasty on femoral artery evaluated with intravascular ultrasound imaging. *Circulation* 1992;86:483-493.

57. Losordo DW, Rosenfield K, Pieczek A, Baker K, Harding M, Isner JM. How does angioplasty work? Serial analysis of human iliac arteries using intravascular ultrasound. *Circulation* 1992;86:1845-1858.

58. Waller BF, Orr CM, Pinkerton CA, van Tassel J, Peters T, Slack JD. Coronary balloon angioplasty dissections: "the Good, the Bad and the Ugly". *J Am Coll Cardiol* 1992; 20:701-706.

59. Yock PG, Fitzgerald PJ, Linker DT, Angelsen BAJ. Intravascular ultrasound guidance for catheter based coronary interventions. *J Am Coll Cardiol* 1991;6:39B-45B.

60. Violaris AG, Linnemeier TJ, Campbell S, Rothbaum DA, Cumberland DC. Intravascular ultrasound imaging combined with coronary angioplasty. *Lancet* 1992; 339:1571-1572.

61. Akasaka T (personal communication).

62. Lee RT, Loree HM, Cheng GC, Lieberman EJ, Jaramillo N, Schoen FJ. Computational structural analysis based on intravascular ultrasound imaging before in vitro angioplasty: prediction of plaque fracture locations. *J Am Coll Cardiol* 1993;21:777-782.

63. Mintz GS, Pichard AD, Kent KM, Satler LF, Popma JJ, Leon MB. Axial plaque redistribution as a mechanism of percutaneous transluminal coronary angioplasty. *Am J Cardiol* 1996;77:427-430.

64. Mintz GS, Kovach JA, Javier SP, Pichard AD, Kent KM, Popma MM, Salter LF, Leon MB. Mechanims of lumen enlargement after excimer laser coronary angioplasty. An intravascular ultrasound study. *Circulation* 1995;92:3408-3414.

65. Mintz GS, Popma JJ, Hong MK, Pichard AD, Kent KM, Satler LF, Leon MB. Intravascular ultrasound to discern device-specific effects and mechanisms of restenosis. *Am J Cardiol* 1996;78:18-22.

66. Mintz GS, Popma JJ, Hong MK, Pichard AD, Kent KM, Satler LF, Leon MB. Intravascular ultrasound to discern device-specific effects and mechanisms of restenosis. *Am J Cardiol* 1996;78:18-22.

67. Slepian MJ. Application of intra luminal ultrasound imaging to vascular stenting. *Int J Cardiac Imaging* 1991;6:285-311.

68. Mudra H, Klauss V, Blasini R, Kroetz M, Rieber J, Regar E, Thiesen K. Ultrasound guidance of Palmaz-Schatz intracoronary stenting with a combined ultravascular ultrasound balloon catheter. *Circulation* 1994;90:1252-1261.

69. Nakamura S, Colombo A, Gaglione A, Almagor Y, Goldberg SL, Maiello L, Finci L, Tobis JM. Intracoronary ultrasound observations during stent implantation. *Circulation* 1994; 89:2026-2034.

70. Goldberg SL, Colombo A, Nakamura S, Almagor Y, Maiello L, Tobis JM. Benefit of intracoronary ultrasound in the deployment of Palmaz-Schatz stents. *J Am Coll Cardiol* 1994;24:996-1003.

71. Colombo A, Hall P, Nakamura S, Almagor Y, Maiello L, Martini G, Gaglione A, Goldberg SL, Tobis J. Intracoronary stenting without anti coagulantia accomplished with intravascular ultrasonic guidance. *Circulation* 1995;91:1676-1688.

72. Post MJ, Borst C, Kuntz RE. The relative importance of arterial remodeling compared with intimal hyperplasia in lumen renarrowing after balloon angioplasty. A study in the normal rabbit and the hypercholesterolemic Yucatan micropig. *Circulation* 1994; 89:2816-2821.

73. Pasterkamp G, Wensing PJ, Post MJ, Hillen B, Mali WP, Borst C. Parodoxical arterial wall shrinkage may contribute to luminal narrowing of human atherosclerotic femoral arteries. *Circulation* 1995;91:1444-1449.

74. Pasterkamp G, Borst C, Post MJ, Mali WP, Wensing PJ, Gussenhoven EJ, Hillen B. *Circulation* 1996;93:1818-1825.

75. Andersen HR, Maeng M, Thorwest M, Falk E. Remodeling rather than neointimal formation explains luminal narrowing after deep vessel wall injury: insights from a porcine coronary (re) stenosis model. *Circulation* 1996;93:1716-1724.

76. Kakuta T, Currier JW, Haudenschild CC, Ryan TJ, Faxon DP. Differences in compensatory vessel enlargement, not intimal formation, account for restenosis after angioplasty in the hypercholesterolemie rabbit model. *Circulation* 1994;89:2809-2815.

77. Shi Y, Pieniek M, Fard A, O'Brien J, Mannion JD, Zalewski A. Adventitial remodeling after coronary arterial injury. *Circulation* 1996;93:340-348.

78. Mintz GS, Popma JJ, Pichard AD, Kent KM, Satler LF, Wing SC, Hong MK, Kovach JA, Leon MB. Arterial remodeling after coronary angioplasty. A serial intravascular ultrasound study. *Circulation* 1996;94:35-43.

79. Painter JA, Mintz GS, Wong SC, Popma JJ, Pichard AD, Kent KM, Satler LF, Leon MB. Serial intravascular ultrasound studies fail to show evidence of chronic Palmaz-Schatz stent recoil. *Am J Cardiol* 1995;75:398-400.

80. Hoffmann R, Mintz GS, Dussaillant GR, Popma JJ, Pichard AD, Satler LF, Kent KM, Griffin J, Leon MB. Patterns and mechanisms of in-stent restenosis. A serial intravascular ultrasound study. *Circulation* 1996;94:1247-1454.

81. Mintz GS, Pichard AD, Kovach JA, Kent KM, Satler LF, Javier SP, Popma JL, Leon MB. Impact of preintervention intravascular ultrasound imaging on transcatheter treatment strategies in coronary artery disease. *Am J Cardiol* 1994;73:423-430.

82. Nishioka T, Luo H, Eigler NL, Tabak SW, Lepor N, Forrester JS, Siegel RJ. The evolving utility of intracoronary ultrasound. *Am J Cardiol* 1995;75:539-541.

83. Alfonso F, Macaya C, Goicolea J, Hernandez R, Segovia J, Zamorano J, Zarco P. Acute coronary closure complicating intravascular ultrasound examination. *Eur Heart J* 1994; 15:710-712.

84. Haussman D, Erbel R, Alibelli-Chemarin MJ, et al The safety of intracoronary ultrasound: a multicenter survey of 2207 examinations. *Circulation* 1995;91:623-630.

85. Nishioka T, Amanullah AM, Luo H, Berglund H, Kim CJ, Nagai T, Hakamata N, Katsushika S, Uehata A, Takase B, Isojima K, Berman DS, Siegel RJ. Clinical validation of intravascular ultrasound imaging for assessment of coronary stenosis severity. *J Am Coll Cardiol* 1999; 33: 1870-1878.

86. Skinner MP, Yan C, Mitsumori L, Hayes CE, Raines EW, Nelson JA, Ross R. Serial magnetic resonance imaging of experimental atherosclerosis detects lesion fine structure, progression and complication in vivo. *Nature Med* 1995;1:69-73.

87. Siegel RJ, Ariani M, Fishbein MC. Histopathologic validation of angioscopy and intravascular ultrasound. *Circulation* 1991;84:109-117.

88. Sherman CT, Litvack F, Grundfest W, Lee M, Hickey A, Chaux A, Kass R, Blanche C, Matloff J, Morgenstern L, Ganz W, Swan HJC, Forrester J. Coronary angioscopy in patients with unstable angina pectoris. *N Engl J Med* 1986;315:913-919.

89. Mizuno K, Satomura K, Ambrose JA. Angioscopic evaluation of coronary artery thrombi in acute coronary syndromes. *New Engl J Med* 1992;326:287-291.

90. Mizuno K, Miyamoto A, Satomura K, Kurita A, Arai T, Sakurada M, Yanagida S, Nakamura H. Angioscopic coronary macromorphology in patients with acute coronary disorders. *Lancet* 1991;337:809-812.

91. White CJ, Ramee SR, Collins TJ, Mesa JE, Jain A. Percutaneous angioscopy of saphenous vein coronary bypass grafts. *J Am Coll Cardiol* 1993;21:1181-1185.

92. Hombach V, Hoher, M, Kochs M, Eggeling T, Schmidt H, Hopp HW, Hilger HH. Pathophysiology of unstable angina pectoris. Correlations with coronary angioscopic imaging. *Eur Heart J* 1988;9:40-45.

93. Neville FN, Yasuhara H, Watanabe BI, Canady J, Duran W, Hobson RW. Endovascular management of arterial intimal defects. An experimental comparison by arteriography, angioscopy and intravascular ultrasonography. *J Vasc Surg* 1991; 13:496-502.

94. White CJ, Ramee SR, Mesa JE, Collins TJ. Percutaneous coronary angioscopy in patients with restenosis after coronary angioplasty. *J Am Coll Cardiol* 1991;17:46B-49B.

95. Teirstein PS, Schatz RA, Wong SC, Rocha-Singh KJ. Coronary stenting with angioscopic guidance. *Am J Cardiol* 1995;75:344-347.

96. De Bruyne B, Bronzwaer JGF, Heyndrickx GR, Paulus WJ. Comparative effects of ischemia and hypoxemia on left ventricular systolic and diastolic function in humans. *Circulation* 1993;88:861-881.

97. Rutishauser W, Simon H, Stucky JP, Schad N, Noseda G, Wellauer J. Evaluation of roentgen cinedensitometry for flow measurement in models and in the intact circulation. *Circulation* 1967;36:951-963.

98. Rutishauser W, Bussmann WD, Noseda G, Meier W, Wellauer J. Blood flow measurement through single coronary arteries by roentgen densitometry. Part I: A comparison of flow measured by a radiologic technique applicable in the intact organism and by electromagnetic flowmeter. *Am J Roentgenol* 1970;109:12-20.

99. Rutishauser W, Noseda G, Bussmann WD, Preter B. Blood flow measurement through single coronary arteries by roentgen densitometry. Part II: Right coronary artery flow in conscious man. *Am J Roentgenol* 1970;109:21-21.

100. Hodgson JM, Legrand V, Bates ER, Mancini GBJ, Aueron FM, O'Neill WW, Simon SB, Beauman GJ, LeFree MT, Vogel RA. Validation in dogs of a rapid digital angiographic tecnhique to measure relative coronary blood flow during routine cardiac catheterization. *Am J Cardiol* 1985;55:188-193.

101. Cusma JT, Toggart EJ, Folts JD, Peppler WW, Hagiandreou NJ, Lee CS, Mistretta CA. Digital subtraction imaging of coronary flow reserve. *Circulation* 1987;75:461-472.

102. Van der Werf T, Heethaar RM, Stegehuis H, Meyler FL. The concept of apparent cardiac arrest as a prerequisite for coronary digital subtraction angiography. *J Am Coll Cardiol* 1984; 4: 239-244.

103. Whiting JS, Drury JK, Pfaff JM, Chang BL, Eigler NL, Meerbaum S, Corday E, Nivatpumin T, Forrester JS, Swan HJC. Digital angiographic measurement of radiographic contrast material kinetics for estimation of myocardial perfusion. *Circulation* 1986;73:789-798.

104. Nissen SE, Elion JL, Booth DC, Evans J, DeMaria AN. Value and limitations of computer analysis of digital subtraction angiography in the assessment of coronary flow reserve. *Circulation* 1986;73:562-571.

105. De Bruyne B, Dorsaz PA, Doriot PA, Meier B, Finci L, Rutishauser W. Assessment of regional coronary flow reserve by digital angiography in patients with coronary artery disease. *Int J Cardiac Imaging* 1987;3:47-55.

106. Zijlstra F, den Boer A, Reiber JHC, van Es GA, Lubsen J, Serruys PW. Assessment of immediate and long-term results of percutaneous transluminal coronary angioplasty. *Circulation* 1988;78:15-24.

107. Legrand V, Mancini GBJ, Bates E, Hodgson JM, Gross MD, Vogel RA. Comparative study of coronary flow reserve, coronary anatomy and result of radionuclide exercise test in patients with coronary artery disease. *J Am Coll Cardiol* 1986;8:1022-1032.

108. Hess OM, McGillem MJ, De Boe SF, Pinto IMF, Gallagher KP, Mancini GBJ. Determination of coronary flow reserve by parametric imaging.*Circulation* 1990; 82: 1438-1448.

109. Pijls NHJ. Maximal myocardial perfusion as a measure of the functional significance of coronary arteriogram. *Kluwer Academic Publishers* 1991.

110. Pijls NHJ, Uijen GJH, Hoevelaken A, Arts T, Aengevaeren WRM, Bos HS, Fast JH, Van Leeuwen KL, Van de Werf T. Mean transmit time for the assessment of myocardial perfusion by videodensitometry. *Circulation* 1990;81:1331-1340.

111. Pijls NHJ, Aengevaeren WRM, Uijen GJH, Hoevelaken A, Pijnenburg T, van Leeuwen K, van de Werf T. The concept of maximal flow ratio of immediate evaluation of percutaneous transluminal coronary angioplasty results by videodensitometry. *Circulation* 1991;83: 854-865.

112. Haude M, Gaspari G, Baumgart D, Brennecke R, Meyer J, Erbel R. Comparison of myocardial perfusion reserve before and after coronary balloon predilatation and after stent implantation in patients with post-angioplasty restenosis. *Circulation* 1996; 94:286-297.

113. Vassalli G, Gallino A, Kiowsky W, Jiang Z, Turina M, Hess OM. Reduced coronary flow reserve during exercise in cardiac transplant recipients. *Circulation* 1997;95:607-613.

114. Wilson RF, Laughlin DE, Ackell PH, Chilian WM, Holida MD, Hartley CJ, Armstrong ML, Marcus ML, White CW. Transluminal subselective measurement of coronary artery blood flow velocity and vasodilator reserve in man. *Circulation* 1985;72:82-92.

115. Sibley DH, Millar HD, Hartley CJ, Whitlow PL. Subselective measurement of coronary blood flow velocity using a steerable Doppler catheter. *J Am Coll Cardiol* 1986; 8:1332-1340.

116. Wilson RF, Marcus ML, White CW. Prediction of the physiological significance of coronary arterial lesions by quantitative lesion geometry in patients with limited coronary artery disease. *Circulation*, 1987;75:723-732.

117. Serruys PW, Juilliere Y, Zijlstra F, Beatt KJ, de Feyter PJ, Suryapranata H, van den Brand M, Roelandt J. Coronary blood flow velocity during percutaneous transluminal coronary angioplasty a s a guide for assessment of the functional result. *Am J Cardiol* 1988; 61:253-259.

118. Wilson RF, Johnson MR, Marcus ML, Aylward PEG, Skorton DJ, Collins S, White CW. The effect of coronary angioplasty on coronary blood flow reserve. *Circulation* 1988;71:873-885.

119. Doucette JW, Corl PD, Payne HM, Flynn AE, Goto M, Nassi M, Segal J. Validation of a Doppler guide wire for intravascular measurement of coronary artery flow velocity. *Circulation* 1992;85:1899-1911.

120. Segal J, Kern MJ, Scott NA, King SB, Doucette JW, Heuser RR, Ofili E, Siegel R. Alterations of phasic coronary artery flow velocity in humans during percutaneous coronary angioplasty. *J Am Coll Cardiol* 1992;20:276-286.

121. Labovitz AJ, Anthonis DM, Cravens TL, Kern MJ. Validation of volumetric flow measurements by means of a Doppler-tipped coronary angioplasty guide wire. *Am Heart J* 1993;126:1456-1461.

122. Di Mario C, Roelandt JRTC, de Jaegere P, Linker DT, Oomen J, Serruys PW. Limitations of the zero-crossing detector in the analysis of intracoronary Doppler. A comparison with fast Fourier transform of basal, hyperemic and transstenotic blood flow velocity measurements in patients with coronary artery disease. *Cath Cardiovasc Diagn* 1992;28:56-64.

123. Gould KL, Lipscomb K, Hamilton GW. Physiological basis for assessing critical coronary stenosis: instanteneous flow response and regional distribution during coronary hyperemia as measures of coronary flow reserve. *Am J Cardiol* 1974;33:87-94.

124. Klocke FJ. Measurements of coronary flow reserve: defining pathophysiology versus making decisions about patient care. *Circulation* 1987;76:245-253.

125. McGinn Al, White CW, Wilson RF. Interstudy variability of coronary flow reserve: influence of heart rate, arterial pressure and ventricular preload. *Circulation* 1990; 81:1319-1330.

126. Rossen JD, Winniford MD. Effect of increases in heart rate and arterial pressure on coronary flow reserve in humans. *J Am Coll Cardiol* 1993;21:343-348.

127. Miller DD, Donohue TJ, Younis LT, Back RG, Aguirre FV, Wittry MD, Goodgold HM, Chaitman BR, Kern MJ. Correlation of pharmacological ^{99m}Tc-sestamibi myocardial perfusion imaging with post-stenotic coronary flow reserve in patients with angiographically intermediate coronary artery stenoses. *Circulation* 1994;89:2150-2160.

128. Moses JW, Shaknovich A, Kreps EM, Undemir C, Lieberman SM. Clinical follow-up of intermediate coronary lesions not hemodynamically significant by Doppler flow wire criteria (abstract). *Circulation* 1994;90:I-227.

129. Kern MJ, Donohue TJ, Aguirre FV, Bach RG, Caracciolo EA, Wolford T, Mechem CJ, Flynn MS, Chaitman B. Clinical outcome of deferring angioplasty in patients with normal translesional pressure-flow velocity measurements. *J Am Coll Cardiol* 1995; 25:178-187.

130. Folts JD, Gallagher K, Rowe GG. Blood flow reductions in stenosed canine coronary arteries: vasospasm or platelet aggregration ? *Circulation* 1982;65:248-253.

131. Goto M, Flynn AE, Doucette JW, Kimura A, Hiramatsu O, Yamamoto T, Ogasawara Y, Tsujioka K, Hoffman JIE, Kaijwa F. Effect of intracoronary nitroglycerin administration on phasic pattern and transmural distribution of flow during coronary artery stenosis. *Circulation* 1992;85:2296-2304.

132. Kajiya F, OgasawaraY, Tsujioka K. Analysis of flow characteristics in post-stenotic regions of the human coronary artery during bypass graft surgery. *Circulation* 1987; 76:1092-1097.

133. Ofili EO, Labovitz AJ, Kern MJ. Coronary flow dynamics in normal and diseased arteries. *Am J Cardiol* 1993;71:3D-9D.

134. Donohue TJ, Kern MJ, Aguirre FV, Bach RG, Wolford T, Bell CA. Assessing the hemodynamic significance of coronary artery stenoses: analysis of translesional pressure-flow velocity relations in patients. *J Am Cardiol* 1993;22:449-458.

135. Mancin i GBJ, McGillem MJ, DeBoe SF, Gallagher KP. The diastolic hyperemic flow vs pressure relation: a new index of coronary stenosis severity and flow reserve. *Circulation* 1989;80:941-950.

136. Mancini GBJ, Cleary RM, DeBoe SF, Moore NB, Gallagher KP. Instanteneous hyperemic flow-vs-pressure slope index. Microsphere validation of an alternative to measures of coronary flow reserve. *Circulation* 1991;84:862-870.

137. Cleary RM, Aron D, Moore NB, De Boe SF, Mancini GBJ. Tachycardia, contractility and volume loading alter conventional indexes of coronary flow reserve, but not the instanteneous hyperemic flow-versus-pressure slope index. *J Am Coll Cardiol* 1992; 20: 1261-1269.

138. Cleary RM, Moore NB, De Boe SF, Mancini GBJ. Sensitivity and reproducibility of the instantenous hyperemic flow-versus-pressure slope index compared to coronary flow reserve for the assessment of stenosis severity. *Am Heart J* 1993;126:57-65.

139. Serruys PW, Di Mario C, Meneveau N, de Jaegere P, Strikwerda S, de Feyter PJ, Emanuelsson. Intra coronary pressure and flow velocity from sensor tip guide wires. A new methodological comprehensive approach for the assessment of coronary hemodynamics before and after interventions. *Am J Cardiol* 1993;71:41D-53D.

140. Di Mario C, Krams R, Gil R, Serruys PW. Slope of the instantaneous hyperemic diastolic coronary flow velocity-pressure relation. A new index for assessment of the physiological significance of coronary stenosis in humans. *Circulation* 1994; 90:1215-1224.

141. Donohue TJ, Kern MJ, Bach K. Examination of the effects of hemodynamic and pharmacologic interventions on coronary collateral flow in a patient during cardiac catheterization. *Cath Cardiovasc Diagn* 1993;28:155-161.

142. Kern MJ, Aguirre FV, Donohue TJ, Bach RG, Caracciolo EA, Flynn MS. Coronary flow velocity monitoring after angioplasty associated with abrupt reocclusion. *Am Heart J* 1994;127:436-437

143. Serruys PW, Di Mario C. Prognostic value of coronary flow velocity and diameter stenosis in assessing the short and long-term outcome of balloon angioplasty: The Debate Study (Doppler Endpoints Balloon Angioplasty Trial Europe). *Circulation* 1996;94:I-317.

144. De Bruyne B and Debate II investigators. A randomized study to evaluate provisional stenting after guided balloon angioplasty. *Circulation* 1998; 98: I-498.

145. Di Mario C and the DESTINI-CFR study group. Doppler and QCA guided aggressive PTCA has the same target lesion revascularization as stent implantation: 6-month-results of the DESTINI-study. *J Am Coll Cardiol* 1999; 33: 47A.

146. Lafont A and the FROST study group. The French optimal stenting trial: a multicenter, prospective, randomized study comparing systematic stenting to angiography/coronary flow reserve guided stenting: 6-month clinical and angiographic follow-up. *J Am Coll Cardiol* 1999; 33: 89A.

147. Bech GJW, Pijls NHJ, De Bruyne B, Peels KH, Michels HR, Bonnier JJRM, Koolen JJ. Usefulness of fractional flow reserve to predict clinical outcome after balloon angioplasty. *Circulation* 1999; 99: 883-888.

148. Baumgart D, Haude M, Goerge G, Ge J, Vetter S, Dagres N, Heusch G, Erbel R. Improved assessment of coronary stenosis severity using the relative flow velocity reserve. *Circulation* 1998; 98: 40-46.

Chapter 4

FRACTIONAL FLOW RESERVE

From Coronary Pressure to Coronary Flow

4.1 Introduction.

As explained in the former chapter, the major disadvantages of absolute coronary flow reserve for clinical decision-making are the variability of normal values, the dependency on hemodynamic loading conditions, and the inability to distinguish the effects of epicardial coronary disease and micro-vascular disease on coronary blood flow[1-5]. As a result, there is a wide variation in normal values and a large overlap between normal and pathologic values, i.e. values associated with inducible ischemia or not[5-7]. Therefore, clinical decision-making based upon absolute coronary flow reserve, remains difficult.

The ideal index of flow reserve should be independent of blood pressure, heart rate, and contractility; it should have an unequivocal normal value irrespective of the individual patient or coronary artery which is being investigated; it should clearly separate lesions which are or are not capable of causing reversible ischemia; and it should include the effects of the collateral circulation. Last but not least, the index should be easy to determine.

These considerations have led to the development of the concept of fractional flow reserve, which has been validated step by step during the last years[7-18]. The easiest way to obtain fractional flow reserve is by coronary pressure measurements. Therefore, before introducing the concept of fractional flow reserve, some prerequisites with respect to the interpretation of coronary pressure measurement have to be made.

4.2   Prerequisites for coronary pressure measurement.

Early attempts to relate transstenotic pressure gradients to the functional significance of a coronary stenosis were made already by Gruentzig but the results were disappointing[19]. No consistent relation between coronary gradients and obstruction to flow could be established at that time. With the development of smaller balloon catheters with 0.014-in lumina, and rapid exchange monorail catheters, coronary pressure as a tool to guide interventions completely disappeared.

There are three reasons why, in the past, coronary pressure measurement has not been useful for assessment of flow.

First, the instrument used (in most cases the balloon catheter) was unsuitable because its size was too large compared with the cross-sectional area of a coronary artery. Even in case of a 50% stenosis in a vessel with a diameter of 3.0 mm, severe overestimation of the pressure gradient may occur when using a 2.2F catheter, and even in normal coronary arteries unpredictable and considerable gradients may be induced by that type of equipment[8,20] (figure 6-4). *Therefore, the first prerequisite for reliable intracoronary pressure recording is to use ultrathin pressure-monitoring guide wires, which are available at present in an 0.014-in size.* It has been demonstrated that such a small wire does not noticeably overestimate gradients, not even in the case of a 80% stenosis in a vessel with a diameter as small as 2.5 mm[8,20].

Second, in the past it was not recognized that meaningful measurement of coronary pressure can only be performed in a maximum hyperemic state. Many coronary stenoses may produce no or minimal gradients at rest, but show considerable gradients at maximum hyperemia. In this context, one should realize that the extent to which a patient is limited by coronary artery disease, is not determined by resting flow or resting gradient, but by maximum hyperemic flow only. As long as maximum flow is sufficient to meet the metabolic demands of the myocardium, there is no ischemia, and the patient has no complaints. As soon as maximum flow, however, is no longer sufficient to meet the metabolic demands of the heart, myocardial ischemia and angina pectoris will occur. *Therefore, to estimate the extent to which a patient is limited by a coronary stenosis, it is only meaningful to study maximum achievable blood flow in that particular artery and to relate this to maximum blood flow in that same coronary artery as it would be if no stenosis were present at all.* As a consequence, pressure measurements are only meaningful at maximum coronary hyperemia. This, in fact, is one of the key concepts in understanding the meaning of fractional flow reserve.

Third, in the initial studies to use transstenotic pressure to predict effects on blood flow, coronary flow or flow impairment has been related to transstenotic pressure gradient itself [21-26]. That approach is fundamentally limited because it fails to recognize that *it is not the gradient, but the remaining distal coronary pressure which determines myocardial perfusion.* This point is further elucidated in the next paragraph and in figure 4.1.

Once these historical limitations have been sufficiently recognized, it is no longer difficult to understand the background and definition of fractional flow reserve.

4.3 Myocardial Fractional Flow Reserve.

The concept of fractional flow reserve is clarified in figure 4.1, which represents a coronary artery and its dependent myocardium. Suppose that this system is studied at maximum vasodilation, corresponding to maximum coronary and myocardial hyperemia when myocardial resistance is minimal (and therefore constant) and blood flow is proportional to driving pressure. If there were no coronary stenosis at all, the perfusion pressure over the myocardium in figure 4.1 would be 100-0 mmHg. Suppose now that there is a coronary stenosis, resulting in a hyperemic gradient of 30 mmHg. To understand the physiologic meaning of such a stenosis, one should *not* look at that gradient but realize, however, that as a result of the stenosis, maximum perfusion pressure over the myocardium has fallen to 70-0 mmHg only. Therefore, maximum attainable blood flow to the myocardium in the presence of the stenosis, is only 70% of normal maximum flow, as it would be in case the artery were completely normal. We say now that the fractional flow reserve of the myocardium supplied by this artery, is 70% or 0.7. *In fact, fractional flow reserve represents that very fraction of maximum flow which can still be maintained in spite of the presence of the stenosis. It is exactly that index which tells to what extent a patient is limited by his coronary artery disease.*

In other words, maximum flow is expressed as a fraction of its normal value.

$$FFR_{myo} = \frac{\underline{\text{Maximum myocardial flow in the presence of a stenosis}}}{\text{Normal maximum flow}}$$

More generally, normal maximum myocardial blood flow (Q^N) is given by:

$$Q^N = \frac{(P_a - P_v)}{R}$$

where R is myocardial resistance at maximum vasodilation and P_a and P_v represent mean aortic pressure and mean central venous pressure, respectively; whereas actual maximum blood flow in the presence of the stenosis is given by:

$$Q = \frac{(P_d - P_v)}{R}$$

where P_d represents hyperemic distal coronary pressure. Because the myocardial vascular bed is maximally vasodilated, its resistance is minimal and constant. Therefore, FFR_{myo}, defined as Q/Q^N, is given by:

$$FFR_{myo} = \frac{P_d - P_v}{P_a - P_v}$$

where P_a, P_d, and P_v represent mean aortic, distal coronary , and central venous pressure, obtained at maximum coronary hyperemia. Because generally, central venous pressure is close to zero, this equation can be further simplified to:

$$FFR_{myo} = \frac{P_d}{P_a}$$

As P_a can be measured in a regular way by the coronary or guiding catheter, and P_d is easily obtainable by crossing the stenosis with a sensor-tipped guide wire, it is clear that FFR_{myo} can be simply obtained, both during diagnostic and interventional procedures, by measuring the respective pressures. From the equations above it is also obvious that, theoretically, FFR_{myo} for a normal coronary artery will equal 1.0.

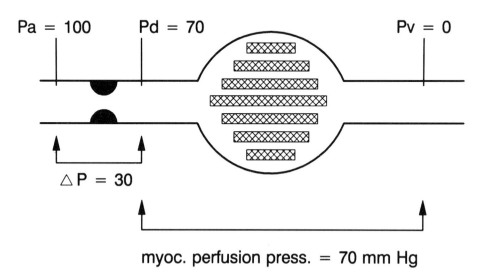

Pa = 100 **Pd = 70** **Pv = 0**

$\triangle$P = 30

myoc. perfusion press. = 70 mm Hg

Figure 4.1 *Simplified representation of a coronary artery and the supplied myocardium to clarify the rationale of FFR_{myo}. In this example at maximum vasodilation, myocardial perfusion pressure would be 100 mmHg if no stenosis were present. Because of the stenosis, this perfusion pressure has decreased to 70 mmHg. Therefore, at maximum vasodilation, the ratio between maximum achievable flow in the presence of that stenosis and normal maximum flow is represented by (70-0)/(100-0). That ratio represents the fraction of normal maximum flow that is preserved despite the presence of the stenosis and is called FFR_{myo}. It may also be clear that it is not the hyperemic pressure gradient (ΔP) that determines the effect of the stenosis on myocardial blood flow, but rather the remaining fraction of myocardial perfusion pressure. P_a, mean aortic pressure; P_d, mean hyperemic distal coronary pressure; P_v, mean hyperemic central venous pressure.*

It is a matter for discussion what is the correct pressure to implement at the exit of the flow system in figure 4.1 It has also been suggested to take left ventricular end-diastolic pressure (which is not correct) or zero-flow pressure. Zero-flow pressure is the arterial pressure at which coronary flow stops during a prolonged diastole. This latter parameter would probably be the best one from a theoretical point of view, but very difficult to determine. Many studies have been performed to assess zero-flow pressure, with

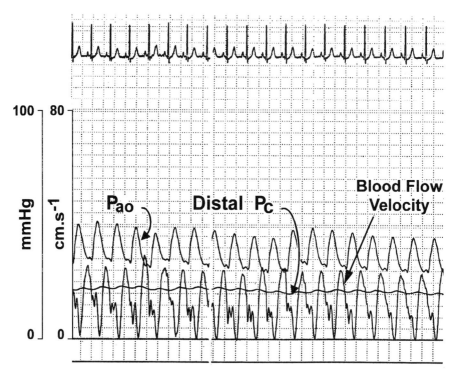

Figure 4.2 *Clinical example illustrating that also in humans zero-flow pressure at maximum hyperemia must be very low. Phasic aortic pressure (P_a), mean distal coronary pressure (P_d), and phasic blood flow velocity are recorded. Despite a mean distal coronary pressure of less than 20 mmHg, the phasic pattern of the flow signal is still maintained, indicating that zero-flow pressure in this patient must be close to zero.*

variable results[27-32]. Although at resting conditions, zero-flow pressure may be as high as 15-40 mmHg, it has been convincingly proved more recently that at maximum coronary vasodilation zero-flow pressure exceeds central venous pressure by only a few mmHg[29], not only in animals but also in the human coronary circulation, as demonstrated in figure 4.2. Assessment of zero-flow pressure in humans is complicated by the curvilinearity of the pressure-flow relation in the low pressure range[32]. Hence, there is concensus that when coronary vasculature is maximally dilated, pressures close to right atrial pressure are present at the cessation of flow. Figure 4.2 illustrates the persistance of phasic coronary blood flow in spite of a distal coronary pressure lower than 20 mmHg. Therefore, because determination of FFR assumes maximum hyperemia, it is acceptable to use central venous pressure instead of zero-flow pressure. In clinical practice, FFR is not affected by doing so because both pressures are generally close to zero and can be neglected. In the case of elevated central venous pressure, the inclusion of this variable is advisable. Also in case of quantification of collateral flow, inclusion of P_v in the calculations is necessary.

The only additional equipment necessary to apply this technique at routine cardiac catheterization, is a sensor-tipped pressure monitoring guide wire and a maximum hyperemic stimulus. By just placing the wire with the

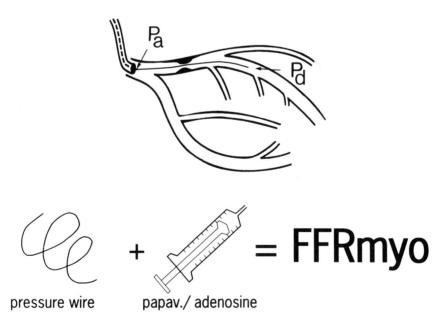

pressure wire   papav./ adenosine

Figure 4.3 *The only additional equipment necessary for calculation of FFR_{myo}, is a sensor-tipped pressure guide wire and an adequate hyperemic stimulus. FFR_{myo} is immediately calculated from the ratio P_d/P_a at maximum hyperemia. P_d = mean hyperemic distal coronary pressure, measured by the pressure wire; P_a = mean aortic pressure, measured by the catheter.*

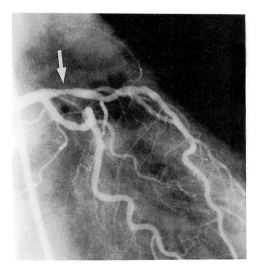

Figure 4.4 *Stenosis of intermediate angiographic severity in the left anterior descending artery in a 77-year-old lady. The pressure recordings are shown in figure 4.5.*

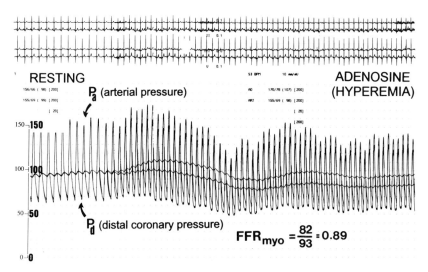

Figure 4.5 *Pressure recordings in the patient of figure 4.4. At maximum coronary hyperemia, induced by i.v. adenosine infusion, FFR_{myo} can be calculated by the ratio of hyperemic distal coronary pressure to aortic pressure.*

sensor across the stenosis, and administering a hyperemic stimulus, FFR_{myo} is known by one single simultaneous measurement of P_a (by the catheter) and P_d (by the wire), as shown in figure 4.3. Practical aspects of set-up and performance of these pressure measurements, are discussed in detail in chapter 5 and 6. A relevant example from the catheterization laboratory is presented in figure 4.4, showing an intermediate proximal LAD-stenosis in a 77-year-old lady with atypical chest pain. A dilemma was present with respect to the question whether this lesion caused the complaints and whether it should be dilated or not. As FFR_{myo} proved to be 0.89 (figure 4.5, far above the critical cut-off point of 0.75, as will be discussed later), no PTCA was performed.

The erroneous conclusions which may be drawn by just looking at gradients are illustrated in figure 4.6. In all three patients (A, B, and C), transstenotic pressure gradient at maximum hyperemia equals 30 mmHg. However, the perfusion pressure over the myocardium greatly varies from 25 to 70 mmHg and FFR_{myo} equals 0.70, 0.56, and 0.45 respectively. Although all the three patients in figure 4.6 have the same hyperemic gradient of 30 mmHg, the physiologic consequence of the 3 stenoses is completely different.

Figure 4.6 (next page) *Illustration why hyperemic transstenotic pressure gradient alone cannot be used as a measure of coronary or myocardial blood flow without taking into account the simultaneously measured arterial pressure. In all three examples in this figure, transstenotic pressure gradient at maximum vasodilation (corresponding with minimal resistance) equals 30 mmHg. However, the driving pressure over the myocardium (which determines myocardial perfusion at maximum vasodilation) largely varies from 25 to 70 mmHg. It is clear from*
this figure that hyperemic myocardial flow is not determined by ΔP but by $(P_d - P_v)/(P_a - P_v)$, which is called the myocardial fractional flow reserve (FFR_{myo}), and represents that fraction of flow reserve that is still present despite the stenosis. If P_v is not elevated, as is usually the case, FFR_{myo} equals hyperemic distal to proximal pressure.

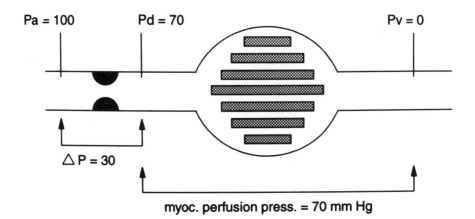

Pa = 100   Pd = 70   Pv = 0

△ P = 30

myoc. perfusion press. = 70 mm Hg

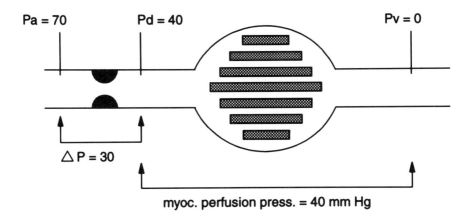

Pa = 70   Pd = 40   Pv = 0

△ P = 30

myoc. perfusion press. = 40 mm Hg

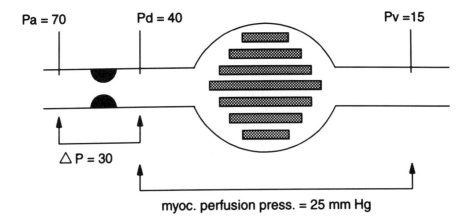

Pa = 70   Pd = 40   Pv =15

△ P = 30

myoc. perfusion press. = 25 mm Hg

4.4   Unique features of myocardial fractional flow reserve.

Myocardial fractional flow reserve is defined as maximum blood flow in the presence of a coronary stenosis, divided by normal maximum flow. It is a lesion-specific index of the functional significance of the epicardial stenosis on maximum perfusion of the myocardium supplied by that particular coronary artery, and has a number of unique features which enable clinical decision-making in the catheterization laboratory. These features are listed in table 4.1 and will be further discussed, validated, and highlighted in the next chapters.

Table 4.1 *Unique features of Myocardial Fractional Flow Reserve.*

- *FFR_{myo} is a lesion-specific index of epicardial stenosis severity.*

- *FFR_{myo} is independent of heart rate, blood pressure, and contractility.*

- *FFR_{myo} has an unequivocal normal value of 1.0 for every patient, every coronary artery, and every myocardial distribution.*

- *FFR_{myo} has clear cut-off points for decision making, both at diagnostic catheterization (0.75) and at coronary intervention (0.90).*

- *FFR_{myo} takes into account the contribution of collateral flow to myocardial perfusion.*

- *FFR_{myo} can be applied in single and multivessel disease. There is no need for a normal control artery to compare with.*

- *FFR_{myo} can be easily obtained, both at diagnostic and interventional procedures, by the ratio of mean hyperemic distal coronary pressure and aortic pressure:*

$$FFR_{myo} = \frac{P_d}{P_a}$$

4.5   Coronary fractional flow reserve and fractional collateral blood flow.

In this paragraph the concepts of coronary fractional flow reserve (FFR_{cor}) and fractional collateral blood flow, will be introduced. It will be shown how the separate contributions of coronary arterial and collateral blood flow to maximum myocardial flow can be obtained by pressure measurements. Because coronary wedge pressure, obtained at occlusion of the coronary artery, is needed in that case, this part of the theory can only be used at coronary interventions.

Although this part of the theory provides a complete description of the distribution of blood flow in all compartments of the coronary circulation, both before and after PTCA and at balloon occlusion, it is not paramount to make the most important clinical decisions, like "to dilate or not ?", "successful PTCA ?", "optimum stent deployment ?". Therefore, reading of the following paragraph may be omitted without affecting the practical ability to use myocardial fractional flow reserve.

In figure 4.7, modified from Gould et al[33], the initial model of figure 4.1 is extended to include the collateral circulation. The coronary circulation is represented now as an arrangement of variable resistances in parallel and in series: R, R_s, and R_c represent the resistances of the myocardial capillary bed, the stenotic artery, and the collateral circulation, respectively at maximum vasodilation. Q, Q_s, and Q_c represent maximum myocardial, coronary, and collateral blood flow. By definition, Q equals the sum of Q_s and Q_c. P_a, P_d, and P_v represent mean hyperemic aortic pressure, transstenotic (distal coronary) pressure, and central venous pressure at maximum coronary hyperemia. At total occlusion of the coronary artery, P_d is called P_w or coronary wedge pressure. In analogy to myocardial fractional flow reserve (FFR_{myo}), also coronary fractional flow reserve (FFR_{cor}) can be defined as maximum coronary artery blood flow in the presence of the stenosis, divided by normal maximum coronary artery flow.

In other words:

$$FFR_{myo} = \frac{\text{Maximum } \mathbf{myocardial} \text{ flow in the presence of a stenosis}}{\text{Normal maximum } \mathbf{myocardial} \text{ flow}}$$

$$FFR_{cor} = \frac{\text{Maximum } \mathbf{coronary} \text{ flow in the presence of a stenosis}}{\text{Normal maximum } \mathbf{coronary} \text{ flow}}$$

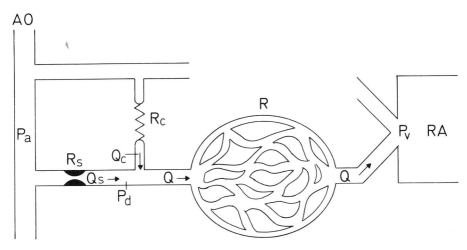

Figure 4.7 *Schematic model representing the coronary circulation. AO, aorta; P_a, arterial pressure; P_d, distal coronary pressure; P_v, venous pressure; Q, blood flow through the myocardial vascular bed; Q_c, collateral blood flow; Q_s, blood flow through the supplying epicardial coronary artery; R, resistance of the myocardial vascular bed; R_c, resistance of the collateral circulation; R_s, resistance of the stenosis in the supplying epicardial coronary artery; RA, right atrium.*

Normal maximum coronary artery flow and normal maximum myocardial flow are equal because the collateral flow in the absence of any stenosis is assumed to be zero. Normal values of Q, Q_s, and Q_c are indicated by the superscript *N*. Therefore, by definition $Q^N = Q_s^N$ and $Q_c^N = 0$. When a coronary stenosis gradually develops, collateral contribution may become important and myocardial flow will become increasingly larger than coronary flow, depending on the development of collaterals. (This effect is illustrated in figure 6.6). As will be demonstrated in the appendix to this chapter, the following pressure-flow equations can be derived now to describe myocardial and coronary fractional flow reserve, respectively, and the contribution of collateral flow to maximum myocardial blood flow (next page):

Maximum recruitable collateral flow at coronary occlusion:

$$(Q_c/Q^N)_{max} = \frac{P_w - P_v}{P_a - P_v} = \text{constant} \qquad \text{(eq. 1)}$$

Coronary Fractional Flow Reserve:

$$FFR_{cor} = \frac{P_d - P_w}{P_a - P_w} \qquad \text{(eq. 2)}$$

Myocardial Fractional Flow Reserve:

$$FFR_{myo} = \frac{P_d - P_v}{P_a - P_v} \qquad \text{(eq. 3)}$$

Fractional Collateral Flow:

$$Q_c/Q^N = FFR_{myo} - FFR_{cor} \qquad \text{(eq. 4)}$$

Equation (1) states the fundamental observation that the ratio of $(P_w - P_v)$ to $(P_a - P_v)$ is constant under conditions of maximum vasodilation. As will be explained in the appendix, equation (1) is used to calculate collateral flow when P_a is not constant.

In equation (1) and (4), Q_c/Q^N represents collateral blood flow as a ratio to normal maximum myocardial flow Q^N. The index Q_c/Q^N is called *fractional collateral flow*. In equation 1, $(Q_c/Q^N)_{max}$ represents maximum recruitable collateral flow as may be encountered during coronary artery occlusion. Equation (1) is also used to calculate the virtual value of P_w before and after PTCA in the case that P_a and/or P_d change during the procedure. Further details and explanations of these equations as well as their mathematical derivation, will be discussed in paragraph 4.7. At first, however, we will present 2 examples how to use these equations:

Example 1.

This first example is based upon a simple case where aortic and venous pressures do not change during the PTCA and where venous pressure is equal to zero. Therefore, according to equation (1), P_w will not change during the procedure. Suppose that P_a is 90 mmHg both before and after PTCA, that P_d equals 40 mmHg before and 80 mmHg after PTCA and suppose that coronary wedge pressure (P_w) at balloon inflation equals 20 mmHg.

	Before PTCA	Balloon occlusion	After PTCA
P_a	90	90	90
P_d	40	-	80
P_v	0	0	0
P_w	(20)	20	(20)

By substituting these values in equation (1), (2), (3), and (4), the next matrix is obtained:

	Before PTCA	Balloon occlusion	After PTCA
FFR_{myo}	0.44	0.22	0.89
FFR_{cor}	0.29	0	0.86
Q_c/Q^N	0.15	0.22	0.03

This matrix completely describes the distribution of flow over the different compartments of the coronary circulation before and after PTCA, and enables the estimation of recruitable collateral flow at occlusion of the coronary artery. In fact, such a matrix indicates that, due to the stenosis in the supplying coronary artery, maximum achievable blood flow to the dependent myocardium was only 44% of what it would be in case of a normal coronary artery. It can also be deduced from the matrix that of every 44 ml of blood flowing to that part of the myocardium, 29 ml was provided by the stenotic artery and 15 ml by collaterals. Furthermore, after successful PTCA of the stenosis, maximum myocardial blood flow has increased to 89% of normal maximum flow, and of every 89 ml blood, 86 ml is provided now by the coronary artery and only 3 ml by the collaterals. At last, maximum recruitable collateral blood flow during occlusion of the epicardial vessel equals 22% of normal maximum myocardial perfusion. This latter index is important, because it has been shown that if $(Q_c/Q^N)_{max}$ is higher than approximately 0.30, the patient is likely to be protected against myocardial infarction, as further discussed in chapter 12 of this book.

At last, as will be shown in paragraph 4.7, the ratio of collateral flow before and after PTCA is proportional to the ratio of hyperemic pressure gradient before and after the procedure (5:1 in this case).

Example 2.

This is an example from real clinical practice, where P_a is not constant during the procedure. The coronary angiograms in this 59-year-old woman are shown in figure 4.8 and the relevant pressure tracings in figure 4.9. Because, by definition, P_w can only be measured at coronary occlusion, equation (1) is used to calculate P_w as it would be at a blood pressure encountered before and after PTCA.

As can be read from figure 4.9, the relevant pressures in this patient are as follows:

	Before PTCA	Balloon occlusion	After PTCA
P_a	101	108	97
P_d	53	-	94
P_v	5	6	5
P_w	(22)	24	(21)

The value of P_w as it would be at P_a and P_v as recorded before and after PTCA, is calculated by using the constancy of equation (1). Because P_a, P_v and P_w are known at the actual balloon occlusion and P_a and P_v are known before and after PTCA, also P_w can be calculated at P_a and P_v encountered before and after PTCA. By substituting the pressure values in equation (2), (3) and (4) the following matrix is obtained:

	Before PTCA	Balloon occlusion	After PTCA
FFR_{myo}	0.50	0.18	0.97
FFR_{cor}	0.39	0.00	0.96
Q_c/Q^N	0.11	0.18	0.01

Again, the matrix completely describes the distribution of blood flow in the different compartments of the coronary circulation. In this patient, the LAD-stenosis was so severe, that maximum achievable blood flow to the dependent myocardium was only 50% of the value achievable if the artery would be completely normal. Of every 50 ml of blood to that part of the myocardium, 39 ml was provided by the stenotic artery and 11 ml by the collateral circulation. After PTCA, maximum achievable myocardial blood flow has increased to 97% of its normal value and almost all that blood is provided by the dilated coronary artery. Maximum recruitable collateral blood flow at coronary artery occlusion equals only 18% of normal maximum flow and therefore it is not surprising that this patient had chest pain and ECG changes during balloon occlusion.

Maximum recruitable collateral blood flow.

As can be appreciated from paragraph 4.7, the mathematical derivation of equation (2) for FFR_{cor} is quite complex. The validity of equation (1), on the other hand, can also be made clear intuitively by looking at figure 4.10.
In that figure, it is clear that at coronary artery occlusion, the remaining perfusion pressure over the myocardial bed equals P_w - P_v ,whereas that driving pressure in the normal case, without occlusion, would have been

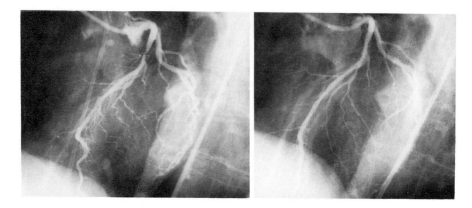

Figure 4.8 *Angiograms before and after PTCA of the LAD artery in a 59-year-old woman. The pressure recordings are shown in figure 4.9*

Figure 4.9 (opposite page) *Tracings showing simultaneous phasic and mean recordings of P_a , P_d and P_v before, during, and after PTCA of a left anterior descending coronary artery stenosis in a 59-year-old woman. For clarity P_v is not displayed in panels B through F. Panel A: Before the pressure wire is introduced into the coronary artery, the tip of the pressure wire is close to the tip of the guiding catheter, and equality of P_a and P_d at that point is verified. B: The pressure wire is advanced into the coronary artery and crosses the stenosis (#). C: After start of intravenous adenosine infusion, steady-state hyperemic pressure curves are obtained, allowing calculation of FFR_{myo} before PTCA. D: The balloon is advanced into the stenosis and inflated. E: The balloon is deflated and withdrawn. The wire remains in the distal coronary artery. Note the large artificial gradient caused by the mere presence of the deflated balloon at the site of the stenosis. F: After intravenous adenosine infusion has been started again, steady-state hyperemic pressure curves are obtained, allowing calculation of FFR_{myo} after PTCA. G: At the end of the procedure, the pressure wire is withdrawn to the tip of the guiding catheter, and it is verified that no drift has occurred during the procedure.*

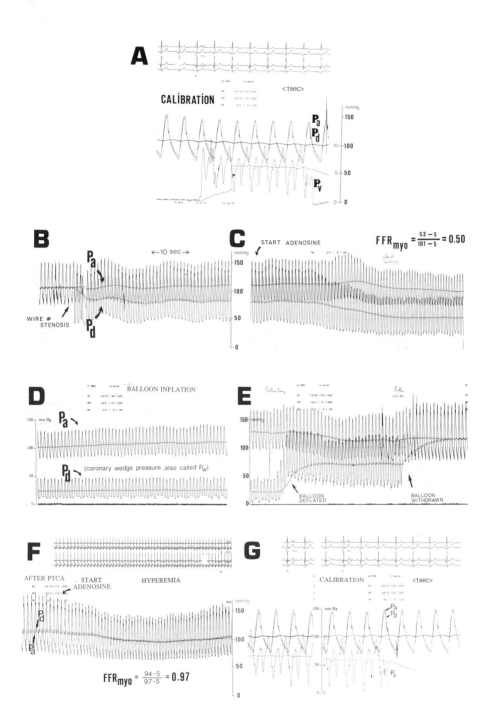

P_a - P_v. In other words, because myocardial resistance is minimal and therefore constant, $(P_w - P_v)/(P_a - P_v)$ represents the fraction of normal maximum myocardial blood flow which can be obtained by collaterals at coronary artery occlusion. It has been shown that fractional collateral blood flow of at least 30%, is predictive to protect against acute myocardial infarction in the case of future occlusion of the coronary artery. Fractional collateral blood flow will be further discussed in chapter 16.

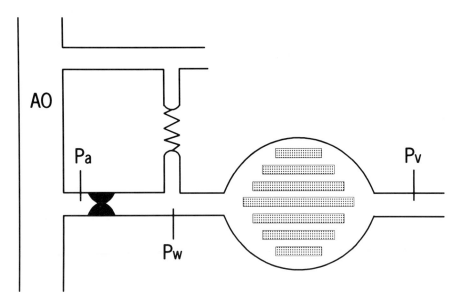

Figure 4.10 *Model of the coronary circulation at total occlusion of the coronary artery. Perfusion pressure over the myocardium, provided by the collaterals, equals* P_w - P_v, *whereas normal perfusion pressure at maximum vasodilation would be* P_a - P_v *.Therefore, recruitable collateral blood flow as a fraction of normal myocardial blood flow, equals* $(P_w - P_v)/(P_a - P_v)$*. That index is called fractional collateral blood flow.*

4.6 Limitations of fractional flow reserve.

4.6.1 Microvascular disease.

An important conceptual limitation of fractional flow reserve, is microvascular disease, distal to the location where P_d is measured.

In the presence of microvascular disease, FFR represents maximum flow in the presence of an epicardial stenosis, expressed as a fraction of maximum flow in the absence of that epicardial stenosis but still not normal because of the presence of the microvascular disease. This can be the case, e.g. in diabetes, but may also play a role after myocardial infarction and in diffuse coronary atherosclerosis. Although this is a limitation from a conceptual point of view, in clinical practice this may turn out to be advantageous when decisions have to be made with respect to dilate or bypass a coronary stenosis: as FFR_{myo} is a specific index of the influence of the epicardial stenosis on myocardial perfusion, also in case of small vessel disease it indicates to what extent maximum blood flow can be increased by relieving the epicardial obstruction. Stated another way, the clinical question: "to what extent are we going to improve this patient by a revascularization procedure ?", can be answered on the basis of fractional flow reserve measurements irrespective of the presence of microvascular disease. This consideration constitutes an essential difference between fractional flow reserve and the classic concept of absolute coronary flow reserve, as is illustrated in figure 11.1. Diminished CFR may indicate epicardial disease, microvascular disease, or both. It cannot separately distinguish between these entities. FFR, on the contrary, more specifically indicates the extent of epicardial coronary disease, but does not account for microvascular disease. To assess both epicardial and microvascular disease, simultaneous measurement of hyperemic intracoronary pressure and blood flow velocity is mandatory[34,35]. If, in that case, the epicardial stenosis and the microvasculature are considered as two serial components of the coronary circulation, diminished hyperemic flow velocity indicates that somewhere in that system an obstruction to flow is present. Subsequently, the decline of hyperemic epicardial coronary pressure, expressed by FFR_{myo}, indicates to what extent the epicardial stenosis and the microvascular disease, if present, each contribute to a reduced flow reserve.

Actually, it is not completely correct to state that FFR is not influenced by microvascular disease. In the presence of an epicardial coronary stenosis and microvascular disease, the latter may limit the maximum blood flow attainable in the coronary artery and therefore the induced pressure drop across the stenosis may be less than it could have been without microvascular disease. As a consequence, FFR_{myo} will be overestimated. Nevertheless, it still indicates to what extent the patient can be improved by eliminating the epicardial stenosis and therefore its usefulness for decision making in the catheterization laboratory is not affected. These issues are further discussed in chapter 13.1 and 13.2.

Similar considerations are applicable to the situation of more than one lesion in the same coronary artery: when assessing the FFR of the first stenosis, this index will be overestimated by the presence of the second one. In chapter 13.4, it will be discussed how, in case of sequential stenoses within one vessel, the true FFR of each individual stenosis after relieve of the other ones, can be predicted.

4.6.2   Extravascular compression, zero-flow pressure, and vascular capacitance.

A unique strength of fractional flow reserve is that pressures are only used as an endpoint and that its calculation is insensitive to all physiologic phenomena which contribute to distal coronary pressure. Therefore, there is no concern about the influence of extravascular compression, critical closing pressure, and capacitance characteristics of the coronary circulation[34-39]. Critical closing pressure or zero-flow pressure, has already been discussed briefly in paragraph 4.3. Pantely et al showed that during maximum coronary hyperemia zero-flow pressure is very low and exceeds central venous pressure by a few mmHg only[29]. Studying zero-flow pressure in humans, is obviously impossible. Accidentally, we observed that zero-flow pressure in humans at maximum coronary hyperemia is very low indeed. During variation of blood pressure, in one patient accidentally an infusion of sodium nitroprusside was administered at a dose 10x as high as usual. During the subsequent (short) period of extremely low distal coronary pressure, the measured blood flow pattern in the distal coronary artery still showed clear phasic pattern, proving that zero-flow pressure in that patient must have been close to zero. (figure 4.2). These issues will be further discussed in chapter 7.

4.6.3   Coronary steal.

Coronary steal is a well-documented pathophysiologic phenomenon, occurring in the case of one critically narrowed or occluded coronary artery, receiving collaterals from another vessel which is stenotic itself (but not critically stenotic)[36,37]. When distal myocardial resistance in the territory of the second vessel decreases (e.g. after administration of a vasodilatory stimulus), blood flow increases and as a result distal coronary pressure decreases, resulting in a lower perfusion pressure over the collaterals and decreased collateral flow to the territory of the first artery (figure 4.11). Hence, in case of distal pressure measurements in collateralized coronary arteries, a steal phenomenon is likely to occur when a stenosis is present in the collateral-supplying artery and when a systemic vasodilating agent is used. When, in the same patient, the vasodilating agent is given only in the vessel under study, no steal phenomenon will occur. As a consequence, theoretically the myocardial fractional flow reserve calculated from pressure measurements will be higher when the vasodilating agent is infused selectively than when it is administered intravenously. In real life circumstances, when exercise is performed, it is likely that not only the vascular bed of the stenotic artery but also the bed of the collateral supplying artery will dilate. Therefore, to precisely assess myocardial

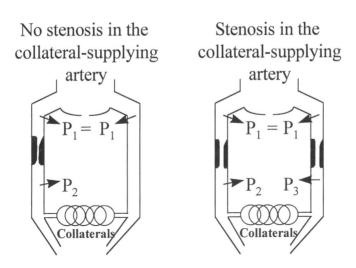

Figure 4.11 *Coronary steal (i.e. decrease of absolute myocardial flow of collateral-dependent myocardium after coronary arteriolar vasodilation) will not occur when collaterals depend on a normal vessel (left panel). Even during maximum vasodilation, the perfusion pressure of the collaterals will remain unchanged. Since P_2 will decrease during coronary vasodilation, the gradient across the collateral vessels will increase and therefore absolute myocardial flow in the collateral-dependent myocardium may even increase. However, when the collaterals depend on a stenotic vessel (right panel), P_3 will decrease during vasodilation and therefore the driving pressure across the collaterals will decrease with a subsequent decrease in myocardial flow in the collateral-dependent area.*

fractional flow reserve in a myocardial region whose collaterals depend on a stenotic vessel, the coronary vasodilator should be given intravenously. Because any decrease in collateral flow, caused by increased conductance in the artery supplying the collaterals, is reflected by a lower P_w in the territory under study, the calculations itself are not affected by coronary steal.

4.6.4   Left ventricular hypertrophy and previous myocardial infarction.

Theoretically, left ventricular hypertrophy and previous myocardial infarction in the investigated distribution may affect FFR. These issues will be more extensively discussed in chapter 13.

4.7 Mathematical derivation and scientific background of the pressure-flow equations.

Note: The next paragraph is provided as a scientific background to proof the mathematical correctness of the pressure-flow equations underlying the concept of Fractional Flow Reserve. Reading of this paragraph is not necessary to use coronary pressure measurements in clinical practice. It can be skipped without affecting the general understanding of this book.

The abbreviations in this paragraph and the numeration of equations refer to paragraph 4.5 and figure 4.7.

It should be kept in mind that all of the theoretical considerations in this appendix apply to a system at maximum vasodilation. Therefore, the resistances R and R_c in figure 4.7 are minimal and constant.

First, it will be proved that the ratio between mean arterial pressure (P_a) and coronary wedge pressure (P_w), both after subtraction of venous pressure (P_v) is constant. For that purpose, suppose in Figure 4.7, at any arbitrary pressures P_a and P_v, that $R_s = \infty$ and $Q_s = 0$, as with total occlusion; then, $Q = Q_c$ and $P_d = P_w$ by definition. In that case:

$$P_a - P_v = Q \cdot (R + R_c)$$

and

$$P_w - P_v = Q \cdot R$$

Therefore

$$\frac{P_a - P_v}{P_w - P_v} = \frac{(R + R_c)}{R} = 1 + \frac{R_c}{R} = C_1 \qquad (1a)$$

Equation 1a can also be rearranged into the following two forms, which will be helpful in later considerations:

$$\frac{P_w - P_v}{P_a - P_w} = \frac{R}{R_c} = C_2 \qquad (1b)$$

and

$$\frac{P_a - P_v}{P_a - P_w} = \frac{R}{R_c} + 1 = C_3 \qquad (1c)$$

where C_1, C_2, and C_3 are all different constants characterizing collateral resistance relative to the resistance of the myocardial bed supplied by the collaterals at maximum vasodilation.

The second step is the calculation of fractional flow reserve of the stenotic coronary artery (FFR_{cor}). By definition,

$$FFR_{cor} = \frac{Q_s}{Q_s^N} = \frac{Q - Q_c}{Q^N - Q_c^N}$$

Because $Q_c^N = 0$:

$$FFR_{cor} = \frac{Q - Q_c}{Q^N}$$

$$= \frac{(P_d - P_v)/R - (P_a - P_d)/R_c}{(P_a - P_v)/R}$$

$$= \frac{(P_d - P_v) - (P_a - P_d) \cdot R/R_c}{(P_a - P_v)}$$

Substitution of the constant value C_2, obtained from Equation 1b, gives the following:

$$FFR_{cor} = \frac{(P_d - P_v)(P_a - P_w) - (P_a - P_d)(P_w - P_v)}{(P_a - P_v)(P_a - P_w)}$$

$$= \frac{P_d - P_w}{P_a - P_w} \tag{2}$$

Next, fractional flow reserve of the myocardium (FFR_{myo}) is calculated as follows:

$$\frac{Q}{Q^N} = \frac{(P_d - P_v)/R}{(P_a - P_v)/R} = \frac{P_d - P_v}{P_a - P_v} \tag{3}$$

Equation (3) has been derived previously by Gould[4]. The contribution of collateral flow to total flow now is calculated as follows. By definition,

$$Q = Q_c + Q_s$$

Therefore:

$$\frac{Q_c}{Q^N} = \frac{Q}{Q^N} - \frac{Q_s}{Q^N}$$

and because $Q_s^N = Q^N$, this can be written as the following:

$$\frac{Q_c}{Q^N} = FFR_{myo} - FFR_{cor} \tag{4}$$

In the case of coronary interventions, it should be realized that flow at maximum vasodilation is directly proportional to the driving pressure (P_a - P_v). Therefore, the ratio between maximum flow through the coronary artery before (situation 1) and after the intervention (situation 2) can be written as follows:

$$\frac{Q_s^{(2)}}{Q_s^{(1)}} = \frac{Q_s^{(2)}}{Q_s^{(2)N}} \cdot \frac{Q_s^{(2)N}}{Q_s^{(1)N}} \cdot \frac{Q_s^{(1)N}}{Q_s^{(1)}}$$

$$= FFR_{cor}^{(2)} \cdot \frac{P_a^{(2)} - P_v^{(2)}}{P_a^{(1)} - P_v^{(1)}} \cdot \frac{1}{FFR_{cor}^{(1)}}$$

$$= \frac{FFR_{cor}^{(2)}}{FFR_{cor}^{(1)}} \cdot \frac{P_a^{(2)} - P_v^{(2)}}{P_a^{(1)} - P_v^{(1)}}$$

By substitution of Equations 1b and 2:

$$\frac{Q_s^{(2)}}{Q_s^{(1)}} = \frac{P_d^{(2)} - P_w^{(2)}}{P_d^{(1)} - P_w^{(1)}} \tag{5a}$$

Note that for evaluation of the functional improvement of a stenotic artery after PTCA, $FFR_{cor}^{(2)}/FFR_{cor}^{(1)}$ theoretically is a better measure than $Q_s^{(2)}/Q_s^{(1)}$ because the first expression is independent of arterial pressure. From Equation 2 it is clear that

$$\frac{FFR_{cor}^{(2)}}{FFR_{cor}^{(1)}} = \frac{P_d^{(2)} - P_w^{(2)}}{P_a^{(2)} - P_w^{(2)}} : \frac{P_d^{(1)} - P_w^{(1)}}{P_a^{(1)} - P_w^{(1)}}$$

$$= \left(1 - \frac{\Delta^{(2)} P}{P_a^{(2)} - P_w^{(2)}} \right) : \left(1 - \frac{\Delta^{(1)} P}{P_a^{(1)} - P_w^{(1)}} \right) \quad (5b)$$

The expression $FFR_{cor}^{(2)}/FFR_{cor}^{(1)}$ represents the improvement of FFR_{cor} of the dilated artery and is identical to what we called pressure-corrected maximum flow ratio (MFR_c) in a previous study[9].

Equation 5a can also be derived directly from figure 4.7 by the following:

$$\frac{Q_s^{(2)}}{Q_s^{(1)}} = \frac{Q^{(2)} - Q_c^{(2)}}{Q^{(1)} - Q_c^{(1)}} = \frac{(P_d^{(2)} - P_v^{(2)})/R - (P_a^{(2)} - P_d^{(2)})/R_c}{(P_d^{(1)} - P_v^{(1)})/R - (P_a^{(1)} - P_d^{(1)})/R_c}$$

and by substituting Equation 1b.

Theoretically, maximum blood flow through the myocardium can be compared before and after the intervention by:

$$\frac{Q^{(2)}}{Q^{(1)}} = \frac{(P_d^{(2)} - P_v^{(2)})/R}{(P_d^{(1)} - P_v^{(1)})/R} = \frac{P_d^{(2)} - P_v^{(2)}}{P_d^{(1)} - P_v^{(1)}} \quad (6a)$$

or, if correction for pressure changes is made, by:

$$\frac{FFR_{myo}^{(2)}}{FFR_{myo}^{(1)}} = \frac{P_d^{(2)} - P_v^{(2)}}{P_a^{(2)} - P_v^{(2)}} : \frac{P_d^{(1)} - P_v^{(1)}}{P_a^{(1)} - P_v^{(1)}}$$

$$= \left(1 - \frac{\Delta^{(2)} P}{P_a^{(2)} - P_v^{(2)}} \right) : \left(1 - \frac{\Delta^{(1)} P}{P_a^{(1)} - P_v^{(1)}} \right) \quad (6b)$$

Finally, the theoretical relation between collateral flow at different degrees of stenosis can be obtained. From figure 4.7, it is clear that $Q_c = (P_a - P_d)/R_c$. Therefore:

$$\frac{Q_c^{(2)}}{Q_c^{(1)}} = \frac{(P_a^{(2)} - P_d^{(2)})/R_c}{(P_a^{(1)} - P_d^{(1)})/R_c} = \frac{\Delta^{(2)}P}{\Delta^{(1)}P} \qquad (7a)$$

or, if correction for pressure changes is made:

$$\frac{Q_c^{(2)}}{Q_c^{(1)}} = \frac{\Delta^{(2)}P}{P_a^{(2)} - P_v^{(2)}} : \frac{\Delta^{(1)}P}{P_a^{(1)} - P_v^{(1)}} \qquad (7b)$$

In fact, Equation 7 states that decrease of hyperemic ΔP by improved stenosis geometry after PTCA induces a proportional decrease of the relative contribution of collateral flow to total myocardial flow.

References.

1. Hoffman JIE: Maximal coronary flow and the concept of coronary vascular reserve. *Circulation 1984; 70: 153-159.*
2. Nissen SE, Gurley JC: Assessment of the functional significance of coronary stenosis: Is digital angiography the answer ? *Circulation 1990; 81: 1431-1435.*
3. Kirkeeide RL, Gould KL, Parsel L: Assessment of coronary stenoses by myocardial perfusion during pharmacologic coronary vasodilation: VIII. Validation of coronary flow reserve as a single integrated functional measure of stenosis severity reflecting all its geometric dimensions. *J Am Coll Cardiol 1986; 7: 103-113.*
4. Gould KL, Kirkeeide RL, Buchi M: Coronary flow reserve as a physiologic measure of stenosis severity. *J Am Coll Cardiol 1990; 15: 459-74.*
5. Hongo M, Nakatsuka T, Watanabe N, Takenaka H, Tanaka M, Kinoshita O, Okubo S, Sekiguchi M: Effects of heart rate on phasic coronary blood flow pattern and flow reserve in patients with normal coronary arteries: A study with an intravascular Doppler catheter and spectral analysis. *Am Heart J 1994; 127: 545-551.*
6. Ofili EO, Labovitz J, Kern MJ. Coronary flow velocity dynamics in normal and diseased arteries. *Am J Cardiol 1993; 71: 3D-9D.*
7. De Bruyne B, Bartunek J, Sys SU, Pijls NHJ, Heyndrickx GR, Wijns W. Simultaneous coronary pressure and flow velocity measurements in humans. *Circulation 1996; 94: 1842-49.*

8. De Bruyne B, Pijls NHJ, Paulus WJ, Vantrimpont PJ, Sys SU, Heyndrickx GR. Transstenotic coronary pressure gradient measurement in humans: in vitro and in vivo evaluation of a new pressure monitoring angioplasty guide wire. *J Am Coll Cardiol* 1993; 22: 119-126.

9. Pijls NHJ, Van Son JAM, Kirkeeide RL, De Bruyne B, Gould KL. Experimental basis of determining maximum coronary, myocardial, and collateral blood flow by pressure measurements for assessing functional stenosis severity before and after percutaneous transluminal coronary angioplasty. *Circulation 1993; 87: 1354-67.*

10. De Bruyne B, Baudhuin T, Melin JA, Pijls NHJ, Sys SU, Bol A, Paulus WJ, Heyndrickx GR, Wijns W. Coronary flow reserve calculated from pressure measurements in man. Validation with positron emission tomography. *Circulation 1994; 89: 1013-1022.*

11. Pijls NHJ, Van Gelder B, Van der Voort P, Peels K, Bracke FALE, Bonnier HJRM, El Gamal MIH. Fractional Flow Reserve. A useful index to evaluate the influence of an epicardial coronary stenosis on myocardial blood flow. *Circulation 1995; 92: 3183-3193.*

12. Pijls NHJ, Bech GJW, El Gamal MIH, Bonnier HJRM, De Bruyne B, Van Gelder B, Michels HR, Koolen JJ. Quantification of recruitable coronary collateral blood flow in conscious humans and its potential to predict future ischemic events. *J Am Coll Cardiol 1995; 25: 1522-1528.*

13. Pijls NHJ, De Bruyne B, Peels K, Van der Voort PH, Bonnier HJRM, Bartunek J, Koolen JJ. Measurement of fractional flow reserve to assess the functional severity of coronary-artery stenoses. *N Engl J Med 1996; 334: 1703-1708.*

14. Van de Voort PH, Van Hagen E, Hendrix G, Van Gelder B, Bech GJW, Pijls NHJ. Comparison of intravenous to intracoronary papaverine for calculation of pressure-derived fractional flow reserve. *Cath Cardiov Diagn* 1996; 39: 120-125.

15. De Bruyne B, Bartunek J, Sys SU, Pijls NHJ, Heyndrickx GR, Wijns W. Simultaneous coronary pressure and flow velocity measurements in humans, feasibility, reproducibility, and hemodynamic dependence of coronary flow velocity reserve, hyperemic flow versus pressure slope index, and fractional flow reserve. *Circulation* 1996; 94: 1843-1849.

16. Bech GJW, De Bruyne B Bonnier HJRM, Bartunek J, Wijns W, Peels K, Heyndrickx GR, Koolen JJ, Pijls NHJ. Long-term follow-up after deferral of percutaneous transluminal coronary angioplasty of intermediate stenosis on the basis of coronary pressure measurement. *J Am Coll Cardiol* 1998; 31: 841-847.

17. Bech GJW, Pijls NHJ, De Bruyne B, Peels KH, Michels HR, Bonnier HJRM, Koolen JJ. Usefulness of fractional flow reserve to predict clinical outcome after balloon angioplasty. *Circulation* 1999; 99: 883-888.

18. Hanekamp CEE, Koolen JJ, Pijls NHJ, Michels HR, Bonnier HJRM. Comparison of QCA, intravascular ultrasound, and coronary pressure measurement to assess optimum stent deployment. *Circulation* 1999; 99: 1015-1024.

19. Aueron FM, Grüntzig AR. Percutaneous transluminal coronary angioplasty. Indication and current status. *Primary Cardiol* 1984; 10: 97-107.

20. De Bruyne B, Sys S, Heyndrickx GR. PTCA catheters versus fluid-filled pressure monitoring guide wires for coronary pressure measurements and correlation with quantitative coronary angiography. *Am J Cardiol* 1993; 72: 1101-1106.

21. Rothman MT, Baim DS, Simpson JB, Harrison DC: Coronary hemodynamics during PTCA. *Am J Cardiol 1982; 49: 1615-1622.*

22. Choksi SK, Meyers S, Abi-Mansour P: Percutaneous transluminal coronary angioplasty: Ten years' experience. *Prog Cardiovasc Dis 1987; 30: 147-210.*

23. MacIsaac HC, Knudtson ML, Robinson VJ, Manyari DE: Is the residual translesional pressure gradient useful to predict regional myocardial perfusion after percutaneous transluminal coronary angioplasty ? *Am Heart J 1989; 117: 783-790.*

24. Kimball BP, Dafopoulos N, Lipreti V: Comparative evaluation of coronary stenoses using fluid dynamic equations and standard quantitative coronary arteriography. *Am J Cardiol 1989; 64: 6-10.*

25. Emanuelsson H, Dohnal M, Lamm C, Tenerz L: Initial experiences with a miniaturized pressure transducer during coronary angioplasty. *Cathet Cardiovasc Diagn 1991; 24: 137-143.*

26. Lamm C, Dohnal M, Serruys PW, Emanuelsson H: High fidelity translesional pressure gradients during percutaneous transluminal coronary angioplasty: correlation with quantitative coronary angiography.

27. Bellamy RF. Diastolic coronary artery pressure-flow relations in the dog. *Circ Research* 1978; 43: 92-101.

28. Satoh S, Klocke FJ, Canty JM. Tone-dependent coronary arterial-venous pressure differences at the cessation of venous outflow during long diastoles. *Circulation* 1993; 88: 1238-1244.

29. Pantely GA, Ladley HD, Bristow JD: Low zero-flow pressure and minimal capacitance effect on diastolic coronary arterial pressure-flow relationships during maximum vasodilation in swine. *Circulation 1984; 70: 485-494.*

30. Dole WO, Alexander GM, Campbell AB, Hixson EL, Bishop VS: Interpretation and physiological significance of diastolic coronary artery pressure-flow relationships in the canine coronary bed. *Circ Res 1984; 55: 215-226.*

31. Klocke FJ, Mates RE, Canty JM, Ellis AK: Coronary pressure-flow relationships: Controversial issues and probable implications. *Circ Res 1985; 56: 310-323.*

32. Di Mario C, Krams R, Gil R, Serruys PW. Slope of the instantaneous hyperemic diastolic coronary flow velocity-pressure relation. A new index for assessment of the physiological significance of coronary stenosis in humans. *Circulation* 1994; 90: 1215-1224.

33. Gould KL: *Coronary Artery Stenosis.* New York, *Elsevier, 1990, pp 79-91.*

34. Mancini GBJ, McGillem MJ, De Boe SF, Gallagher KP: The diastolic hyperemic flow versus pressure slope index: microsphere validation of an alternative to measures of coronary reserve. *Circulation 1991; 84: 862-870.*

35. Di Mario C, Krams R, Gil R, Meneveau N, Serruys PW: The instanteneous hyperemic pressure-flow relationship in conscious humans. In: Reiber JHC, Serruys PW, eds.: *Progress in quantitative coronary arteriography.* Dordrecht, NL: *Kluwer Academic Publishers; 1994: 247-268.*

36. Gross GJ, Warltier DC. Coronary steal in four models of single or multiple vessel obstruction in dogs. *Am J Cardiol* 1981; 48: 84-92.

37. Demer L, Gould KL, Kirkeeide R. Assessing stenosis severity; coronary flow reserve, collateral function, quantitative coronary arteriography, positron imaging, and digital subtraction angiography. A review and analysis. *Prog CV Dis* 1988; 30: 307-322.

Chapter 5

PRACTICAL SET-UP OF CORONARY PRESSURE MEASUREMENT

The present chapter aims at providing the reader with the practical aspects of coronary pressure measurements in humans. The technical requirements, equipment, "tips and tricks" of the procedure itself, and methods to induce hyperemia are reviewed. Potential pitfalls to be aware of, are discussed in chapter 6.

5.1   Set-up in the catheterization laboratory.

To measure coronary pressure in the catheterization laboratory, no major technical adaptations are needed as compared with a regular diagnostic procedure.

5.1.1. Pressure transducers.

A regular pressure transducer is necessary for aortic pressure (P_a), recorded through the guiding catheter or through the diagnostic catheter as usual. In some cases, a second pressure transducer may be needed for central venous pressure (P_v) recordings. However, as explained in chapter 4, central venous pressure can most often be neglected so that in routine clinical practice P_v is no longer measured.

There are two types of pressure measuring guide wires: microsensor-tipmanometer wires and fluid-filled hollow guide wires. The sensor-tipped wires are connected to a small interface, without the need for a conventional pressure transducer. This will be described in detail in the next paragraph. All fluid-filled systems can be connected directly to any conventional pressure transducer. This additional transducer should then be placed as close as possible to the patient's groin because the quality of the pressure tracing will depend, among other factors, on the distance from the coronary artery to the pressure transducer.

All fluid-filled pressure transducers must be zeroed at the right atrial level. For the sensor-tipped wires, the measurements are not affected by the height of the interface.

Many pressure monitoring systems presently available allow for the simultaneous recording of phasic and mean pressures. This capability is highly recommended when intracoronary pressure recordings are made. The mean pressure is needed to calculate the pressure gradient and the pressure-derived fractional flow reserve. The phasic pressure signal is useful to detect mild changes in the morphology of the signal and thus to validate the quality of the recorded data, and reliably reflects a number of physiologic and pathologic phenomenon which may occur during cardiac catheterization or intervention and are important to be recognized for a correct interpretation of coronary pressure measurements.

In some centers an extra pressure transducer is used to monitor femoral pressure (P_{fem}) through the side arm of the arterial introduction sheath. Continuous monitoring of the phasic signal of the femoral artery is convenient for 2 reasons: *first,* the pressure signal of the central aorta (guiding or diagnostic catheter) is interrupted when contrast medium or any other drug is injected or when the balloon catheter is manipulated. The recording of the femoral pressure allows uninterrupted monitoring of systemic blood pressure; *second*, simultaneous recording of central aortic pressure and femoral pressure is often an easy way to detect "wedging" of the catheter in the coronary ostium as illustrated in paragraph 6.4.

5.1.2 Medications.

When the decision is made to perform coronary pressure measurements, intracoronary nitrates, intravenous heparin and an intracoronary or intravenous coronary vasodilator should be available.

Intravenous heparin must be given before the pressure guide wire enters the coronary tree, whether or not an angioplasty is scheduled after the pressure measurements. Heparin can be administered according to local routine as during angioplasty. Some centers give a bolus of 10.000 U at the start of the procedure, repeated by 5000 U after every hour; other centers prefer to measure ACT and to have this value > 250 s. At the end of the measurements, when no angioplasty is performed, heparin may be neutralized by intravenous protamine.

As in all other intracoronary procedures, intracoronary nitrates should be given before advancing the pressure wire through the stenosis to avoid any mechanically induced coronary spasm. More details about medications used to obtain maximal coronary vasodilation are given in paragraph 5.4.

5.1.3 Catheters.

In general, pressure wires can be advanced through 6F diagnostic catheters. However, the use of a 6F (or larger) angioplasty guiding catheter is strongly recommended since the better inner coating of these catheters allow for better torque control of the wire in the coronary tree. In addition, an angioplasty can be performed, when indicated by the measurements, without pulling back the wire.

When the evaluation of the functional severity of a coronary lesion by means of intracoronary pressure measurements is planned, guiding catheters with side holes should be avoided as will be discussed in paragraph 6.5.

5.2 Pressure-monitoring guide wires.

The field of pressure monitoring guide wires is evolving rapidly. They can be subdivided in fluid-filled wires (the distal coronary pressure is transmitted through a tiny fluid column to an external pressure transducer), and in high-fidelity tip-manometer pressure wires (a micro manometer is implemented close to the tip of the wire). The technical characteristics of these wires are briefly presented below.

5.2.1 Fluid-filled pressure-monitoring guide wires.

Although the initial experience with coronary pressure and FFR was achieved by fluid-filled hollow guide wires, the use of this type of wires has been largely abandoned and replaced by the electronic sensor-tipped wires which are easier to use and allow superior registrations of both phasic and mean pressure. The only wire based upon the fluid-filled concept which is still used, is the Scimed Informer wire.

Scimed Informer wire (Scimed Incorporated, Minneapolis, Minnesota). The Scimed Pressure Wire is a 0.014-in (0.36mm) fluid-filled wire based pressure measuring tool. The pressure is sensed at openings just proximal to the spring tip and communicates through the fluid column to the sensing electronics at the proximal end of the wire. The wire transitions from a stiff stainless steel support section to a flexible nitinol section that terminates distally in a flexible and shapeable spring tip. The proximal end of the wire docks into a plastic housing which incorporates the fluid path that transmits pressure to a silicon pressure sensor and associated electronics. This pressure transducer interfaces directly with the existing catheterization laboratory equipment through an eight foot disposable cable and a reusable monitor cable to display phasic wave forms on the catheterization laboratory monitors. The Scimed pressure wire has a signal fidelity comparable to the regular invasive blood pressure systems.

Like regular blood pressure systems, the pressure wire system needs to be prepared prior to use. The preparing sequence involves flushing the wire and the transducer with heparinized saline using a 10 cc syringe. The pressure transducer is then zeroed with no pressure and calibrated manometrically, as defined by the catheterization laboratory monitoring system. The wire is now ready to measure coronary pressures. The plastic housing can be detached to use or manipulate the wire. To measure pressure again at any time the wire can be simply docked in the plastic housing and be flushed with heparinized saline. The wire characteristics in terms of steerability and torquability, are close to regular guide wires and well enough to use the wire as a first line guide wire.

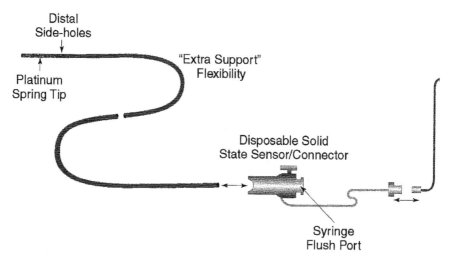

Figure 5.1 *Fluid-filled 0.014-in pressure-monitoring guide wire (Informer^{TM}, Scimed Inc, Minneapolis, MN). Due to a solid state sensor which can be connected to the proximal part of the wire, both phasic and mean pressure recordings are possible.*

5.2.2 Micromanometer-tipped guide wires.

Presently, 2 FDA-approved electronic systems are available, based on high-fidelity sensor-tipped wire technology. These are both 0.014-in wires with the pressure sensor located at 3 cm from the floppy tip.

PressureWire[TM] *(Radi Medical Systems, Uppsala, Sweden).* This pressure wire is most frequently used at present and has a worldwide experience of over 30.000 cases. Although the torquability was suboptimal in the original wire, this was largely improved in the new so-called *Pressure Wire XT* (extra torque) which can be used as a first line guide wire in almost every case. Presently, the *Pressure Wire XT-2* is tested which has a further improved torquability similar to a high torque floppy wire. The sensor in this wire is a piezo resistive pressure sensor coupled in a Wheatstone bridge. The linear working range of the sensor is from -30 to 300 mmHg, with a frequency range between 0 and > 200 Hz. The pressure sensor is located just proximal to the junction between the radiopaque distal tip and the non-radiopaque part of the wire. The proximal end of the wire is disconnectable and can be plugged into a special connector (figure 5.2, lower panel). The signal is transmitted to a small interface which, in turn, can be connected to an ordinary pressure monitoring system in the cardiac catheterization laboratory. The interface calibrates each sensor individually. This calibration procedure takes approximately 5 seconds only. Temporal and thermal drift are extensively tested clinically and are less than 5 mmHg/hour. Once the wire has been calibrated, further calibrations are generally not necessary, even not during long procedures. When the wire is disconnected from the interface connector-cable, all regular balloon catheters, IVUS catheters, and other interventional equipment can be advanced as in normal routine. To measure pressure again at any time, the wire can be easily plugged into the connector.

Recently, a pressure sensor has been developed with multiple functions, including temperature measurement with an accuracy up to 0.05 °C. That sensor allows simultaneous determination of FFR (by pressure), CFR (by thermodilution using 2 cc of saline), and coronary temperature. Validation studies for those multiple functions are performed presently.

Wavewire[TM] *(Endosonics Inc., Rancho Cordova, CA).*

The second system is the Wavewire[TM] (Endosonics Corp, Rancho Cordova, CA). The torquability of this wire is excellent. Although the initial wires suffered from a lack of stability of the pressure signal, requiring repeated re-

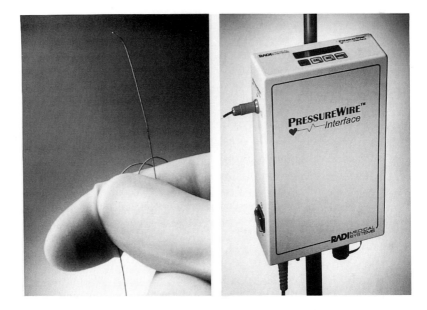

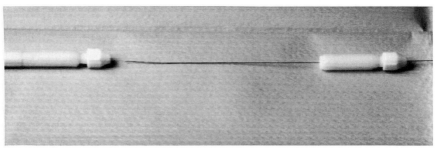

Figure 5.2   *Electronic sensor-tipped 0.014-in high-fidelity pressure guide wire (PressureWire XT ^{TM}, Radi Medical Systems, Uppsala, Sweden) and corresponding interface (upper panels). The proximal end of this flexible wire is disconnectable and can be plugged into a special connector (lower panel).*

Figure 5.4 and 5.5 (opposite page) *Examples of simultaneous mean and phasic tracings of aortic pressure (P_a, measured by a 7F guiding catheter) and transstenotic coronary pressure (P_d, measured by a sensor-tipped pressure wire, Radi Medical Systems, Uppsala, Sweden). In the patient in figure 5.4 (top), only a slight diastolic gradient is present at rest, reflecting that resting coronary blood flow in the left coronary artery predominantly occurs during diastole. In figure 5.5 (bottom), hyperemic tracings are shown in the presence of a significant LAD-stenosis. A large gradient is present throughout the heart cycle, but still largest at diastole, resulting in a typical distal pressure curve, representative of a severe stenosis.*

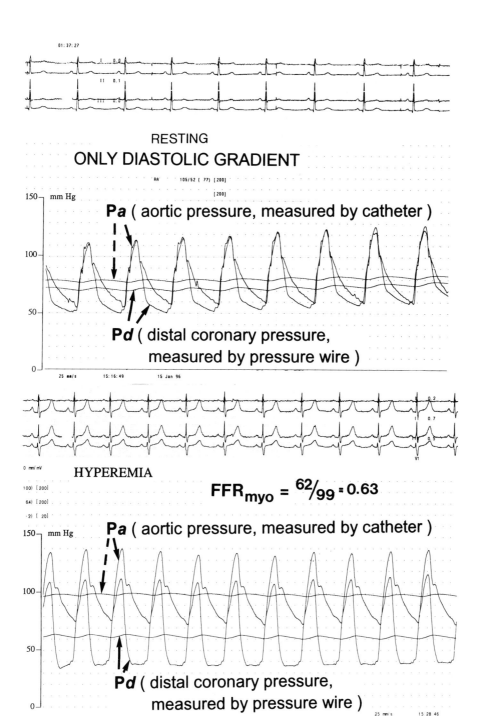

RESTING

ONLY DIASTOLIC GRADIENT

Pa (aortic pressure, measured by catheter)

Pd (distal coronary pressure,
measured by pressure wire)

HYPEREMIA

$$FFR_{myo} = \frac{62}{99} = 0.63$$

Pa (aortic pressure, measured by catheter)

Pd (distal coronary pressure,
measured by pressure wire)

calibrations during the procedure, the stability has been considerably improved and in many of these wires no intraprocedural recalibrations are necessary anymore. The interface of this system gives an option for electronic re-calibration, called "normalization". It should be emphasized, however, that re-calibration can only be made after having pulled back the pressure sensor into the guiding catheter, which can be problematic for decisions during interventions.

From current experience the perfect electronic pressure wire does not yet exist. Further improvement of wire characteristics, to become equal to a high torque floppy wire, and complete elimination of any drift and reconnection problems, should be achieved. Having seen the developments over the last year and the endeavors of both manufacturers, such improvements are likely to be achieved within the next year.

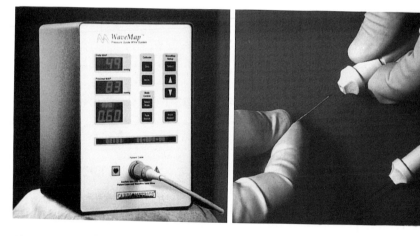

Figure 5.3   *Electronic sensor-tipped 0.014-in high-fidelity pressure guide wire (Wavewire^{TM}, Endosonics Inc., Rancho Cordova, CA) and corresponding interface. The proximal end of this flexible wire is disconnectable and can be connected to a special rotating connector (lower panel).*

5.3   Performance of the procedure.

As already mentioned, it is recommended that guiding catheters are used when coronary pressure measurements are performed. The inner coating of diagnostic catheters is rather rough and the lumen smaller, which may result in friction when any intracoronary device is advanced. Every guiding catheter, from 6F on, can be used. However, in interventional procedures one should realize that generally some damping of the aortic pressure signal occurs when a balloon catheter is advanced into a 6F guiding catheter.

All pressure wires presently available are 0.014-in in diameter and can be used in combination with every regular balloon catheter, IVUS catheter, or any intracoronary device. In most interventional cases, the current pressure wires can be used as first line wires and all necessary manipulations and exchange procedures can be performed in a regular way. The pressure transducer of the fluid-filled guiding catheter, should be fixed to the table to avoid misreadings of aortic pressure due to changing height of this transducer. All consecutive steps of coronary pressure recordings and determination of fractional flow reserve, are described and illustrated below and can also be followed in figure 4.9.

5.3.1 Verification of equal pressures in the ascending aorta.

While the guiding catheter is positioned in the coronary ostium and reference images are obtained, the pressure wire can be connected to its interface and adequately zeroed and calibrated, as described in paragraph 5.2 for the different specific pressure wires.

Thereafter, the wire is introduced into the guiding catheter and advanced to a location where the sensor is close to the tip of the guiding catheter. This can be just inside the guiding catheter or in the very proximal part of the coronary artery. At that location, it is verified that two completely identical pressure signals are obtained (figure 5.6). If a small difference is present at this site, this is probably due to an incorrect height of the pressure transducer of the fluid-filled guiding catheter (paragraph 6.2; figure 6.5 and 6.6). By decreasing the height of that transducer a few centimeters, P_a will increase a few mmHg and vice versa. We do not recommend to equalize pressures at this point by an electronic normalization procedure because, once this has been done, it can lead to confounding later on during the procedure and to incorrect interpretation of data. If the difference between the guiding pressure and the pressure recorded by the wire exceeds 10 mmHg, we recommend to take the wire out and to repeat the calibration. If a guiding catheter with side holes is used, a small difference in pressure may also be present. In that case, verification of equal pressures should be performed with the catheter out of the coronary ostium.

Verification of two equal pressure signals by the wire and by the guiding catheter at that location, is extremely important and should always be performed before and at the end of every procedure. If drift has occurred during the procedure (which should be < 5 mmHg/hour with the present equipment) this can be observed at the end of the procedure and corrections can be made if appropriate.

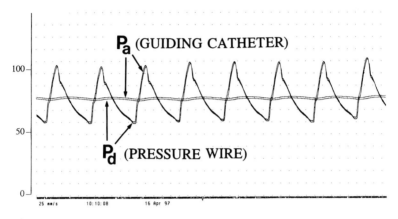

Figure 5.6 *A pressure wire is advanced until the sensor is close to its tip. At that location 2 identical signals should be obtained: P_a by the guiding catheter and P_d by the pressure wire. If a small difference is present, the height of the transducer of the fluid-filled guiding catheter should be slightly adjusted. (of figure 6.5 and 6.6)*

5.3.2   Crossing the stenosis.

Next, the wire is advanced into the coronary artery and crosses the stenosis. In the ideal case, this can be done during continuous registration of pressure either at full or at a low paper speed (figure 5.7). However, if the vessel is tortuous or the stenosis difficult to cross, the operator may prefer to disconnect the wire temporarily in order to have a better steerability of the wire. In that case, the wire can be connected again after the stenosis has been crossed. In the latter case, the recordings of the "pressure-drop" when the sensor crosses the stenosis, is not possible. However, the pressure is actually recorded 3 cm proximal to the tip. Therefore, once the wire has been positioned distal to the stenosis, the sensor can be pulled back and advanced across the stenosis time and again, leaving the tip of the wire distal to the lesion. In this way, the exact location of the pressure-drop can be detected exactly, safely, and reproducibly (figure 5.8). Such a "pull-back curve" is even more illustrative if performed at maximum hyperemia.

5.3.3 Induction of maximum hyperemia.

Once the sensor is distal to the stenosis, a maximum hyperemic stimulus should be administered for complete evaluation of the physiologic significance of the lesion and for calculation of fractional flow reserve.

Even if no or only a slight gradient is present at rest, hyperemia will unmask the true effect of the stenosis on coronary blood flow (figure 5.4 and 5.5; and figure 5.10 to 5.13).

The different intracoronary and intravenous maximum hyperemic stimuli which can be used as well as the pitfalls associated with their use, are described in detail in the next paragraph and in chapter 6. Knowledge about the characteristics and limitations of these stimuli is essential to be able to interpret coronary pressure measurements correctly.

It is important to be aware that when a short-acting, intracoronary stimulus is used (such as i.c. adenosine), the aortic pressure should be interrupted as short as possible for administration of the drug. The drug should be rapidly and completely delivered, followed by a few cc of saline, and phasic and mean pressure signals should be recorded again. Especially if the mean signal is averaged over a few seconds or more (and therefore is not rapid enough), the peak pressure gradient may be underestimated and FFR_{myo} overestimated by up to 0.10 (figure 5.13). It should also be stated that intracoronary administration of an hyperemic stimulus will be incomplete, if a guiding catheter with sideholes is used. In that case, intravenous infusion of an hyperemic drug is mandatory.

At maximum hyperemia, FFR_{myo} can be calculated immediately by the ratio of distal coronary pressure, measured by the wire, and proximal aortic pressure, measured by the catheter. If FFR_{myo} is < 0.75, the particular lesion can be held responsible for reversible ischemia and PTCA can be performed subsequently. Generally, it is not necessary to measure central venous pressure, unless there are clinical indications that this pressure is markedly increased, or specific studies of collateral blood flow are performed.

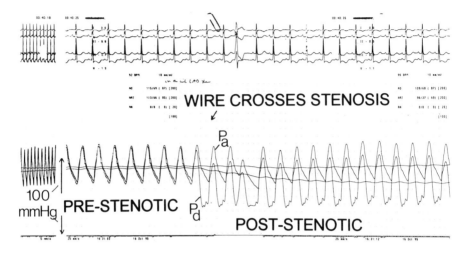

Figure 5.7 *The pressure wire crosses the stenosis, resulting in a sudden decrease of coronary pressure. Note the change in the phasic distal coronary pressure curve with a large diastolic and a smaller systolic gradient. In the lower panel, the curve is written at a lower paper speed (5 mm/s).*

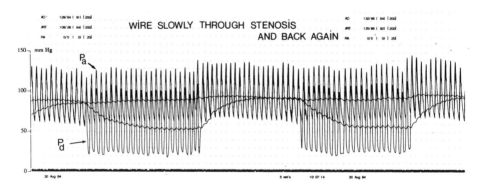

Figure 5.8 *So called pull-back curve: at a low paper speed, the pressure sensor is advanced and pulled back across the stenosis. Especially when a wire is used with its sensor a few cm from the tip, this can be repeated time and again very safely (without crossing the lesion again with the tip of the wire) and enables exact location of the stenosis, even when the angiogram is difficult to interpret.*

5.3.4 Pull-back curve.

The most convincing and reproducible demonstration of the exact location and severity of a coronary stenosis, is the so-called pull-back curve (figure 5.8). Ideally, such a curve should be recorded at maximum hyperemia and at a paper speed of 5-10 mm/s. Because intracoronary adenosine is too short-acting, intravenous adenosine or ATP, or intracoronary papaverine (which has a hyperemic plateau of approximately 30 seconds) is necessary. During maximum hyperemia, the sensor is slowly pulled back and advanced again across the stenosis, which can be safely done by wires with the sensor a few centimeters from its tip. If a large gradient is already present at rest and the main purpose of the pull-back curve is to determine the exact location of lesion, the additional hyperemia is not necessary per se during the pull-back curve. The pull-back curve also enables registration of more lesions within one vessel, or the presence of diffuse disease (see chapter 17, case 16, 17, 18, and 19, respectively). In fact, the pressure pull-back recording during maximum hyperemia is an unique and powerful method to analyze every particular segment of a coronary artery.

After a coronary intervention, the severity of any residual stenosis or plaque can be precisely determined by the pull-back curve. At last, the pressure pull-back curve under maximum hyperemia enables recognition of almost every pitfall which may occur and a possibility to correct for unforeseen drift, as will be discussed in paragraph 6.6.

5.3.5 PTCA and stenting.

If it is decided to perform an intervention, either based upon the calculation of FFR_{myo} or because the indication was clear anyhow, any monorail balloon catheter can be advanced as usual and the intervention can be performed. As a matter of fact, generally the gradient will increase when the balloon is placed in the stenosis and distal pressure will further decrease at balloon inflation. During balloon occlusion of the coronary artery, distal coronary wedge pressure (P_w) can be recorded continuously (figure 5.9) and also coronary fractional flow reserve (FFR_{cor}) and fractional collateral blood flow can be calculated now, as explained in paragraph 4.5.

Sometimes, an increase in P_w/P_a over time will be observed, indicating recruitment of collaterals or an increase of left ventricular diastolic pressure during ischemia. If P_w/P_a remains constant and if this value is less than 0.25, chest pain and ECG changes will often be present. If that ratio exceeds 0.30, ischemia at rest is rare (chapter 16).

After the balloon has been deflated, P_d usually increases rapidly. Often, a gradient will still be present but will decrease after withdrawal of the empty balloon from the stenosis (figure 4.9E). After a satisfactory angiogram has been obtained, post-PTCA FFR_{myo} can be determined by another administration of an hyperemic stimulus.

The interpretation of FFR_{myo} post-PTCA, is described in detail in chapter 14. If FFR_{myo} is still < 0.75, the result of the intervention is unacceptable anyhow (even if the angiogram looks satisfactory). If $0.75 < FFR_{myo} < 0.90$, stenting or another additional treatment, should be considered. If FFR_{myo} is $\geq$ 0.90 and the angiogram is satisfying, it has been demonstrated that restenosis rate is low and in the magnitude of 10% in the first year. Additional treatment like stenting can be mostly avoided in those cases[1].

If stent implantation is performed, post-stent FFR_{myo} should be at least 0.90 (a result achievable in 85-90% of the patients), whereas it has been demonstrated that $FFR \geq 0.94$ corresponds with optimal employment according to the most stringent IVUS criteria[2]. Of course, in case of a residual intracoronary pressure gradient after PTCA or stenting, it should be verified if this is due to the treated lesion itself or to disease elsewhere in the vessel. It should be emphasized that after treatment of a severe lesion and restoration of a higher achievable flow, a gradient across another lesion in the same vessel may become apparent which was masked previously by the presence of the first stenosis (paragraph 13.4 and case 17 and 19 in chapter 17). It will be clear that these issues can be best evaluated by a pull-back curve at maximum hyperemia. By use of a short-acting intracoronary

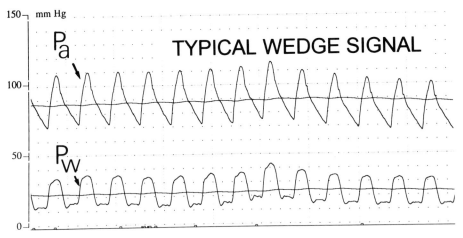

Figure 5.9   *Example of distal coronary pressure at balloon occlusion of the coronary artery (coronary wedge pressure, P_w).*

stimulus this information may be missed.

In case of more lesions within the same vessel, no significant hyperemic pressure drop should be present anymore across the stented segment (hyperemic distal to proximal pressure ratio ≥ 0.94).

5.3.6 Control for drift or other mistakes.

As already described above, at the end of the procedure the wire is slowly pulled back, the sensor is placed close to the tip of the guiding catheter, and it is confirmed again that equal pressures are recorded by the wire and the catheter at that location, or in other words, that no drift has occurred during the procedure. A drift of at most 5 mmHg/hour is considered acceptable. The issue of drift as well as how to recognize it and how to deal with it, is further discussed in paragraph 6.6.

5.4   Maximum hyperemic stimuli.

As outlined in chapter 4, for complete evaluation of the functional significance of a coronary stenosis, it is mandatory to perform pressure measurements under conditions of maximum coronary and myocardial hyperemia, corresponding with minimal myocardial resistance and minimal distal coronary pressure. Achievement of maximum hyperemia is essential for the interpretation of coronary pressure measurement and the calculation of FFR. If maximum hyperemia is not completely achieved, the actual severity of the lesion will be underestimated and patients may be undertreated. Therefore, if there is any doubt whether true maximum hyperemia was achieved, it is necessary to check carefully the composition and dosage of the drug used, to check if all stopcocks of the manifold are in the right position, and if there is no leakage. If uncertainty persists, a higher dosage of the respective drug or another hyperemic stimulus (i.v. instead of i.c.) should be tried. A number of pharmacological hyperemic stimuli have been described and their use, advantages, limitations, and pitfalls will be discussed below.

5.4.1 Intracoronary versus intravenous stimuli.

From a practical point of view, the use of short-acting intracoronary vasodilators like papaverine or adenosine is attractive. No venous line or

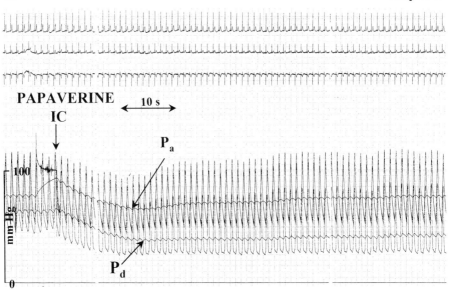

Figure 5.10 *Induction of maximum hyperemia by intracoronary administration of papaverine. Peak hyperemia corresponds with maximum transstenotic gradient and minimal distal coronary pressure. Note the proportionality between P_a and P_d at maximum hyperemia.*

Table 5.1 ***Intracoronary Papaverine***

♦ 1 ampul = 1 ml = 50 mg
  add 9 ml of saline → solution of 5 mg/ml

♦ intracoronary administration
  10 mg right coronary artery; 15 mg left coronary artery

♦ gold standard for maximum hyperemia

♦ peak hyperemia between 30-60 seconds after administration and
  lasts for 30-60 seconds

♦ side effects : QT-prolongation and T-wave changes
  very seldom : ventricular dysrhytmias/torsade des pointes

♦ opalescence when used in combination with ionic contrast agents and
  hexabrix. Non-ionic contrast agent must be used

♦ pitfalls: do not use guiding catheter with sideholes

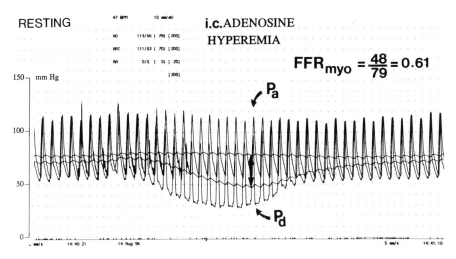

Figure 5.11 *Induction of maximum hyperemia by intracoronary administration of 20µg of adenosine in the left coronary artery. To avoid interruption of arterial pressure (P$_a$) by injection of the drug, P$_a$ was recorded by the side channel of the femoral arterial sheath. P$_d$: coronary pressure distal to the stenosis.*

Table 5.2 **Intracoronary Adenosine or ATP Intracoronary Bolus Administration**

- ◆ Dosage: 20-40 µg LCA; 15-30 µg RCA
- ◆ Rapid and short hyperemia after 5-10 sec, no steady state
- ◆ Effect disappears within 30 sec.
- ◆ Effect slightly prolonged if flushed by contrast agent.
- ◆ No side-effects: sometimes AV-block during a few seconds after injection in RCA.

- ◆ Pitfalls: - submaximum stimulus in some patients.
    - interruption of aortic pressure → peak hyperemia already passed before arterial pressure has adjusted.
    - maximum gradient underestimated when calculated from mean signal, unless it is taken on beat-to-beat basis.
    - no pull-back curve possible.
    - large guidings and guiding catheters with side-holes confound calculation and may underestimate maximum gradient.

In summary: risk of overestimation of FFR, underestimation of stenosis severity.

sheath is necessary and the measurements can be performed quickly and repeated with short intervals, if desired. However, some important restrictions should be recognized:

First: One should realize that the recording of the aortic pressure signal has to be interrupted for administration of the drug. Therefore, the drug should be administered rapidly, followed by a few cc of saline, whereafter the stopcock of the manifold should be switched back to its original position to register P_a again. Even then, it may take a few more seconds before P_a is displayed reliably, depending on the quality of the recording equipment. Care should be taken to be sure that the correct value is taken for P_a at the correct moment (peak hyperemia, minimal distal pressure). This is especially important when i.c. adenosine is used with the peak effect very early after its administration (10 seconds) and a short duration of hyperemia (5-10 seconds)[3]. For intracoronary papaverine, with a hyperemic plateau 30-60 seconds after its administration, this point is less critical[4].

Second: In many pressure recording systems, especially older types, the mean pressure signal is often averaged over many seconds and displayed as a flat signal. Therefore, rapid changes induced by i.c. adenosine, are not adequately monitored. Consequently, ΔP_{max} may be underestimated and FFR_{myo} overestimated if only the mean signal is studied. Therefore, we strongly recommend taking the mean signal averaged over one heart cycle only and to record both the mean and phasic signals simultaneously. If this issue is not taken into account well, overestimation of FFR by at least 10% can easily occur (figure 5.12) As a matter of fact, we further recommend using a rather large part of the monitor-display and paper for pressure recording, to demonstrate the pressures as well as possible. Presently, the importance of reliable pressure measurement is better recognized by most monitor equipment companies and more attention is paid to these issues.

Third: If a guiding catheter with sideholes is used, one should be aware that an unpredictable part of the hyperemic drug will be spilled in the ascending aorta. As a consequence, the measurements are unreliable, ΔP_{max} may be underestimated and FFR_{myo} overestimated. Therefore, we recommend not using guiding catheters with sideholes. If their use is unavoidable, an intravenous maximum hyperemic stimulus should be used and the catheter should be slightly pulled back from the ostium during the measurements, as mentioned before.

Fourth: If for any reason doubt may be present about the reliability of the pressure tracings, after intracoronary administration of a short-acting stimulus, continuous intravenous infusion of adenosine or ATP in the femoral vein will result in prolonged and safe steady-state hyperemia and enable unequivocal recognition of the relevant pressures.

5.4.2 Intracoronary papaverine.

Intracoronary papaverine is considered as the gold standard for induction of maximum coronary and myocardial hyperemia[4-5]. A steady state maximum hyperemic plateau is reached between approximately 30 and 60 seconds after its administration (figure 5.10). In the USA, some concern exists about intracoronary papaverine with respect to QT-prolongation and polymorphic ventricular tachycardia[5-7]. Although QT-prolongation is very common, in our experience in more than 1000 cases ventricular fibrillation occurred only 3 times (which is not significantly different from the incidence of ventricular fibrillation after regular contrast injections). Papaverine should not be used in combination with hexabrix and some other contrast agents, because opalescence and salt deposits may appear. Therefore, we recommend using papaverine in combination with true non-ionic contrast agents only. The dosage, preparation, advantages, and limitations of i.c. papaverine are summarized in table 5.1.

5.4.3 Intracoronary adenosine.

Intracoronary adenosine is an extremely safe agent to induce maximum hyperemia[3], without noticeable side-effects and with the possibility of repeating the measurements within minutes (figure 5.11 and 5.12). Its very rapid onset (within 10 seconds) and short peak hyperemia (a few seconds only, no plateau) can be a considerable limitation as discussed in paragraph 5.4.1. As explained, no pressure pull-back curve can be made, which means that only a gradient is obtained between the location of the sensor and the ostium of the coronary artery without the detailed spatial information about the specific site within the coronary artery where this pressure drop originates. If intracoronary adenosine is used, care should be taken to restore the aortic pressure signal as rapidly as possible. Sometimes, we have connected the arterial pressure line of the guiding catheter to the side channel of the femoral sheath to maintain the arterial signal during administration of i.c. adenosine (figure 5.11). A number of pitfalls associated with the use of intracoronary adenosine, should be recognized and are already discussed here above in paragraph 5.4.1. These pitfalls may result in overestimation of FFR and underestimation of true stenosis severity (figure 5.12). A specific concern is that in our experience, in some of patients intracoronary adenosine induces submaximal hyperemia only. In those patients, FFR may be overestimated up to 0.10. This is especially important because the ischemic threshold value of 0.75 has been validated by i.c. papaverine and i.v. adenosine, creating true maximum hyperemia. Therefore, if the reliability of the pressure tracings after intracoronary administration of a short-acting stimulus is questioned, a continuous intravenous infusion of adenosine or ATP will result in prolonged and safe steady-state hyperemia and enable unequivocal recognition of the relevant pressures.

In summary, when i.c. adenosine is used, the peak pressure gradient and FFR should be calculated from beat-to-beat mean signals and not from the delayed mean signals as indicated in a display, which may underestimate the gradient with a corresponding overestimation of FFR, and one should keep in mind that in some patients only submaximum hyperemia will be induced which can result in overestimation of FFR up to 10% in some patients. A last point in this context is to mention that the use of theophylline or large amounts of caffeine-containing beverages, should be avoided the last 20 hours before studies using adenosine or ATP.

Finally, the dosage of i.c. adenosine can be safely increased to 40 µg in the left and 20-30 µg in the right coronary artery. If AV-block occurs, which is not often the case, this is transient within seconds. The dosage, preparation, advantages and limitations of i.c. adenosine, are summarized in table 5.2

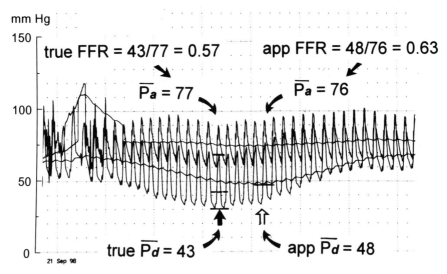

Figure 5.12: *Illustration how FFR can be overestimated (and the significance of the stenosis underestimated) by use of intracoronary adenosine. Because of the very short peak hyperemia, the mean pressure signal does not adequately reflect the peak gradient and the phasic coronary pressure signal is necessary to make correct calculations. The dashed line indicates true minimal mean coronary pressure (P_d), calculated from the phasic recording.*

5.4.4 Intravenous adenosine.

If adenosine is infused into a central vein at a rate of 140 µg/kg/min, steady state maximum hyperemia is reached within 1-2 minutes without a significant influence on AV-conduction[8,10]. Mostly, a slight increase of the PR-interval is observed, whereas second or third degree block is extremely rare. A reproducible steady-state maximum hyperemia is achieved by i.v. adenosine, which disappears within one minute after cessation of administration (figure 5.13).

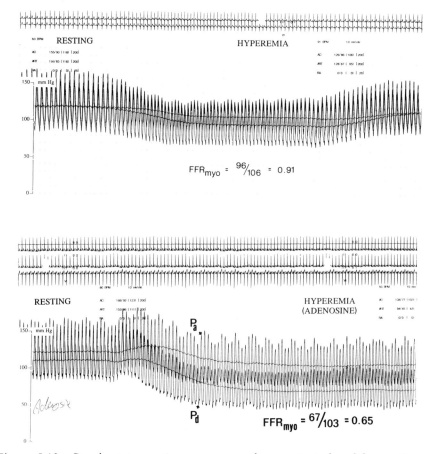

Figure 5.13 *Steady state maximum coronary hyperemia induced by continuous infusion of adenosine (140 µg/kg/min) in the femoral vein. Upper panel: mild stenosis in the LAD-artery; lower panel: angiographically intermediate (but functionally significant) stenosis in the right coronary artery. The paper speed is 5 mm/s to visualize the pressure changes more clearly.*

Intravenous adenosine can also be administered into a large anticubital vein, provided that the forearm is extended and uninterrupted venous return to the heart is guaranteed[11]. If administered in this way, it takes slightly longer before steady state maximum hyperemia is achieved.

As shown by Wilson et al, by Kern et al, and by Van der Voort et al, the hyperemic effect of i.v. adenosine is equivalent to intracoronary papaverine (figure 5.14)[3,8,9].

Intravenous infusion of adenosine is mostly accompanied by a burning, angina-like sensation on the chest or in the throat and sometimes by flushing. It should be emphasized that this is completely harmless and only caused by stimulation of free nerve fibers in the heart, which are stimulated by adenosine as this agent is one of the intrinsic transmitters of angina pectoris. If the patient is warned for this unpleasant sensation, and if it is explained to him that this is really harmless and will only last for a few minutes, a vast majority of them will sustain this sensation quite easily[9]. If such a sensation is not present at all, one should question if the drug is really being delivered well. Adenosine is rapidly de-aminated and de-activated by whole blood. Therefore, uninterrupted venous return to the heart should be guaranteed and Valsalva-like manoeuvres with increase of intrathoracic pressure and corresponding decrease of venous return, should be avoided.

Table 5.3 *Adenosine Intravenous Continuous Infusion*

- ♦ Femoral vein or large anticubital vein.
- ♦ Dosage: 140 - 160 µg/kg/min.
- ♦ Safe steady-state hyperemia achieved ≤ 1-2 min.
- ♦ Beautiful pull-back curve; best stimulus to obtain physiologic information about complete coronary artery; enables direct comparison of pressure just distal and proximal to stenosis or stent.
- ♦ Effect disappears within 1-2 minutes after cessation of administration.
- ♦ Side-effects: - decrease of blood pressure by 10-15%.
  - burning or angina-like chest pain during infusion. This is *harmless* and does *not* indicate ischemia.
  - not to be used in patients with severe obstructive lung disease (bronchospasm).

- ♦ Pitfalls: - if peripheral vein is used, avoid kinking of arm/elbow
  - avoid Valsalva manoeuvres.
  - withdraw guiding catheter slightly out of ostium if any sign of obstruction of the ostium is observed, or if guiding catheter with side-holes is used.

In case of any doubt, achievement of maximum hyperemia may be checked by either an additional bolus of intracoronary adenosine or by papaverine administration, or by increasing the i.v. infusion rate of adenosine to 160-180 µg/kg/min.

In our experience in more than 800 patients in whom i.v. adenosine was infused, no serious complications have been observed, no case of allergy was encountered, and only a few patients had second or third degree AV-block which always disappeared spontaneously within 20-30 seconds after cessation of the administration.

Intravenous adenosine infusion at a rate of 140 µg/kg/min, is accompanied by a decrease of blood pressure of about 10-15% and an increase in heart rate of 10-15%[3,9,10]. Remarkably, at the very start of its action, a short transient increase of blood pressure is often seen.

Many physicians feel somewhat uncomfortable when using intravenous adenosine (or ATP) infusion in their first cases. The presence of chest pain or discomfort in the patient makes them nervous which in turn is often felt by the patient. However, once having become familiar with i.v. adenosine, its unique advantage to make a pressure pull-back curve and to analyze the complete coronary artery will be appreciated and be a stimulus for further use, especially in cases with multiple abnormalities or diffuse disease. A last issue with i.v. adenosine is its price, which is unjustified high. In Europe, in many hospitals, i.v. adenosine is prepared by the hospital pharmacy at a price of less than 5% of the commercial price. The dosage, preparation, advantages and limitations are summarized in table 5.3

5.4.5. Intracoronary ATP.

In Japan, intracoronary ATP is often used as an alternative to intracoronary adenosine. Its dosage, effect, properties, advantages, and possible pitfalls are completely identical to intracoronary adenosine and will not be discussed separately[11].

5.4.6 Intravenous ATP.

The use of i.v. ATP as an alternative to adenosine, was first described by Japanese investigators and also confirmed at our laboratories[11,13]. It should be accompanied by less chest discomfort as adenosine. As is the case for i.v. adenosine, blood pressure mostly decreases by 10-15% and heart rate increases by 10-15%. Just as adenosine, ATP can be administered in either the femoral or a large peripheral vein. On its way to the heart, it will be metabolized to adenosine. The dosage, preparation, advantages and limitations of i.v. ATP, are summarized in table 5.4

Table 5.4 *ATP intravenous continuous infusion*

♦ Femoral vein or large anticubital vein.
♦ Dosage: 140 - 160 µg/kg/min.
♦ Safe steady-state hyperemia achieved ≤ 1-2 min.
♦ Beautiful pull-back curve; best stimulus to obtain physiologic information about complete coronary artery; enables direct comparison of pressure just distal and proximal to stenosis or stent.
♦ Effect disappears within 1-2 minutes after cessation of administration.
♦ Side-effects: - decrease of blood pressure by 10-15%.
                        - burning or angina-like chest pain during infusion. This is *harmless* and does *not* indicate ischemia.
                        - not to be used in patients with severe obstructive lung disease (bronchospasm).

♦ Pitfalls: - if peripheral vein is used, avoid kinking of arm/elbow
              - avoid Valsalva manoeuvres.
              - withdraw guiding catheter slightly out of ostium if any sign of obstruction of the ostium is observed, or if guiding catheter with side-holes is used.

5.4.7   Intravenous dipyridamole.

Administration of intravenous dipyridamole at the usual dosage of 0.56 mg/kg over 4 minutes, results in a long-lasting hyperemic state, which, however, is submaximal in a number of patients. The higher dosage, which is 0.75 mg/kg over 4 minutes, results in maximum hyperemia in almost every patient but is often accompanied by marked decrease of blood pressure or other side effects[14,15].
The hyperemia lasts for at least 20 minutes and can be directly counteracted by 250 mg aminophylline intravenously. Although this long action is an advantage in nuclear imaging methods with a long acquisition time, it is a major disadvantage in the catheterization laboratory, where measurements are mostly repeated with short intervals. Allergic reactions are more common than with adenosine and ATP. We do not recommend the use of dipyridamole, because the hyperemia, safety and side-effects are inferior to adenosine and because repeated measurements are precluded by its long action.

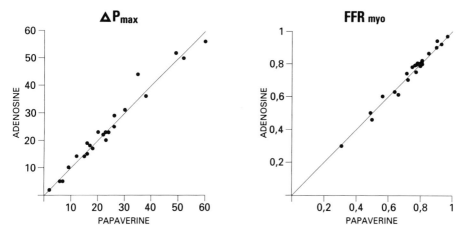

Figure 5.14 *Maximum transstenotic pressure gradient (left) and myocardial fractional flow reserve (right) after intracoronary administration of papaverine (horizontal axis) and during intravenous adenosine infusion in the femoral vein (vertical axis).*

5.4.8 Intravenous dobutamine.

High-dose dobutamine (up to 40µg/kg/min) is increasingly used to detect and evaluate coronary artery disease. As illustrated in figure 5.15, we have recently shown that dobutamine, in addition to its positive inotropic and chronotropic effects, induces a decrease in myocardial resistance equal to that observed with intracoronary adenosine despite a less-than-maximal increase in rate-pressure product (figure 5.16 and 5.17). In addition, myocardial resistance did not further decrease at dobutamine doses > 20 µg/kg/min suggesting a direct effect of dobutamine on resistance vessels[27].

5.5 Influence of the presence of a guide wire across the lesion on stenosis hemodynamics.

Because the cross-sectional area of a guide wire is small, one would expect no further increase in pressure gradient when the wire is passed through a coronary narrowing. This was tested for a 0.015-in guide wire in an in vitro model of stenosis as illustrated in figure 5.18, with stenoses ranging from 50% to 90% area reduction and the flow varying from 1 to 5 ml/s[18]. In mild stenoses (50% area stenosis) the difference in pressure gradient measured without and with the

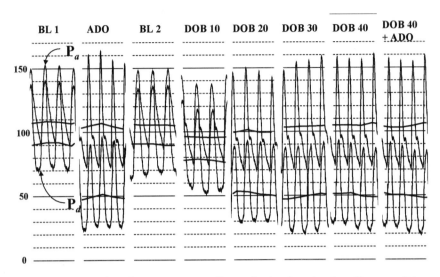

Figure 5.15 *Example of pressure recordings obtained under baseline conditions, after intracoronary administration of adenosine, during incremental dosages of intravenous dobutamine and after an additional intracoronary bolus of adenosine at peak dose of dobutamine. (ADO: adenosine; BL1 and BL2: baseline 1 and 2, respectively; DOB10, DOB20, DOB30, DOB40: during intravenous infusion of dobutamine at 10, 20, 30 and 40 μg/kg/min, respectively; DOB40 + ADO: during intravenous infusion of dobutamine at 40μg/kg/min and an additional intracoronary bolus of adenosine).*

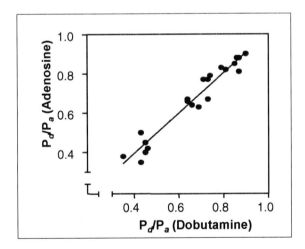

Figure 5.17 *Plots of the values of P_d/P_a observed after intracoronary administration of adenosine (ADO) and during the peak dose of dobutamine (DOB).*

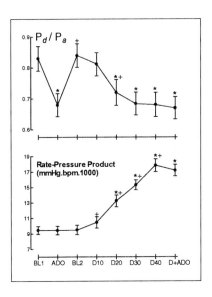

Figure 5.16 *Mean values (± SEM) of P_d/P_a (upper panel) and rate-pressure product (lower panel). Beyond the dose of 20 μg/kg/min of dobutamine P_d/P_a achieves a plateau while rate-pressure product continues to increase significantly. (ADO: adenosine; BL1 and BL2: baseline 1 and 2, respectively; DOB10, DOB20, DOB30, DOB40: during intravenous infusion of dobutamine at 10, 20, 30 and 40 μg/kg/min, respectively; DOB40 + ADO: during intravenous infusion of dobutamine at 40 μg/kg/min and an additional intracoronary bolus of adenosine; Rate-pressure product; * p < 0.05 versus preceding value; + p < 0.05 versus BL1).*

0.015-in guide wire through the lesion remained small (< 5 mmHg) even at high flow rates (5 ml/s). In severe stenoses (≥ 90% area stenosis), overestimation of the true gradient was induced by the presence of the guide wire itself through the stenotic segment at flow rates of ≥ 2 ml/s which are almost never encountered in such a tight stenosis. For example, in a stenosis of 90% area reduction at a flow rate of 2 ml/s, the pressure gradient measured across the lesion was 23 mm Hg with the guide wire compared with only 16 mmHg without the guide wire. In intermediate lesions, some overestimation was present only at very high flow rates. For example, in an 80% area stenosis, the measured gradient was 5.9 versus 4.8 mmHg for a 3 ml/s flow. At the extremely high flow rate of 5ml/s, the gradient was 36 mmHg with the wire versus 27 mmHg without the wire (figure 5.19). In interpreting these numbers, one should keep in mind that normal resting flow in an unaffected LAD-artery is approximately 1.0 ml/s and maximum flow up to 5.0 ml/s. In the presence of an 80% stenosis, therefore, the flow rates mentioned above are not readily achieved in real life. In summary, these results suggest that in mild and moderate stenoses, the overestimation in pressure gradient produced by the presence of the guide wire itself can be neglected. In tight lesions (≥ 90% area stenosis) a moderate overestimation is observed when blood flow exceeds 3 ml/s. However, this overestimation is of little clinical relevance: *first*, the mean pressure necessary to increase the flow above 3 ml/s through a 90%

area stenosis exceeds the physiological range (> 190 mmHg). Maximal coronary flow is limited in tight stenoses and no major increase in flow is to be expected once the stenosis exceeds 90% area stenosis; *second*, in clinical practice, these tight lesions do not require sophisticated measurements to be considered critical and to trigger an appropriate clinical decision.

Hence, in lesions of intermediate severity and in post-angioplasty segments where angiography often fails to be conclusive, the guide wire should provide a true pressure gradient value that reliably reflects epicardial resistance and can be helpful in clinical decision making.

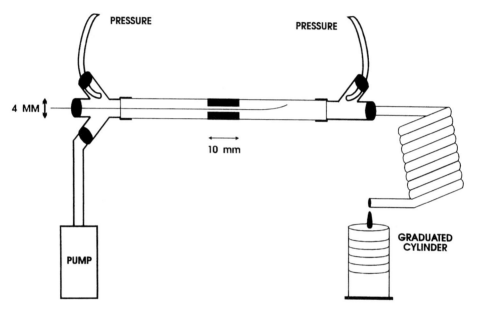

Figure 5.18 *In vitro model of coronary stenosis. Seven 10-mm long narrowings were created in rigid plastic tubes with an inner diameter of 4 mm and a length of 12 cm. The percent area reduction of the stenosis ranged from 50 to 95% (50%, 60%, 70%, 80%, 90%, 95%). One end of the tube was attached to a connector with three side arms. A high fidelity pressure monitoring catheter was advanced through one valve of this connector. The 0.015-in (0.038 cm) pressure monitoring wire was placed through the valve of the second arm and the third arm was connected to a power injector (Mark IV, Medrad Inc.). The other end of the tube was attached to a conventional angioplasty Y connector. A second high fidelity pressure monitoring catheter was introduced through the valve of this connector, and the other arm was left open. The power injector was filled with saline solution and constant flow rates of 0.5, 1, 1.5, 2, 3, 4 and 5 mL/s were infused in the stenosis model. The accuracy and constancy of the flow rates were controlled with a graduated cylinder placed under the distal opening of the system. For each level of stenosis severity, pressures were recorded proximal and distal to the stenosis for the different flow rates. Each measurement was performed successively without and with the guide wire through the narrowing.*

5.6 Safety of intracoronary pressure measurement.

To obtain FFR$_{myo}$ at a diagnostic procedure, introduction of a floppy guide wire into a coronary artery is necessary. It has been repeatedly demonstrated that introduction of such wires, both for measuring pressure or blood flow

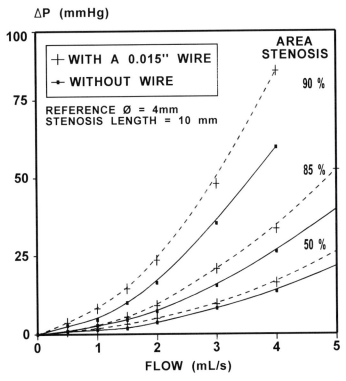

Figure 5.19 *Plot of the in vitro measured pressure gradient (ΔP) for varying stenosis severities (50%, 85% and 90% area stenosis) at incremental flow rates. Each measurement was obtained with (continuous line) and without (broken line) the 0.015-in. guide wire through the stenosis.*

velocity, can be safely performed by well-trained operators and that the very small risk is counterbalanced by the valuable information obtained in case of ambiguity about the functional significance of a stenosis[10,21-26]. In our own experience in more than 600 cases with the first generation of wires, we have observed possible complications due to the specific manipulations with these wires in only 2 cases. With the new wires available at present with markedly improved wire characteristics, we did not encounter any guide wire related complication in the first 300 diagnostic cases performed so far.

In interventional procedures, the question is trivial because introduction of a wire into the coronary artery is mandatory in those cases anyway and the technical manipulations are exactly the same as in routine PTCA.

Using a pressure guide wire at PTCA enables continuous monitoring of distal coronary pressure throughout the procedure. Not only can the FFR be calculated and the result better assessed, but also the phasic intracoronary pressure curve can be continuously studied, providing instantaneous feedback during intracoronary manipulations, contrast injections, etc., and enabling early recognition of ischemic or hemodynamic problems. The safety of a PTCA, therefore, is increased by using such a pressure wire.

References.

1. Bech GJW, Pijls NHJ, De Bruyne B, Peels KH, Michels HR, Bonnier HJRM, Koolen JJ. Usefulness of fractional flow reserve to predict clinical outcome after balloon angioplasty. *Circulation* 1999; 99: 883-888.
2. Hanekamp CEE, Koolen JJ, Pijls NHJ, Michels HR, Bonnier JJRM. Comparison of QCA, intravascular ultrasound, and coronary pressure measurement to assess optimum stent deployment. *Circulation* 1999; 99: 1015-1021.
3. Wilson RF, Wyche K, Christensen BV, Zimmer S, Laxson DD: Effects of adenosine on human coronary arterial circulation. *Circulation* 1990; 82: 1595-1606.
4. Wilson RF, White CW: Intracoronary papaverine: An ideal coronary vasodilator for studies of the coronary circulation in conscious humans. *Circulation* 1986; 73: 444-451.
5. Wilson RF, White CW: Serious ventricular dysrhythmias after intracoronary papaverine. *Am J Cardiol* 1988; 62: 1301-1302.
6. Talman CL, Winniford MD, Rossen JD, Simonetti I, Kienzle MG, Marcus ML: Polymorphous ventricular tachycardia: A side effect of intracoronary papaverine. *J Am Coll Cardiol* 1990; 15: 275-278.
7. Kern MJ, Deligonul U, Tatineni S, Serota H, Aguirre F, Hilton TC: Intravenous adenosine: continuous infusion and low dose bolus administration for determination of coronary vasodilator reserve in patients with and without coronary artery disease. *J Am Coll Cardiol* 1991; 18: 718-729.
8. Kern MJ, Deligonul U, Serota H, Gudipati C, Buckingham T: Ventricular arrhythmia due to intracoronary papaverine: Analysis of QT intervals and coronary vasodilator reserve. *Cathet Cardiovasc Diagn* 1990; 19: 229-236.
9. Van der Voort P, Van Hagen E, Hendrix G, Van Gelder B, Bech GJW, Pijls NHJ. Comparison of intravenous adenosine to intracoronary papaverine for calculation of pressure-derived fractional flow reserve. *Cath Cardiov Diagn* 1996; 39: 120-125.

10. Pijls NHJ, Van Gelder B, Van der Voort P, Peels CH, Bracke FALE, Bonnier JJRM, El Gamal MIH: Fractional Flow Reserve: a useful index to evaluate the influence of an epicardial coronary stenosis on myocardial blood flow. *Circulation* 1995; 92: 3183-3193.

11. Pijls NHJ, Kern MJ, Yock PG, De Bruyne B. Practice and potential pitfalls of coronary pressure measurement. *Cath Cardiov Interv* 1999; (in press).

12. Kinoshita K, Suzuki S, Shindou A. The accuracy and side effects of pharmacologic stress thallium myocardial scintigraphy with ATP infusion in the diagnosis of coronary artery disease. *Kaku Igaku* 1994; 31: 935-941.

13. Miyagawa M, Kumano S, Sekiya M, Watanabe K, Akutzu H, Imachi T, Tanada S, Hamamoto K. Thallium-201 myocardial tomography with intravenous infusion of ATP in diagnosis of coronary artery disease. *J Am Coll Cardiol* 1995; 26: 1196-1201.

14. Homma S, Gilliland Y, Guiney TE, Strauss HW, Boucher CA. Safety of intravenous dipyridamole for stress testing with thallium imaging. *Am J Cardiol* 1987; 59: 152-154.

15. Pijls NHJ, Aengevaeren WRM, Uyen GJH, Hoevelaken A, Pijnenburg T, Van Leeuwen K, Van der Werf T. Concept of maximal flow ratio for immediate evaluation of PTCA result by videodensitometry. *Circulation* 1991; 83: 854-865.

16. De Bruyne B, Sys SU, Heyndrickx GR. Percutaneous transluminal coronary angioplasty catheters versus fluid-filled pressure monitoring guide wires for coronary pressure measurements and correlation with quantitative coronary angiography. *Am J Cardiol* 1993; 72: 1101-1106.

17. Serruys PW, Wijns W, Reiber JHC. Values and limitations of coronary pressure during percutaneous coronary angioplasty. *Herz* 1985; 10: 337-342.

18. De Bruyne B, Pijls NHJ, Paulus WJ, Vantrimpont PJ, Sys SU, Heyndrickx GR. Transstenotic coronary pressure gradient measurements in humans: in vitro and in vivo evaluation of a new pressure monitoring angioplasty guide wire. *J Am Coll Cardiol* 1993; 22: 119-126.

19. Tron C, Donohue TJ, Bach RG, Aguirre FV, Carracciolo EA, Wolford TL, Miller DD, Kern MJ. Comparison of pressure-derived fractional flow reserve with poststenotic coronary flow velocity reserve for prediction of stress myocardial perfusion imaging results. *Am Heart J* 1995; 130: 723-733.

20. De Bruyne B, Stockbroeckx J, Demoor D, Heyndrickx GR, Kern MJ. Role of sideholes in guide catheters; observations on coronary pressure and flow. *Cath Cardiov Diagn* 1994; 33: 145-152.

21. Pijls NHJ, De Bruyne B, Peels K, Van der Voort PH, Bonnier JJRM, Bartunek J, Koolen JJ. Measurement of fractional flow reserve to assess the functional severity of coronary artery stenosis. *N Engl J Med* 1996; 334: 1703-1708.

22. De Bruyne B, Bartunek J, Sys SY, Heyndrickx GR: Relation between myocardial fractional flow reserve calculated from coronary pressure measurements and exercise-induced myocardial ischemia. *Circulation* 1995; 92: 39-46.

23. Ofili EO, Labovitz J, Kern MJ. Coronary flow velocity dynamics in normal and diseased arteries. *Am J Cardiol* 1993; 71: 3D-9D.

24. Serruys PW, Di Mario C, Meneveau N, De Jaegere P, Strikwerda S, De Feyter PJ, Emanuelsson H. Intracoronary pressure and flow velocity with sensor-tip guide wires: a new methodologic approach for assessment of coronary hemodynamics before and after coronary interventions. *Am J Cardiol* 1993; 71: 41D-53D.

25. Kern MJ, Donohue TJ, Aguirre FV, Bach RG, Garaccido EA, Ofili E, Labovitz AJ. Assessment of angiographically intermediate coronary artery stenosis using the Doppler Flowire. *Am J Cardiol* 1993; 71: 26D-33D.

26. Anderson HV, Kirkeeide RL, Stuart Y, Smaling RW, Heibig J, Willerson JT. Coronary artery flow monitoring following coronary interventions. *Am J Cardiol* 1993; 71: 62D-69D.

27. Bartunek J, Wijns W, Heyndrickx GR, De Bruyne B. Effects of dobutamine on coronary stenosis physiology and morphology. Comparison with intracoronary adenosine. *Circulation* 1999; 100: 243-249.

Chapter 6

PITFALLS IN CORONARY PRESSURE MEASUREMENT

As with every new technique, the cardiologist starting to perform coronary pressure measurements by wire technology will face some potential pitfalls which may lead to erroneous results or misinterpretation of data. Most of these pitfalls are easily recognized, a few are more tricky. There are some pitfalls specifically related to the equipment, to the guiding catheter used, to the use of the different hyperemic stimuli, and to specific physiologic or pathophysiologic conditions. Most of these pitfalls are easily avoided once the operator is aware of them.

The purpose of this chapter is to discuss these pitfalls systematically and to suggest methods on how to deal with them.

Pitfalls associated with the use of the different hyperemic stimuli, have already been discussed in paragraph 5.4.

Specific pathologic conditions influencing the interpretation of data, like left ventricular hypertrophy, previous myocardial infarction, and sequential stenoses within one artery, are discussed in chapter 13.

6.1 Use of balloon catheters or hypotubes instead of wires.

Early interventional cardiologists used balloon catheters to measure distal coronary pressure. This was unreliable. Figure 6.1 schematically illustrates why an overestimation in transstenotic pressure drop is to be anticipated when distal coronary pressure is measured with an angioplasty balloon catheter. Comparative data of transstenotic pressure gradients measured with a pressure-monitoring guide wire versus an angioplasty balloon catheter confirm that a uniform overestimation is induced by the presence of the balloon catheter in the lesion[1,2]. In a series of 34 patients, we measured distal coronary pressure by a 0.015-in pressure measuring guide wire and by a 2.7 - 3.0F balloon catheter in the stenosis. Both before and after PTCA, the mean pressure gradient measured with the wire was significantly lower than the

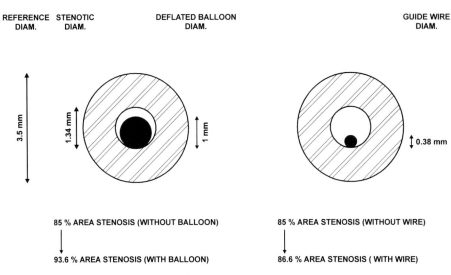

REFERENCE STENOTIC   DEFLATED BALLOON   GUIDE WIRE
    DIAM.   DIAM.   DIAM.   DIAM.

85 % AREA STENOSIS (WITHOUT BALLOON)   85 % AREA STENOSIS (WITHOUT WIRE)

93.6 % AREA STENOSIS (WITH BALLOON)   86.6 % AREA STENOSIS (WITH WIRE)

Figure 6.1 *Schematic illustration of the room occupied in an 85% area stenosis (72% diameter stenosis) in a 3.5 mm vessel by a balloon catheter and by an 0.014-in guide wire, respectively.*

mean transstenotic pressure gradient with the balloon catheter (figure 6.2). Finally, the relative overestimation in pressure gradient induced by the presence of the balloon catheter was small in severe lesions, while a major and unpredictable overestimation was observed in mild and moderate lesions, i.e. precisely in those lesions in which functional information is most desirable (figure 6.3).

Taken together, these data suggest that coronary pressures measured with balloon catheters are useless, both for the evaluation of the severity of coronary stenoses and for the assessment of functional results after angioplasty. In the more recent past, especially in the USA where pressure wires were not available until recently, some investigators used 2.2-3.5F infusion catheters, and similar equipment for intracoronary pressure recordings. However, large artificial and unpredictable transstenotic gradients may be created in that way and even in normal coronary arteries large intracoronary gradients may be induced (figure 6.4)[1-3].

As the occurrence of the overestimation is unpredictable, it is impossible to correct for these artifacts. Therefore, previous studies where intracoronary pressures were measured with infusion catheters, may have lead to erroneous results and should be interpreted with the greatest caution[3]. A clear illustration of this problem is shown in figure 6.4.

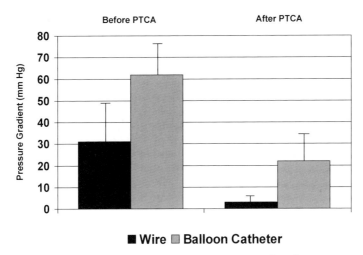

Figure 6.2 *Transstenotic pressure gradient as assessed with a pressure-monitoring guide wire or with an angioplasty balloon catheter, before and after angioplasty.*

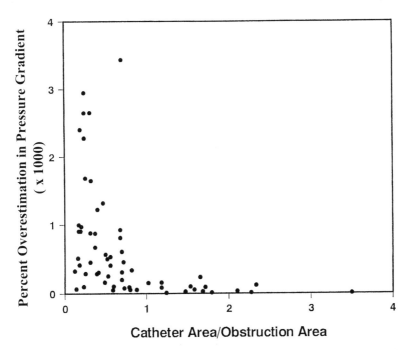

Figure 6.3 *Relation between the percent overestimation of the actual pressure gradient due to the superimposition of the balloon catheter into the stenosis and the relative dimensions of the balloon catheter as compared with the stenotic cross-sectional area.*

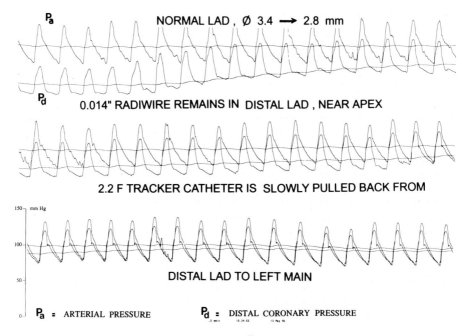

Figure 6.4 *Illustration how a large artificial intracoronary pressure gradient is created by measuring coronary pressure by a small catheter instead of a pressure wire. Aortic pressure (P_a) and distal coronary pressure (P_d) in a normal left anterior descending (LAD) artery are measured simultaneously during continuous steady state maximum hyperemia, induced by intravenous adenosine infusion. P_a is measured by a 6F guiding catheter and P_d by an 0.014" sensor-tipped pressure guide wire. A 2.2F Tracker catheter (Ø 0.7 mm) was advanced over the wire into the distal LAD, and a large intracoronary gradient is present (upper left). When the Tracker catheter is pulled back slowly during maximum hyperemia (leaving the pressure wire with the sensor in the distal part of the LAD), the gradient gradually decreases and after the Tracker catheter has been pulled back completely into the guiding catheter, no hyperemic gradient is present anymore. This example shows that coronary pressure measurements with small catheters instead of guide wires, are unreliable.*

6.2 Incorrect height of the pressure transducer.

When coronary pressure is measured by a sensor-tipped guide wire, its value is compared to aortic pressure, measured by the fluid-filled guiding catheter. The pressure transducer of that guiding catheter is generally fixed to the catheterization table at a height of 5 cm below the sternum, which is estimated to be the location of the aortic root. One should realize, however, that this estimation may be incorrect by a few centimeters and therefore, real aortic pressure may be incorrectly recorded by a few mmHg. As a result, when the sensor is close to the tip of the guiding catheter a small difference between both signals may be present. If this difference is only 1 or 2 mmHg, it is convenient because it allows better visualization of the two separate signals. When it is more, it should be corrected by adjusting the height of the fluid-filled pressure transducer (figure 6.5 and 6.6). Decreasing the transducer level will increase aortic pressure and vice versa. Note that this issue emphasizes the need to verify equal pressures when the sensor is close to the tip of the guiding catheter. It makes also clear that old systems, where the pressure transducer was not fixed to the table, should not be used. If, at the start of the procedure, the difference between guiding pressure and the pressure recorded by the wire, exceeds 10mmHg, we recommend to repeat the calibration instead of performing an electronic normalization procedure, because, in our experience, this may lead to confounding later on during the procedure.
At last, the hollow Informer Wire matches two external pressure transducers, which are placed at the same height, resulting in the absence of any difference between both pressures.

6.3 Use of a guide wire introducer.

A guide wire introducer is often put into the Y-connector to facilitate wire manipulations in the coronary artery. The space around the wire within the introducer may leak and decrease aortic pressure (P_a) by 0-10 mmHg, depending on the type of introducer. Therefore, if such an introducer with "leakage" is used, for all measurements including the verification of equal pressures, the measurement of FFR, and the verification for drift at the end of a procedure, the introducer should be taken out of the Y-connector and the Y-connector closed. Of course, when FFR is clearly in a normal or pathologic range, these differences are not so important, but when FFR is

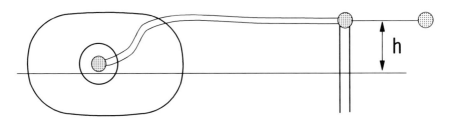

Figure 6.5   *Improper height of the pressure transducer of the guiding catheter, results in over- or underestimation of aortic pressure.*

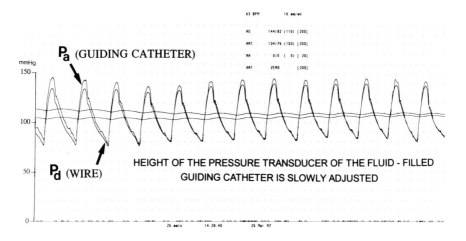

Figure 6.6   *Adjustment of the height of the pressure transducer of the guiding catheter, corrects the mistake illustrated in figure 6.5.*

close to a cut-off value (0.75 at diagnostic procedure;   0.90 after an intervention), meticulous awareness of these confounders is necessary. As there is quite a difference in this respect between different introducers, it is recommended to check this issue when starting coronary pressure measurement in a particular cathlab for the first time.

6.4 Damping of pressure by the guiding catheter.

When performing coronary pressure measurements, it is advisable to use a 6F or 7F guiding catheter. If using a larger guiding, an additional gradient between the aorta and the proximal coronary artery will be created either at rest or during maximum hyperemia by the presence of the guiding catheter (figure 6.7). This situation is recognized by some change in shape (damping) of the pressure signal recorded by the guiding catheter. *It is important to stress that this "damping" is often only unmasked by hyperemia (figure 6.8).* This can lead to underestimation of the hyperemic gradient across the coronary artery stenosis and a corresponding overestimation of FFR, and subsequently underestimation of the functional significance of the interrogated stenosis. Reason for this is, that a large guiding catheter can blunt maximum blood flow through the artery, resulting in a lower gradient and higher FFR than is truly the case. This pitfall can be prevented by pulling back the guiding catheter carefully from the ostium, leaving the pressure wire in the distal vessel, and using an intravenous instead of an intracoronary hyperemic stimulus.

Another potential problem related to the use of a large guiding catheter with some wedging in the coronary ostium, is a decrease of proximal pressure

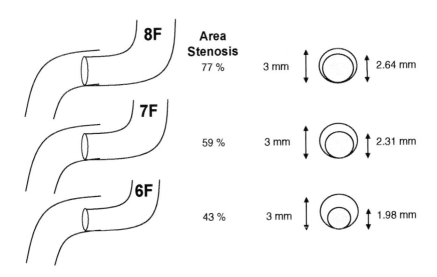

Figure 6.7   *Schematic representation of the room occupied in the right coronary ostium by several sizes of guiding catheters.*

below the autoregulatory range. This risk of being below the autoregulatory range, can also be present when measurements are performed in patients with very low systemic blood pressure. Therefore, if P_a has a mean value below 60 mmHg in the presence of a severe stenosis, increasing mean blood pressure by volume expansion to at least 70 or 80 mmHg before measuring FFR will increase measurement accuracy.

In summary, the use of large guiding catheters should be avoided and if that cannot be done, it is strongly advisable to withdraw the guiding catheter during the measurement and to use an intravenous hyperemic stimulus.

6.5 Guiding catheter with sideholes.

If a guiding catheter with sideholes is used in a small coronary ostium, one should realize that the pressure signal recorded through the catheter does not necessarily correspond to the pressure at its tip but may be determined both by coronary pressure (through the distal end of the catheter) and by aortic pressure (through the sideholes). Because of the presence of the catheter, the actual coronary pressure may be lower than the value recorded by the catheter[4,5]. In most instances, the sideholes are large enough to maintain a normal flow at rest without pressure drop. However, during arteriolar vasodilation a significant pressure drop may occur. This pressure drop is often not, or only partially, reflected by the pressure recorded through the guiding catheter. Therefore, measured P_a may exceed the actual proximal coronary pressure. This gradient, however, will not be detected if a guiding catheter with sideholes is used. (figure 6.9 and 6.10). As a result, FFR_{myo} of a more distal stenosis will be underestimated (as ΔP_{max} will be overestimated). Therefore, if a guiding catheter with sideholes is used, it is mandatory to pull it back out of the coronary ostium before the measurements for FFR calculation are made[5].

This emphasizes the second problem, associated with a guiding catheter with sideholes: no intracoronary hyperemic stimulus can be used because part of the drug will be delivered into the aorta and one can never be sure that true maximum vasodilation of the distal myocardial bed is achieved. Intravenous administration of an hyperemic stimulus, is necessary in those cases (paragraph 5.4.1).

In summary: when a guiding catheter with sideholes is used, the catheter should be slightly pulled back out of the ostium during the measurements (leaving the wire distal to the stenosis) and an intravenous infusion of a hyperemic stimulus is mandatory.

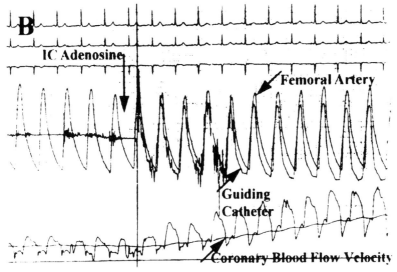

Figure 6.8 *Damping of the pressure recorded by an 8F guiding catheter at hyperemia illustrated by simultaneous measurement of femoral artery pressure. True stenosis severity may be underestimated. Removal of the guiding from the coronary ostium and use of i.v. adenosine is necessary for reliable assessment of true stenosis severity.*

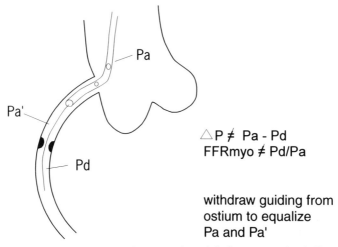

$\triangle P \neq P_a - P_d$
$FFRmyo \neq P_d/P_a$

withdraw guiding from
ostium to equalize
Pa and Pa'

Figure 6.9 *When a guiding catheter with sideholes is used, ΔP_{max} may be overestimated and FFR_{myo} underestimated because $P_a > P_a'$. Such a guiding catheter should be pulled back from the coronary ostium before the measurements are made.*

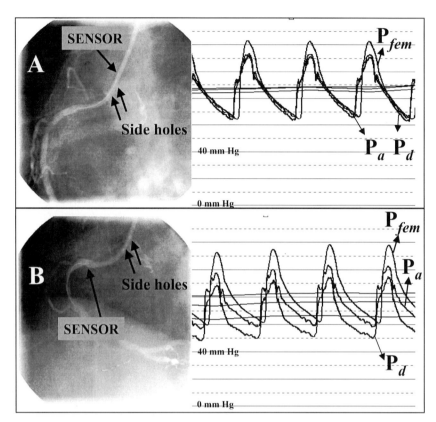

Figure 6.10 *Confounding effect of guiding catheter with side-holes. In the upper part of the figure, the pressure sensor (located at the transition of the radiopaque and radiolucent part of the wire) is positioned close to the side-holes of a 7F JR guiding catheter. Completely identical pressure signals are obtained (P_a by the side-holes, P_d by the sensor). Femoral artery pressure (P_{fem}) is also recorded by the side-arm of the arterial sheath.*

In the lower part of the figure, the sensor is advanced just to the tip of the guiding catheter, and hyperemia is induced by intravenous adenosine infusion. A gradient of 7 mmHg develops between P_{fem} en P_a , and an even larger gradient of 12 mmHg develops between P_a and P_d . Therefore, confounding will occur when evaluating distal coronary pressure in the RCA. In fact, P_{fem} represents true arterial blood pressure, P_a is the pressure recorded by the side-holes (a mixture of true arterial pressure and proximal coronary pressure), and P_d is the true pressure at the ostium of the coronary artery. If a guiding catheter with side-holes is unavoidable, the only way for correct interpretation of coronary pressure is to use intravenous adenosine and to withdraw the guiding catheter slightly from the coronary ostium during the measurements.

6.6 Signal drift during procedure.

Ideally, no drift during a procedure should occur. In our opinion, the maximum acceptable drift is ≤ 5 mmHg/hour. Repeat calibrations during the studies should be unnecessary. Re-calibration is time-consuming and potentially harmful because the wire has to be pulled back into the guiding catheter and then re-cross the stenosis again. When performing coronary pressure measurement, it is important to recognize potential drift and to know how to avoid confounding of data[5]. Drift occurring during the procedure can often be recognized by the shape of the pressure signal recorded in the distal coronary artery (figure 6.11). In a left coronary artery blood flow at rest occurs predominantly during diastole. Therefore, in case of a stenosis there will be a diastolic gradient but almost no or a much smaller systolic gradient and therefore the shape of the pressure curve recorded by the wire is different from the aortic pressure curve. During hyperemia, diastolic blood flow increases with a lesser increase in systolic flow, further accentuating the specific shape of the distal pressure signal (figure 6.11). Therefore, a true pressure gradient within a left coronary artery will demonstrate this typical shape of the distal signal. When a difference (gradient) between the proximal and distal signal is present but the shape of the curves is almost identical, one should consider this as clear evidence of drift (figure 6.12).

When performing transstenotic pressure measurement in the right coronary artery, there is not such a typical shape of the distal pressure curve (flow in a RCA is often balanced between systole and diastole). Recognizing drift by the shape of the curve is more difficult in that case. Maintenance of the aortic notch in the distal pressure signal in the presence of a considerable gradient, should raise suspicion that drift has occurred (figure 6.12). If drift is suspected, one solution is pulling the sensor back to the guiding catheter and rechecking the calibration, obviously an unattractive option because the procedure has to be interrupted. Another way to deal with this problem is making the *pull-back recording at maximum hyperemia,* which is *the most powerful and accurate way under any circumstances to establish the true severity of a stenosis.* The technique of making a pull-back curve has already been mentioned in paragraph 5.3.4. *The pull-back curve helps to overcome almost every possible pitfall.* Even when drift has occurred during the procedure, making a pull-back curve during steady state hyperemia enables reliable calculation of FFR, by comparing the pressure just distal to the stenosis of interest to the pressure proximal to that stenosis. A correction can be made and FFR of the respective lesion is known.

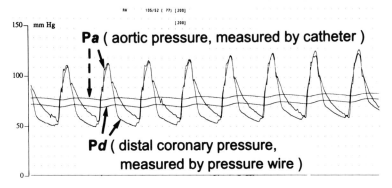

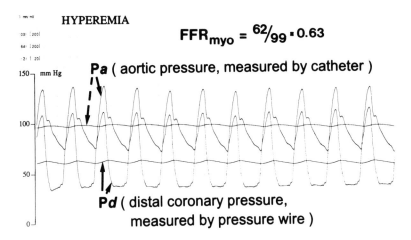

Figure 6.11 *Example of true gradient in the LCA. At rest, there is no systolic gradient and only a small diastolic gradient, whereas the systolic aortic and distal coronary pressures are almost identical, reflecting the almost exclusive diastolic flow in the left coronary artery at rest. At hyperemia, the diastolic gradient increases and also a systolic gradient occurs, resulting in a typical "ventricularized" shape of the distal coronary pressure curve, reflecting a true stenosis.*

Note by the way, that a pressure difference between a location just proximal to the lesion and the ascending aorta does not necessarily indicate drift. There is also the possibility of additional lesions - even if not visible on the angiogram - or diffuse disease in the remaining part of the blood vessel. But also these conditions will be recognized by pulling back the sensor slowly to the coronary ostium during hyperemia after the intervention has been done. In addition, especially after successful PTCA and stenting of a severe stenosis, it may happen that an apparently "new" gradient appears elsewhere in the vessel. This does not necessarily indicate drift but is often due to the increased blood flow, unmasking the hemodynamic effects of plaques and other abnormalities more proximal or distal in the vessel (cf. chapter 17, case 25). In summary, a pull-back curve at maximum hyperemia is the most accurate, most convincing, and most reliable way to study the functional status of every part of a coronary artery. *The pull-back curve under hyperemia never lies !*

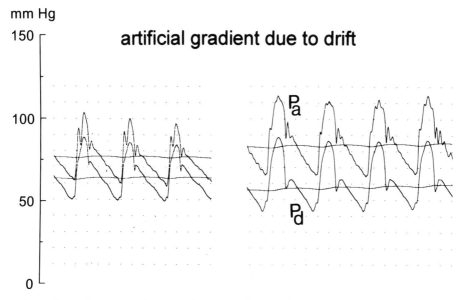

Figure 6.12 *Two examples of drift: Although a gradient is present, the shape of the aortic and distal coronary curve is completely identical and, despite an apparent gradient, the aortic notch is maintained in the distal curve. Both signs are indicative for drift.*

6.7   Proportionality of P_d and P_a.

As may be clear from chapter 4, ΔP_{max} and P_d are proportional to P_a. Therefore, changes in systemic blood pressure during maximum hyperemia are accompanied by changes in ΔP_{max}. This is not an artifact but an physiologic phenomenon and does not affect FFR_{myo} as clarified in figure 6.13 and figure 9.9.

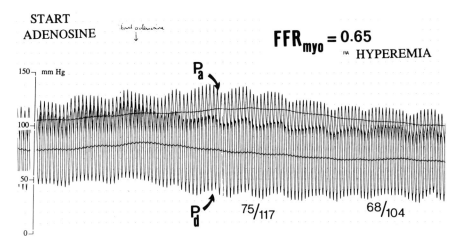

Figure 6.13   *Illustration of the proportionality between P_a and P_d. As can be observed, FFR_{myo} is not affected by the pressure changes.*

6.8   Reversed or paradoxical gradient.

Sometimes, when the sensor-tipped guide wire is advanced into the distal part of a normal artery, P_d will exceed P_a by a few mmHg. This is due to the fact that the atmospheric level of the ascending aorta (where P_a is measured) may be different from that of the distal coronary artery. In that case, an additional fluid column of some centimeters H_2O influences the pressure sensor and a small paradoxical or "reversed" gradient may occur (figure 6.14). In fact, this is not a real pitfall but a normal physiologic phenomenon.

The opposite, decrease of P_d by a few mmHg if the atmospheric level of the distal coronary artery is higher than that of the ascending aorta, will mostly not be recognized because the small (extra) gradient is ascribed to decline of pressure along the coronary artery. Generally, these differences are small and do not confound the interpretation of data or clinical decision making.

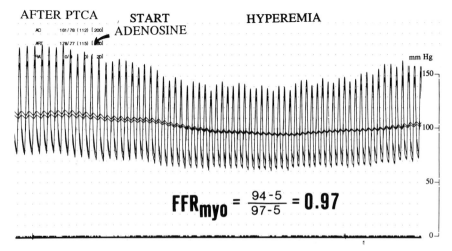

Figure 6.14 *A small paradoxical gradient is sometimes observed when the pressure wire is distal in the coronary artery. This is caused by a different atmospheric level of the location where P_d is measured and the aortic root, where P_a is measured. In this example, at hyperemia P_d decreases slightly and the gradient seems to disappear paradoxically.*

6.9 Inadequate registration of aortic pressure by the guiding catheter.

It is often taken as a matter of fact that the signal produced by the guiding catheter is the correct recording of aortic pressure. However, that is not always the case. In paragraph 6.2, the importance of a correct height of the guiding catheter has already been mentioned. Moreover, during a longer procedure we sometimes observe that the guiding catheter signal not only becomes somewhat damped but also shows some decrease over time as compared to true aortic pressure. Vigorous flushing of the guiding catheter by saline mostly restores the original signal. Finally, in rare cases the guiding catheter signal may be affected by dynamic pressure changes superimposed on the true aortic pressure. A better alignment of the guiding catheter with the coronary ostium mostly solves that problem.

References.

1. De Bruyne B, Sys SU, Heyndrickx GR. Percutaneous transluminal coronary angioplasty catheters versus fluid-filled pressure monitoring guide wires for coronary pressure measurements and correlation with quantitative coronary angiography. *Am J Cardiol* 1993; 72: 1101-1106.
2. De Bruyne B, Pijls NHJ, Paulus WJ, Vantrimpont PJ, Sys SU, Heyndrickx GR. Transstenotic coronary pressure gradient measurements in humans: in vitro and in vivo evaluation of a new pressure monitoring angioplasty guide wire. *J Am Coll Cardiol* 1993; 22: 119-126.
3. Tron C, Donohue TJ, Bach RG, Aguirre FV, Carracciolo EA, Wolford TL, Miller DD, Kern MJ. Comparison of pressure-derived fractional flow reserve with poststenotic coronary flow velocity reserve for prediction of stress myocardial perfusion imaging results. *Am Heart J* 1995; 130: 723-733.
4. De Bruyne B, Stockbroeckx J, Demoor D, Heyndrickx GR, Kern MJ. Role of sideholes in guide catheters; observations on coronary pressure and flow. *Cath Cardiov Diagn* 1994; 33: 145-152.
5. Pijls NHJ, Kern MJ, Yock PG, De Bruyne B. Practice and potential pitfalls of coronary pressure measurement. *Cath Cardiov Interv* 2000; in press.

Chapter 7

VALIDATION OF FRACTIONAL FLOW RESERVE IN ANIMALS

7.1 Introduction.

As outlined in the previous chapter, fractional flow reserve (FFR) expresses maximum achievable blood flow in the presence of a coronary stenosis as a ratio to normal maximum flow. In other words: maximum flow in a stenotic coronary artery and maximum flow to the myocardium supplied by that artery are expressed as a fraction of normal maximum coronary and myocardial blood flow (FFR_{cor} and FFR_{myo}, respectively). The main aim of this animal study in dogs was to validate experimentally the basic pressure-flow equations as described in chapter 4.

Maximum recruitable collateral flow at coronary occlusion:

$$(Q_c/Q^N)_{max} = \frac{P_w - P_v}{P_a - P_v} \qquad \text{(eq. 1)}$$

Coronary Fractional Flow Reserve:

$$FFR_{cor} = \frac{P_d - P_w}{P_a - P_w} \qquad \text{(eq. 2)}$$

Myocardial Fractional Flow Reserve:

$$FFR_{myo} = \frac{P_d - P_v}{P_a - P_v} \qquad \text{(eq. 3)}$$

Fractional Collateral Flow:

$$Q_c/Q^N = FFR_{myo} - FFR_{cor} \qquad \text{(eq. 4)}$$

In the present study, the equation for pressure-derived FFR_{cor} is directly validated against measured maximum coronary blood flow, as assessed by an epicardial Doppler probe, and indirect evidence is obtained to prove the validity of the equation for FFR_{myo} and fractional collateral flow. The constancy of the expression

$$\frac{P_w - P_v}{P_a - P_v}$$

in equation (1), irrespective of the value of P_a and P_v, is also experimentally proved in this chapter. The numeration of the equations in this chapter refers to the numeration in paragraph 4.7. Also, the abbreviations used are identical to those in that chapter. In chapter 8, direct validation of pressure-derived FFR_{myo} is performed in conscious humans, using positron-emission tomography.

7.2   Methods.

7.2.1   The Pressure-Flow Model.

The pressure-flow model of the coronary circulation underlying this experimental study, and the abbreviations used are similar to the schematic model in figure 4.7, modified from Gould et al [5]. The coronary circulation is schematically represented as an arrangement of variable resistances in parallel and in series. In the presence of maximum vasodilation obtained by a sufficient vasodilatory stimulus, the resistances of the myocardial capillary bed (R) and the collateral circulation (R_c) are minimal and constant, and in that case the flow-dependent stenosis resistance (R_s) is maximal and therefore also constant. R_s may be changed by an intervention, such as PTCA. Mean arterial pressure (P_a), central venous pressure (P_v), and coronary pressure distal to the stenosis (P_d), are defined as before, whereas the coronary wedge pressure (P_w) is defined as the pressure distal to the stenosis during coronary artery occlusion. ΔP is defined as $P_a - P_d$. The total blood flow through the myocardial bed (Q) is the sum of the blood flow through the supplying stenotic artery (Q_s), also called coronary artery flow, and collateral flow (Q_c). If no stenosis is present, Q and Q_s are called Q^N and Q_s^N, respectively, and are assumed to be equal. In other words, Q^N and Q_s^N

represent maximum myocardial and coronary blood flow in the case that the supplying coronary artery is completely normal.

As stated before, FFR is defined as the maximally achievable flow in the presence of a stenosis divided by the maximum flow expected in the same distribution in the absence of a stenosis. In analogy to Q_s and Q, fractional coronary artery flow reserve (FFR_{cor}) and fractional myocardial flow reserve (FFR_{myo}) are defined as Q_s/Q_s^N and Q/Q^N, respectively. As shown in paragraph 4.5, by using this model of the coronary circulation, the relations among Q, Q_s, and Q_c can be elucidated, and both FFR_{cor} and FFR_{myo} can be calculated by performing pressure measurements under maximum vasodilated conditions using equations 2 and 3.

7.2.2 Animal instrumentation.

After premedication with 0.1 mg fentanyl, 5.0 mg droperidol,and 0.5 mg atropine i.m., five mongrel dogs (weight 24 - 36 kg) were anesthetized with 25 mg/kg sodium pentobarbital i.v. and ethrane. A left thoracotomy was performed, and the proximal left circumflex artery was dissected free. A perivascular ring-mounted 20-MHz pulsed Doppler transducer (Crystal Biotech Inc., Holliston, Mass.) was placed around the artery, and a circular balloon occluder (R.E.Jones, Silver Spring, Md.) was placed just distal to the Doppler probe. A femoral vein and two femoral arteries were dissected free. An 8F Millar manometer catheter (Millar microtipped-catheter transducer SPC-780 C) was introduced into the femoral vein and positioned into the right atrium for measurement of central venous pressure. Another 8F Millar manometer catheter was introduced into the left femoral artery and positioned in the ascending aorta, just above the aortic valve, for measurement of arterial pressure. A 6F left Judkins coronary arteriography catheter was introduced into the right femoral artery and advanced into the ostium of the left main coronary artery. Finally, a pressure-monitoring device was advanced through the Judkins catheter into the left circumflex artery and positioned with its tip 3-5 cm distal to the balloon occluder (figure 6.1). This pressure-monitoring device consisted of a flexible synthetic tube with a length of 75 cm and an outer diameter of 0.028-in, connected to the distal 15 cm of an 0.015-in hollow guide wire. Only the distal part of this device (i.e. the guide wire) entered the coronary artery. The time constant of this device was determined in advance according to a protocol described earlier[7], and never exceeded 1 second. ECG, venous pressure (P_v), aortic pressure (P_a), distal coronary pressure (P_d), and phasic and mean coronary blood flow velocities in the left circumflex artery were continuously recorded on an eight-channel recorder.

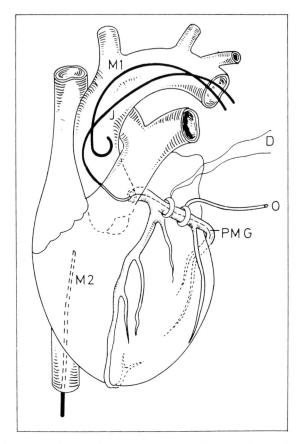

Figure 7.1   *Schematic of animal instrumentation. D, Doppler probe; J, 6F left Judkins catheter; M_1, Millar catheter in ascending aorta; M_2, Millar catheter in right atrium; O, balloon occluder; PMG, pressure-monitoring guide wire with its tip 3 - 5 cm distal to the balloon occluder.*

Figure 7.2   (opposite page) *Example of hemodynamic recordings in one series of one dog. Central venous pressure (P_v), distal coronary pressure (P_d), mean aortic pressure (P_a), and phasic and mean blood flow velocity (Q_s) in the left circumflex artery are recorded before vasodilation (first column), after intracoronary papaverine administration (second column), in the presence of a moderate stenosis (third column) and a severe stenosis (fourth column) induced at papaverine-induced maximum hyperemia, and at coronary artery occlusion (fifth column). O, occlusion of the coronary artery; P, intra-coronary administration of 8 mg papaverine; R, release of stenosis; S, induction of stenosis.*

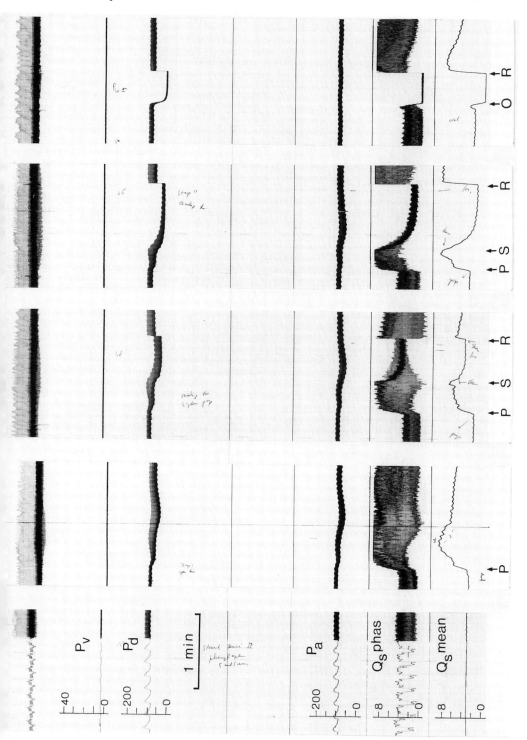

7.2.3   Experimental protocol.

In all dogs, experiments were performed at three different levels of mean arterial pressure called the normotensive, hypertensive, and hypotensive states. After stabilization of all hemodynamic parameters, maximum coronary blood flow velocity in the left circumflex artery was measured after intracoronary (i.c.) administration of 8 mg papaverine through the guiding catheter into the left main coronary artery. This value was compared with maximum hyperemic blood flow velocity after a 20-second occlusion period to confirm that maximum arteriolar vasodilation was obtained by that dose of papaverine. Also, P_w was recorded at the end of that 20-second occlusion of the left circumflex artery. Thereafter, 12 different degrees of stenosis were induced in the left circumflex artery by partial inflation of the balloon occluder[17]. Each stenosis was applied after an 8 mg papaverine i.c. injection through the guiding catheter. Next, P_a, P_d, and P_v were measured at the moment of maximum transstenotic pressure gradient, corresponding to peak coronary hyperemia (figure 6.2). Measurement of P_w during occlusion of the coronary artery was repeated halfway through and at the end of the series of stenoses.

Intravenous infusion of phenylephrine (0.05 mg/ml) then was started to achieve a steady-state mean arterial pressure of approximately 25 - 50 % above the normotensive state. After the desired steady hypertensive state was achieved, another series of 12 measurements at 12 different degrees of stenosis was performed, preceded and followed by registration of P_w during total occlusion in a way identical to that described before.

Finally, intravenous administration of sodium nitroprusside (1 mg/ml) was started to create hypotension at an arterial pressure of approximately 25 - 50 % below the initial value, and another series of measurements at 12 different degrees of stenosis was performed, again preceded and followed by determination of P_w respectively.

7.2.4   Data processing and statistical analysis.

With this experimental protocol, in each dog values for P_a, P_d, and P_v during maximum vasodilation were determined for 36 different stenoses at three different pressure states. At first, P_a, P_v, and P_w as measured during the different coronary artery occlusions were substituted in equation 1 to test the constancy of this equation. Thereafter, FFR_{cor} and FFR_{myo} were calculated according the equations 2 and 3, and these calculated values were compared with fractional coronary flow reserve (Q_s/Q_s^N) as measured directly by the epicardial Doppler probe. Correlation coefficients were calculated for each dog. Finally, at every degree of stenosis and at every pressure state, the contribution of collateral blood flow was calculated according to equation 4. All hemodynamic data are expressed as mean ± SD.

7.3   Results.

7.3.1 Hemodynamic observations and the relation between mean arterial pressure and coronary wedge pressure.

No serious complications and no technical problems occurred in performing the pressure measurements. In every dog, maximum coronary blood flow in the presence of the different degrees of stenosis ranged from near 0% to 100% of the initial control value in the absence of a stenosis, thereby indicating that the complete spectrum of stenosis severities was represented. The ratio between maximum blood flow velocity after intracoronary papaverine injection (8 mg) and post-occlusional maximum blood flow velocity at the start of each series was 0.99 ± 0.03 (range, 0.95 - 1.03), confirming that the presence of maximum arteriolar vasodilation was obtained by this dose of papaverine. In figure 7.2, examples of the hemodynamic recordings at a number of steps in one series of stenoses for one dog are demonstrated. In all dogs, the three levels of arterial blood pressure were achieved (table 7.1). In one dog, at the end of the hypertensive series, diffuse intrathoracic bleeding occurred and led spontaneously to arterial hypotension, which was controlled thereafter by fluid infusion to obtain a steady-state hypotensive level for completion of the third series of stenoses. No sodium nitroprusside was administered in this case.

The relation between (P_a - P_v) and (P_w - P_v) is shown for the individual dogs in figure 7.3. As expected from theory (equation 1), the experimentally observed relation is constant. The correlation coefficient is 0.97 ± 0.03 with a slope of 4.4 ± 1.2 and an intercept of 9.5 ± 13.3 mmHg (table 7.1). This intercept is not significantly different from 0 (Student's t test). The slope of the regression line equals $1 + R_c/R$ and therefore can be considered to be a measure of the extent of collateral circulation. The resistance of the collateral circulation as a percentage of the resistance of the myocardial bed can be calculated directly from this slope.

From the data presented in figure 7.3, it is also possible to prove the pressure independency of fractional collateral blood flow on arterial pressure. That relation is presented in figure 7.4.

Table 7.1 *Mean arterial blood pressure in the five experiments without medication, during infusion of phenylephrine and nitroprusside, respectively, as well as individual correlation coefficients, slope, and intercepts of regression lines of relations investigated in this study.*

Experiment	P_a (mmHg)			FFR$_{cor}$ vs Q_s/Q_s^N			FFR$_{myo}$ vs Q_s/Q_s^N			$(P_a{-}P_v)$vs $(P_w{-}P_v)$		
	0	Ph	N	r	sl	int	r	sl	int	r	sl	int
1	77	97	59	0.99	0.95	0.05	0.98	0.68	0.31	0.99	3.0	14.9
2	72	115	40	0.97	0.97	0.00	0.95	0.71	0.25	0.98	4.9	13.8
3	67	98	50	0.99	0.94	0.05	0.99	0.64	0.36	0.98	3.5	-9.8
4	92	131	55	0.99	0.97	0.02	0.98	0.78	0.22	0.99	4.5	25.5
5	110	125	77	0.98	1.05	-0.01	0.99	0.84	0.18	0.92	6.0	3.1

P_a *mean arterial blood pressure; 0, no medication; Ph, infusion of phenylephrine; N, nitroprusside; sl, slope; int, intercept; P_v, venous pressure; P_w, coronary wedge pressure; FFR$_{cor}$, coronary fractional flow reserve calculated from pressure measurements; FFR$_{myo}$, myocardial fractional flow reserve calculated from pressure measurements; Q_s , blood flow through the coronary artery at maximum vasodilation in the presence of a stenosis, Q_s^N, blood flow through the coronary artery at maximum vasodilation in the absence of a stenosis. The ratios Q_s/Q_s^N were measured directly by perivascular Doppler.*

7.3.2   Calculated versus measured FFR and contribution of of collateral flow to total flow.

FFR$_{cor}$ as directly measured by the Doppler transducer (Q_s/Q^N) was compared with FFR$_{cor}$ as calculated from pressure measurements by $(P_d - P_w)/(P_a - P_w)$ at maximum hyperemia according to equation 2. This relation is shown in figure 7.5, with excellent correlation in all dogs and a correlation coefficient of 0.98 ± 0.01, a slope of 0.98 ± 0.04, and an intercept of almost 0 (0.02 ± 0.03; table 7.1). If these data of all dogs and all pressure levels are combined, the correlation coefficient is 0.98, the slope 0.97, and the intercept is 0.03. These data validate the basic, essential equation 2 and prove the correctness of this part of the theoretical model experimentally.

The major goal of this study was to validate the basic concepts expressed in equations 1 and 2 using multiple Doppler and pressure measurements over a wide range of flows and pressures as shown in figures 7.3, 7.4, and 7.5.

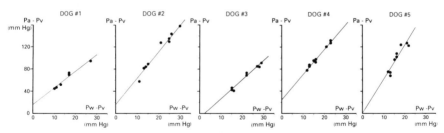

Figure 7.3 *Plots of relation between (P_a - P_v) and (P_w -P_v) in the five dogs. The solid line indicates the least squares best fit of the data. P_a , mean aortic pressure; P_v , central venous pressure; P_w , coronary wedge pressure. The slope of the regression line is inversely proportional to maximum recruitable collateral blood flow.*

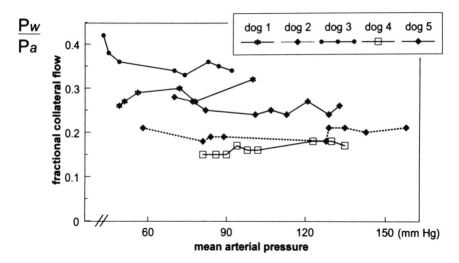

Figure 7.4 *Fractional collateral blood flow, represented by the ratio (P_w-P_v)/P_a-P_v), as a function of mean arterial blood pressure. It can be observed how this index of collateral flow is almost independent of arterial perfusion pressure over a large range. If the $P_w.P_a$ index is taken, almost similar plots are obtained.*

We did not use radiolabeled microspheres for myocardial perfusion because large numbers of flow measurements cannot be made with that technique. Consequently, we could not validate directly the prediction of FFR$_{myo}$ from pressure measurements (i.e. equation 3). However, we obtained indirect support for the validity of equation 3 by comparing FFR$_{myo}$ predicted from pressure measurements by the expression (P_d - P_v)/(P_a - P_v) according to

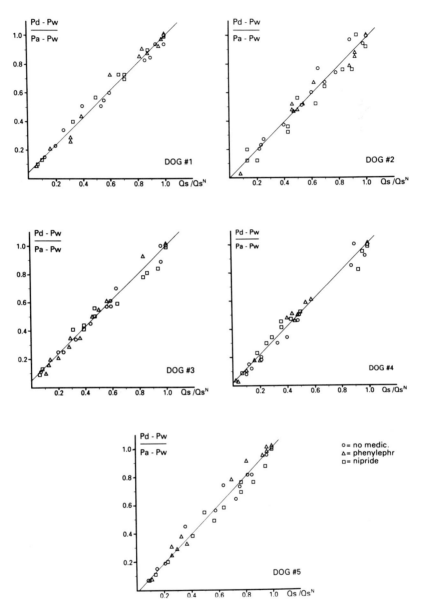

Figure 7.5 *Plots of relation between* $(P_d - P_w)/(P_a - P_w)$ *(pressure-derived* FFR_{cor}*), and* Q_s/Q_s^N *(directly measured* FFR_{cor}*) at different arterial pressures and different stenoses in the five experiments.* P_a, *mean aortic pressure;* P_d, *hyperemix coronary pressure distal to the stenosis;* P_v, *central venous pressure;* P_w, *coronary wedge pressure.*

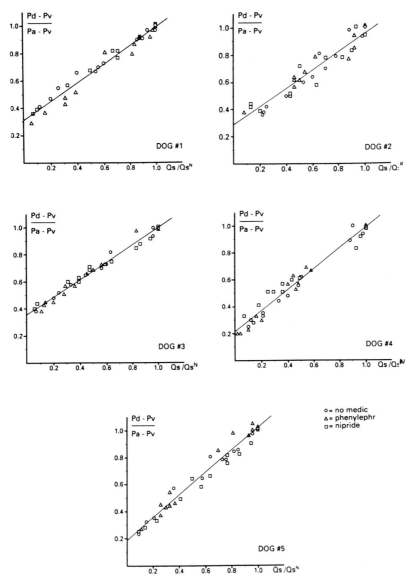

Figure 7.6 *Plots of relation between $(P_d - P_v)/(P_a - P_v)$ (pressure-derived FFR_{myo}), and Q_s/Q_s^N (directly measured FFR_{cor}) at different arterial pressures and different stenoses in the five experiments. At increasing stenosis severity, corresponding with decreasing maximum blood flow through the supplying epicardial artery, $(P_d - P_v)/(P_a - P_v)$ progressively exceeds Q_s/Q_s^N (or: FFR_{myo} progressively exceeds FFR_{cor}), indicating an increasing contribution of collateral blood flow to myocardial blood flow. The intercept of the regression line with the y-axis represents the collateral flow achievable at total occlusion and expressed as a fraction of normal maximum myocardial flow. Abbreviations as in figure 7.5.*

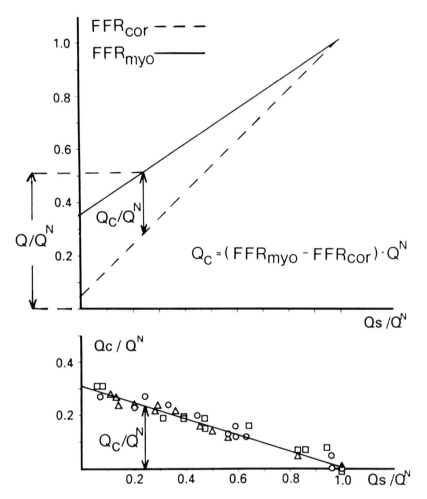

Figure 7.7 *Diagram from one of the experiments, illustrating how at every arbitrary degree of stenosis the contribution of coronary (Q_s) and collateral blood flow (Q_c) to myocardial blood flow (Q) can be estimated from the regression lines of FFR_{cor} (fractional coronary artery flow reserve) and FFR_{myo} (fractional myocardial flow reserve) (top panel). Pressure-derived collateral blood flow is presented in the bottom panel. In the absence of a stenosis, $Q_s = Q$, whereas $Q_c = 0$. At total occlusion, $Q_s = 0$ and $Q_c = Q$. In the bottom panel, the intercept of the regression line with the y-axis represents the collateral flow achievable at total occlusion, expressed as a fraction of normal myocardial flow (Q^N).*

equation 3, with Q_s/Q^N measured directly by Doppler. This relation is shown in figure 7.6. For mild or no stenosis, Q_s/Q^N is equal to the calculated value $(P_d - P_v)/(P_a - P_v)$ because collateral flow is negligible in that case. With more severe stenoses, FFR_{myo} and FFR_{cor} are both reduced, and $(P_d - P_v)/(P_a - P_v)$, representing calculated FFR_{myo}, is related to but larger than measured FFR_{cor} to the extent that collateral flow contributes to myocardial perfusion. As shown in figure 7.6, a good correlation is present between Q_s/Q^N, measured by Doppler, and $(P_d - P_v)/(P_a - P_v)$, representing FFR_{myo} from pressure measurements (r = 0.98 ± 0.02, slope = 0.73 ± 0.08, intercept = 0.26 ± 0.07). With total occlusion, Q_s/Q_s^N is 0, and the y intercept theoretically indicates the relative contribution of collateral flow to the myocardium, achievable during total occlusion. In figure 7.6, this intercept ranges from 0.18 to 0.36, indicating that collateral flow achievable during coronary artery occlusion under conditions of maximum vasodilation was 18 - 36% of normal maximum perfusion in the absence of a stenosis (table 7.1).

Finally, at every degree of stenosis corresponding to a certain level of diminished maximum blood flow through the epicardial artery, the contribution of collateral flow can be determined from the regression lines of FFR_{myo} and FFR_{cor} or calculated by equation 4. For one of the dogs, this estimation of collateral flow is illustrated in figure 7.7.

7.4 Discussion.

7.4.1 Advantages of fractional flow reserve.

In our model of a stenotic arterial system at maximum arteriolar vasodilation, the flow expressed as a fraction of normal maximum flow in the absence of a stenosis can be calculated from measurements of the relevant pressures, provided that vascular resistances are constant as is the case theoretically at maximum vasodilation. These calculated values of FFR correspond closely to those directly measured by an epicardial Doppler velocity meter, thereby confirming the validity of the concept that pressures alone under conditions of maximum vasodilation are related to maximum flow.

The basis for coronary flow reserve or maximum flow as a measure of stenosis severity has been well established[1-5,12,17]. Since the introduction of the concept of (absolute) coronary flow reserve (CFR), this index has been considered the standard for the functional status of a coronary artery for many years[22]. In clinical practice, however, measuring absolute coronary flow reserve has limited applications largely due to methodological limitations[1,16,23-26]. In the first place, CFR is strongly dependent on changes in blood pressure, heart rate and contractility. In addition, because coronary flow reserve is defined as a ratio, diminished coronary flow reserve can reflect decreased maximum flow, increased resting flow, or both. Because all methods proposed for absolute coronary flow reserve determination in humans, except positron emission tomography, require invasive manipulations or intracoronary contrast injections, true resting conditions in clinical situations are difficult to obtain, which increases the variability of absolute CFR. Furthermore, several physiological and pathological conditions unrelated to the stenosis itself, including microvascular disease, may result in altered absolute coronary flow reserve for a given fixed stenosis[1-4,25,26].

In contrast to absolute coronary flow reserve, determining maximum flow in a stenotic coronary artery as a fraction of normal maximum flow without a stenosis avoids the problem of variability in resting flow and is independent of loading conditions. Therefore, it is a complementary, independent measure of stenosis severity. Determining FFR from pressure measurements alone has the additional advantage of being applicable to three-vessel disease because, as shown in this experimental study, pressure measurements are made only in the stenotic artery, not in comparison to adjacent normal coronary arteries. In contrast to assessment of relative flow reserve by imaging techniques, no adjacent normally perfused reference distribution is necessary in the present approach. Finally, FFR from pressure measurements in theory incorporates effects of collateral flow through its effects on P_w. The influence of other physiological phenomena, such as compression and zero flow pressure, are all accounted for through their effects on measured P_d and P_w. Thus, assessing impairment of maximum flow or, in case of PTCA, assessing increase in maximum flow after the intervention, is a straightforward way of evaluating the functional significance of a stenosis or the improvement by PTCA. In chapter 11, an excellent correlation between increase of fractional flow reserve after PTCA and improved exercise test results will be demonstrated emphasizing the value of maximum flow as a clinically relevant endpoint.

7.4.2   From coronary pressure to coronary flow.

For assessing the functional significance of coronary artery disease by pressure measurements, most previous studies have measured transstenotic pressure gradient or this gradient in relation to arterial pressure[1,9-11,15,27].

Equations 1 to 4, indicate that measuring gradients only is an incomplete approach. Our model and results show that with increasing severity of stenosis, the contribution of collateral flow increases considerably, even in dogs studied acutely. Corresponding FFR of the coronary artery is overestimated when based on equation 3 instead of equation 2. Thus, coronary FFR should be calculated using equation 2 rather than equation 3, as initially proposed by Gould et al[1,5] but incomplete in failing to account for collateral flow. Myocardial FFR, on the other hand, can be correctly addressed by equation 3.

In the present study, the separate contributions of flow through the supplying coronary artery and collateral flow to myocardial blood flow can be quantified differentially. According to our calculations, the maximum recruitable collateral flow, as encountered during coronary artery occlusion, ranged from 18% to 36% of normal maximum myocardial blood flow. These data are compatible with a former study by Schaper in chronic instrumented dogs[28]. In that study, maximum collateral flow was approximately 30% of maximum myocardial blood flow.

Our model also shows that reduction of a transstenotic pressure gradient (e.g., from 40 to 10 mmHg) by PTCA does not carry the same meaning in different patients, even when arterial pressure is identical in both patients, The extent of collateral flow represents a significant associated variable, where the effects of collaterals are not represented exclusively by P_w at coronary occlusion but also significantly depend on simultaneously measured P_a and P_v. equation 1 states that maximum recruitable collateral blood flow at total occlusion of the coronary artery, expressed as a fraction of normal maximum myocardial blood flow, is given by:

$$Q_c/Q^N = (P_w - P_v)/(P_a - P_v).$$

Therefore, according to our theory, $P_w = 20$ mmHg in an individual with $P_a = 90$ mmHg and $P_v = 10$ mmHg indicates a collateral contribution of only 12.5% of maximum myocardial perfusion, whereas the same P_w in another individual with a simultaneously measured $P_a = 70$ mmHg and $P_v = 0$ mmHg, results in a collateral contribution of 29% of maximum myocardial perfusion. This example illustrates why P_w alone does not reliably reflect the extent of collateral circulation, as assumed in previous studies[8,13].

7.4.3 Limitations of the model.

Our model applies only to maximally dilated conditions when all resistances are constant and the derivation of flow reserve from pressure is possible. In this study, maximum arteriolar vasodilation and the resulting constant resistances were achieved by intracoronary administration of papaverine.

Papaverine has been shown to induce maximum coronary and myocardial hyperemia within 30 seconds after intracoronary administration. The duration of maximum vasodilation, approximately 30 seconds, is long enough to permit reliable pressure measurements after which the effect completely vanishes within minutes so that repeated measurements may be made[19,21]. Although polymorphic ventricular tachycardia associated with prolongation of the QT interval has been described in humans[29], in our experience with more than 1000 cases, serious dysrhythmias occurred in only 3 patients. Also other pharmacological stimuli such as intravenous or intracoronary adenosine may be used[20]. However, the peak hyperemia after an intracoronary bolus of adenosine in a recommended dose of 20-40 µg is quite short (often less than 5 seconds), and no steady-state distal coronary pressure may be reached, whereas, because the drug is administered through the coronary catheter, the arterial pressure signal has to be interrupted. More recently, it has also been shown by Kern et al and Van der Voort et al, that i.v. adenosine at a rate of 140 mg/kg/min., is an excellent and safe alternative to induce beautiful steady-state maximum coronary hyperemia. Also intravenous ATP has been documented by Japanese investigators to induce maximum hyperemia. The different ways to induce maximum hyperemia, are extensively discussed in chapter 5.

In the present study, flow ratios were assessed by a Doppler velocity meter, which could have been influenced by changes in luminal diameter of the coronary artery associated with the arteriolar vasodilation. However, as shown by Wilson and White[21] in a previous study, no significant changes in epicardial luminal diameter occur after intracoronary papaverine injection. Therefore, it is assumed that ratios of flow were accurately represented by ratios of flow velocity measured epicardially.

A prerequisite for correct pressure measurements is a sufficiently small catheter or guide wire that has a negligible effect on the transstenotic pressure gradient. Standard PTCA catheters do not meet this criterion, and severe overestimation of ΔP may have occurred in former studies. In earlier studies, we demonstrated that for a wide range of stenosis severity, ΔP decreased significantly if pressure was measured by a small pressure-monitoring guide wire with a cross-sectional area of only 0.11 mm^2 compared with measurements by a standard balloon catheter with a cross-sectional area of 0.72 - 1.0 mm^2. The device used for measuring distal coronary pressure in this study was of comparable small size and occupies only 25% of the area of a 90% area stenosis in a moderate-sized coronary artery with a diameter of 2.5 mm. It consisted of a main proximal part with a length of 75 cm and diameter of 0.71 mm (0.028 in.) connected to the distal

15 cm of a hollow pressure-monitoring guide wire with a diameter of 0.38 mm (0.015 in.) Only the distal part of this device - the guide wire - entered the coronary artery. The guide wire-tipped device was a prototype to test our concept. In the mean time, several much better pressure-monitoring wires have been developed, as described in paragraph 5.2.

Our model was not intended to address or separately account for a number of phenomena affecting pressure and flow, such as extravascular compression and critical closing presssure, because the model deals with flow and pressure as endpoints affected by net accumulation of these phenomena lumped together[30-35]. Our results give only some indirect support to former observations that in maximally vasodilated beds, critical closing pressure exceeds coronary venous pressure by only a few millimeters Hg[32]. A unique observation, supporting that position in a living human, was made unintendedly in the patient shown in figure 4.2. To whatever extent these factors affect pressure and flow, they are accounted for through the pressure measurements at maximal vasodilation.

The capacitance characteristics of the coronary vascular bed may affect its instantaneous, phasic pressure flow patterns[36,37]. In this study, however, the end points measured are mean pressures at steady-state maximum flow or at steady-state levels after coronary occlusion. Therefore, because capacitance effects cancel out over diastole and systole, mean pressure measurements theoretically are not affected. Furthermore, because pressures at coronary occlusion were measured only after reaching a steady state, venous capacitance effects are also avoided in our study. Consequently, we believe that potential effects of capacitance are not germane and do not have to be accounted for in our model or in its potential clinical applications.

Our model assumes that maximum recruitable flow in collaterals remains constant throughout the procedure of a number of brief total occlusions for measuring P_w. The literature indicates different and sometimes longer time constants for opening collateral channels compared with our measurement period[27,38-43] subject to further experimental validation. The excellent correlation between pressure-derived FFR and directly measured FFR provide strong indirect evidence for the correctness of our equations in measuring collateral flow. However, further confirmation of the details of our model for collateral flow is warranted and requires a different animal model in which arterial flow and separate collateral and myocardial perfusion are measured by radiolabeled microspheres. Because large numbers of flow measurements could not been made with that technique, we used the simpler animal model described here to compare FFR calculated from pressure measurements to direct measurements of maximum coronary flow, thereby validating the essential concept and the most complex equation 2 directly.

Our results raise some conceptual questions that need further investigations in carefully controlled animal and human studies. Strictly speaking, we have validated the model in figure 4.7 by experimental one-vessel disease with collateral flow that enters at the pre-arteriolar level. Theoretically our equations are also true with repetitive units of the model in figure 4.7. This is further clarified and validated both experimentally and clinically in chapter 13.

Assessment of relative flow reserve by imaging techniques becomes problematic in diffuse or balanced three-vessel disease where relative flow reserve may erroneously appear normal despite extensive coronary artery disease[1]. Pressure, however, is a universal measure of the function of the coronary vascular system for different sizes or regional coronary vascular beds with and without coronary artery disease. Therefore, our approach predicts FFR accurately even in the presence of balanced three-vessel disease.

Another important qualification is necessary in the presence of small vessel disease distal to the location where P_d and P_w are measured, as occurs in diabetes. In that case, equations 2 and 3 represent maximum flow in the presence of an epicardial stenosis, expressed as a fraction of maximum flow in the absence of that epicardial stenosis, but still not normal because of the distal small vessel disease. The value of this method for clinical decision making with respect to the need of a coronary intervention or assessing the increase of maximum flow by PTCA would not be affected by that limitation as already extensively discussed in paragraph 4.6.1.

A final issue that should be addressed in this context is coronary steal, a clearly recognized, well-documented phenomenon occurring in a number of patients with collateral circulation during maximum vasodilation[44,45]. In our opinion, however, this phenomenon is already accounted for in our model because any decrease in Q_c caused by increased conductance of the artery supplying the collaterals, is reflected by a lower coronary wedge pressure (P_w). Coronary steal is further discussed in paragraph 4.6.3.

7.4.4 Clinical implications.

The methods used in this animal study are applicable in humans both at diagnostic catheterization (FFR_{myo}) and at PTCA (all indexes), provided that a pressure-monitoring guide wire is used with a small size similar to that of the distal part of our device. No simplifications, adaptations, or additional hypotheses are necessary. The guide wire should be positioned across the stenosis as usual and after administration of a maximum vasodilatory stimulus, P_a and P_d can be measured by the guiding catheter and the pressure-wire, respectively. FFR_{myo} is known then and a decision to perform or avoid an intervention, can be made. If PTCA is indicated, during balloon inflation, P_a and P_w are recorded again. After the last balloon inflation, when the balloon has been pulled back but the guide wire remains distal of the dilated lesion, P_a and P_d are measured again after administration of an hyperemic stimulus. P_v can be measured directly with a Swan-Ganz catheter or estimated from the neck veins. If venous pressure is not elevated and one is only interested in increase of maximum coronary or myocardial blood flow after the PTCA (which is most important from the point of view of the interventional cardiologist), the venous pressure may be neglected because its influence on equation 2 or 3 is minimal in that case. The complete pressure-measuring sequence can be implemented during routine PTCA with prolongation of the procedure by only a few minutes. Other than a pressure-monitoring guide wire, no special equipment is needed. No special instructions to the patient or extra contrast injections or other manipulations are necessary. Therefore, coronary and myocardial FFR of the instrumented artery and its dependent myocardium as well as the contribution of collateral flow are readily obtainable before and after the intervention.

Despite its importance for understanding coronary artery disease[46-51], a clinically feasible method for quantitative assessment of collateral blood flow was not described before this animal study was performed. This study has provided the theory and experimental basis for a potential clinical method for assessing FFR and collateral flow during PTCA, which will be further worked out in chapter 16 and which has also been the basis for further studies by other groups, although the index was named differently[52].

Thus, this experimental study validates the accuracy of the pressure-flow model and corresponding equations as presented in chapter 4, and provides a firm experimental basis of the concept of fractional flow reserve. Validation in conscious humans will be presented in the next chapter.

References.

1. Gould KL, Kirkeeide RL, Buchi M: Coronary flow reserve as a physiologic measure of stenosis severity. *J Am Coll Cardiol* 1990; 15: 459-474.
2. Gould KL: Functional measures of coronary stenosis severity at cardiac catheterization. *J Am Coll Cardiol* 1990; 16: 198-199.
3. Kirkeeide RL, Gould KL, Parsel L: Assessment of coronary stenoses by myocardial perfusion imaging during pharmacologic coronary vasodilation: VIII. Validation of coronary flow reserve as a single integrated functional measure of stenosis severity reflecting all its geometric dimensions. *J Am Coll Cardiol* 1986; 7: 103-113.

4. Gould KL: Identifying and measuring severity of coronary artery stenosis: Quantitative coronary arteriography and positron emission tomography. *Circulation* 1988; 78: 237-245.
5. Gould KL: *Coronary Artery Stenosis*. New York, Elsevier, 1990, pp 79-91.
6. Gould KL, Kelley KO: Experimental validation of quantitative coronary arteriography for determining pressure-flow characteristics of coronary stenoses. *Circulation* 1982; 66: 930-937.
7. De Bruyne B, Pijls NHJ, Paulus WJ, Vantrimpont PJV, Stockbroeckx J, DeMoor D, Nelis O, Heyndrickx JR: In vitro and in vivo evaluation of a new 0.015" fluid-filled guide wire for distal pressure monitoring during PTCA. *J Am Coll Cardiol* 1993; 22: 119-126.
8. Meier B, Luethy P, Finci L, Steffenino L, Rutishauser W: Coronary wedge pressure in relation to spontaneously visible and recruitable collaterals. *Circulation* 1987; 75: 906-913.
9. Rothman MT, Baim DS, Simpson JB, Harrison DC: Coronary hemodynamics during PTCA. *Am J Cardiol* 1982; 49: 1615-1622.
10. Choksi SK, Meyers S, Abi-Mansour P: Percutaneous transluminal coronary angioplasty: Ten years' experience. *Prog Cardiovasc Dis* 1987; 30: 147-210.
11. MacIsaac HC, Knudtson ML, Robinson VJ, Manyari DE: Is the residual translesional pressure gradient useful to predict regional myocardial perfusion after percutaneous transluminal coronary angioplasty ? *Am Heart J* 1989; 117: 783-790.
12. Pijls NHJ, Aengevaeren WRM, Uijen GJH, Hoevelaken A, Pijnenburg T, Van Leeuwen K, Van der Werf T: The concept of maximal flow ratio for immediate evaluation of percutaneous transluminal coronary angiography result by videodensitometry. *Circulation* 1991; 83: 854-865.
13. De Bruyne B, Meier B, Finci L, Urban P, Rutishauser W: Potential protective effect of high coronary wedge pressure on left ventricular function after coronary occlusion. *Circulation* 1988; 78: 566-572.
14. Anderson HV, Roubin GS, Leimgruber PP, Cox WR, Douglas JS, King SB, Gruentzig AR: Measurement of transstenotic pressure gradient during percutaneous transluminal coronary angioplasty. *Circulation* 1986; 73: 1223-1230.
15. Kimball BP, Dafopoulos N, Lipreti V: Comparative evaluation of coronary stenoses using fluid dynamic equations and standard quantitative coronary arteriography. *Am J Cardiol* 1989; 64: 6-10.
16. Nissen SE, Gurley JC: Assessment of the functional significance of coronary stenoses: Is digital angiography the answer ? *Circulation* 1990; 81: 1431-1435.
17. Pijls NHJ, Uijen GJH, Hoevelaken A, Arts T, Aengevaeren WRM, Bos HS, Fast JH, Van Leeuwen KL, Van der Werf T: Mean transit time for the assessment of myocardial perfusion by videodensitometry. *Circulation* 1990; 81: 1331-1340.
18. Wilson RF, Laughlin DE, Ackell PH, Chilian WM, Holida MD, Hartley CJ, Armstrong ML, Marcus ML, White CW: Transluminal subselective measurement of coronary artery blood flow velocity and vasodilator reserve in man. *Circulation* 1985; 72: 82-92.
19. Zijlstra F, Serruys PW, Hugenholtz PG: Papaverine: The ideal coronary vasodilator for investigating coronary flow reserve ? A study of timing, magnitude, reproducibility and safety of the coronary hyperemic response after intracoronary papaverine. *Cathet Cardiovasc Diagn* 1986; 12: 298-299.
20. Wilson RF, Wyche K, Christensen BV, Zimmer S, Laxson DD: Effects of adenosine on human coronary arterial circulation. *Circulation* 1990; 82: 1595-1606.
21. Wilson RF, White CW: Intracoronary papaverine: an ideal coronary vasodilator for studies of the coronary circulation in conscious humans. *Circulation* 1986; 73: 444-451.

22. Gould KL, Lipscomb K, Hamilton GW: Physiologic basis for assessing critical coronary stenosis: Instantaneous flow response and regional distribution during coronary hyperemia as measures of coronary flow reserve. *Am J Cardiol* 1974; 33: 87-94.

23. Klocke FJ: Measurements of coronary flow reserve: Defining pathophysiology versus making decisions about patient care. *Circulation* 1987; 76: 1183-1189.

24. White CW, Wright CB, Doty DB, Hiratza LF, Eastham CL, Harrison DG, Marcus ML: Does visual interpretation of the coronary arteriogram predict the physiological importance of a coronary stenosis ? *N Engl J Med* 1984; 310: 819-824.

25. Hoffman JIE: Maximal coronary flow and the concept of coronary vascular reserve. *Circulation* 1984; 70: 153-159.

26. Klein LW, Agarwal JB, Schneider RM, Hermann G, Weintraub WS, Helfant RH: Effects of previous myocardial infarction on measurements of reactive hyperemia and the coronary vascular reserve. *J Am Coll Cardiol* 1986; 8: 357-363.

27. Rentrop KP, Thornton JC, Feit F, Van Buskirk M: Determinants and protective potential of coronary arterial collaterals as assessed by an angioplasty model. *Am J Cardiol* 1988; 61: 667-684.

28. Schaper W: Influence of physical exercise on coronary collateral blood flow in chronic experimental two-vessel occlusion. *Circulation* 1982; 65: 905- 912.

29. Wilson RF, White CW: Serious ventricular dysrhytmias after intracoronary papaverine. *Am J Cardiol* 1988; 62: 1301-1302.

30. Ellis AK, Klocke FJ: Effects of preload on the transmural distribution of perfusion and pressure flow relationships in the canine coronary vascular bed. *Circ Res* 1979; 46: 68-77.

31. Marcus ML: Autoregulation in the coronary circulation, in Marcus ML(ed): *The Coronary Circulation in Health and Disease*. New York, McGraw-Hill, 1983, pp 102-107.

32. Pantely GA, Ladley HD, Bristow JD: Low zero-flow pressure and minimal capacitance effect on diastolic arterial pressure-flow relationships during maximum vasodilation in swine. *Circulation* 1984; 70: 485-494.

33. Dole WP, Alexander GM, Campbell AB, Hixson EL, Bishop VS: Interpretation and physiological significance of diastolic coronary artery pressure-flow relationships in the canine coronary bed. *Circ Res* 1984; 55: 215-226.

34. Klocke FJ, Mates RE, Canty JM, Ellis AK: Coronary pressure-flow relationships: Controversial issues and probable implications. *Circ Res* 1985; 56: 310-323.

35. Klocke FJ, Ellis AK, Canty JM: Interpretation of changes in coronary flow that accompany pharmacologic interventions. *Circulation* 1987; 75 (suppl V): V-34-V-38.

36. Marcus ML: Coronary anatomy, in Marcus ML (ed): *The Coronary Circulation in Health and Disease*. New York, McGraw-Hill, 1983, pp 4-5.

37. Spaan JAE, Breuls NPW, Laird JD: Diastolic-systolic coronary flow differences are caused by intramyocardial pump action in the anesthetized dog. *Circ Res* 1981; 49: 584-593.

38. Pupita G, Maseri A, Kaski JC, Galassi AR, Gavrielides S, Davies G, Crea F: Myocardial ischemia caused by distal coronary artery constriction in stable angina pectoris. *N Engl J Med* 1990; 323: 514-520.

39. Fujia M, McKown DP, McKown MD, Hartley JW, Franklin D: Evaluation of coronary collateral development by regional myocardial function and reactive hyperemia. *Cardiovasc Res* 1987; 21: 377-384.

40. Yamamoto H, Tomoike H, Shimokawa H, Nabeyama S, Nakamura M: Development of collateral function with repetitive coronary occlusion in a canine model reduces myocardial reactive hyperemia in the absence of significant coronary stenosis. *Circ Res* 1984; 55: 623-632.

41. Yamanishi K, Fujita M, Ohno A, Sasayama S: Importance of myocardial ischemia for recruitment of coronary collateral circulation in dogs. *Cardiovasc Res* 1990; 24: 271-277.

42. Mohri M, Tomoike H, Noma M, Inoue T, Hisano K, Nakamura M: Duration of ischemia is vital for collateral development: Repeated brief coronary artery occlusions in conscious dogs. *Circ Res* 1989; 64: 287-296.

43. Sasayama S, Fujita M : Recent insights into coronary collateral circulation. *Circulation* 1992; 85: 1197-1204.

44. Gould KL: Coronary steal: Is it clinically important ? *Chest* 1989; 96: 227-229.

45. Demer LL, Gould KL, Goldstein RA, Kirkeeide RL: Noninvasive assessment of coronary collaterals in man by PET perfusion imaging. *J Nucl Med* 1990; 31: 259-270.

46. Gensini GG, DaCosta BCB: The coronary collateral circulation in living man. *Am J Cardiol* 1969; 24: 393-400.

47. Schaper W: The role of the collateral circulation in human ischemic heart isease, in Black DAK (ed): *The Collateral Circulation of the Heart.* New York, Elsevier, 1971, pp 261-269.

48. Patterson RE, Jones-Collins BA, Aamodt R, Ro Y: Differences in collateral myocardial blood following gradual vs abrupt coronary occlusion. *Cardiovasc Res* 1983; 17: 207-214.

49. Feldman RL, Pepine CJ : Evaluation of coronary collateral circulation in conscious humans. *Am J Cardiol* 1984; 53: 1233-1238.

50. Schaper W, Goerge G, Winkler B, Schaper J: The collateral circulation of the heart. *Prog Cardiovasc Dis* 1988; 31: 57-77.

51. Hirai T, Fujita M, Nakajima H, Asanoi H, Yamanishi K, Ohno A, Sasayama S: Importance of collateral circulation for prevention of left ventricular aneurysm formation in acute myocardial infarction. *Circulation* 1989; 79: 791-796.

52. Seiler C, Fleisch M, Garachamani A, Meier B. Coronary collateral quantitation in patients with coronary artery disease using intravascular flow velocity or pressure meaurements. *J Am Coll Cardiol* 1998; 32: 1272-1279.

Chapter 8

VALIDATION OF FRACTIONAL FLOW RESERVE IN HUMANS

During maximum vasodilation, which corresponds with minimal myocardial resistance, distal coronary pressure divided by aortic pressure equals maximum myocardial blood flow divided by the normally expected value as it would be if no epicardial lesion were present[1,2]. The theoretical background of the concept of fractional flow reserve and its experimental validation have been provided in the preceding chapters. So far, however, pressure-derived fractional flow reserve was validated in an open chest dog model against the ratio of epicardial hyperemic flow velocity in the presence of a stenosis to hyperemic flow velocity in the absence of a stenosis.

As coronary pressure measurements and pressure-derived fractional flow reserve calculations are methods intended to be applied in humans, it was also of crucial importance to determine first, whether fractional flow reserve indeed serves as an index of *myocardial* flow and second, whether this pressure-derived information reflects the effect of an epicardial lesion on myocardial flow better than coronary angiography which is currently the most widely available technique used to assess the severity of coronary artery disease. Therefore, a study was conducted to compare pressure-derived fractional flow reserve to relative myocardial flow reserve determined by positron emission tomography and to angiographic indexes in patients with an isolated stenosis in the proximal left anterior descending coronary artery.

8.1 Study design.

8.1.1 Study population.

The study population consisted of 22 patients (18 men; mean age 56 ± 8 years; range 36 to 78 years), admitted because of anginal chest pain due to an isolated, discrete lesion in the proximal- or mid - anterior descending coronary artery, without other lesions in the epicardial coronary arteries. All patients had a normal ECG and normal global and regional left ventricular systolic function on a biplane left ventricular angiogram. They were scheduled for an elective percutaneous transluminal coronary angioplasty (PTCA) because of significant ST-depression either during a bicycle stress test or during a spontaneous episode of angina pectoris. Patients were selected on the basis of the ideal suitability of their lesion for quantitative coronary angiography. All cardiac medications were stopped at least 48 hours before admission. Molsidomine 4 mg t.i.d. was started on the day of admission.

All patients underwent successively a positron emission tomographic study (PET) on day 1 and cardiac catheterization on day 2 with quantitative coronary angiography and intracoronary pressure measurements. On day 1, all patients also underwent bidimensional echocardiography at rest and during adenosine infusion (140 µg/kg/min) to test their tolerance to adenosine and to rule out left ventricular cavity dilatation and wall thinning which could lead to a erroneous sampling during PET studies.

8.1.2 Positron emission tomographic studies.

Preparation of radionuclides. ^{15}O-water was produced by irradiating natural oxygen with 28 MeV protons from the Cyclotron (Cyclone 30). ^{38}K was produced by the ^{40}Ar-^{38}K reaction on Argon gas. Irradiation was carried out with a 18 mA beam of 30 MeV protons.
Tomographic procedure. Myocardial perfusion images were obtained with an ECAT III (911/01 CTI Inc., Knoxville) one-ring device, the characteristics of which have been previously described[3]. Measurements were performed with a stationary ring, and images were reconstructed with an Hann filter giving an in-plane resolution of 8 mm full-width at half-maximum (FWHM). The collimator aperture was set at 30 mm, resulting in a slice thickness of 15 mm FWHM. Regular calibration of the tomography versus a well counter was performed by measuring a uniform cylindrical phantom (diameter, 20 cm) filled with a solution of ^{68}Ge. All patients were studied after overnight fasting. The patients were carefully positioned in the tomograph. Serial transmission scintigrams at different levels were obtained to select an adequate mid-ventricular cross-sectional plane and to allow for subsequent correction for photon attenuation. All transmission scintigrams were viewed before collection of emission data to verify proper positioning of the patient. The selected imaging plane corresponded to a mid-ventricular plane. Correct positioning was maintained throughout the study with the use of a light beam and indelible felt-pen marks on the patient's torso. Soon after transmission scintigrams were recorded, 15 mCi of H_2^{15}O was administered intravenously as a slow bolus over a 30-second period with an infusion pump (model 351, Sage Instruments). Thirty serial images were acquired during 180 seconds (15 during 2 seconds and 15 during 10 seconds). The use of water for quantifying myocardial blood flow necessitates the injection of another isotope because water is a freely diffusible tracer taken up by both the ventricular walls and the blood pool. Five minutes after the end of the H_2^{15}O acquisition, 5 to 8 mCi of ^{38}K ($T_{1/2}$: 462 seconds) was injected intravenously over a 20-second period with an infusion pump. Beginning with tracer injection, 35 serial images

were acquired in a decay-compensated mode for 20 minutes. The three last images of 240 s each were used to delineate the regions of interest which will be used for the $H_2^{15}O$ imaging processing. Thirty minutes after the end of the ^{38}K acquisition, adenosine was infused intravenously (140μg/kg/min). ECG, heart rate, and invasive brachial arterial pressure were recorded and digitized on-line. Then, the same sequence of tomographic acquisition as the one previously described was performed during arteriolar vasodilation: $H_2^{15}O$ injection and acquisition followed by ^{38}K injection and acquisition.

Analysis of tomographic data and calculation of myocardial perfusion. After random coincidence subtraction, normalization of sinograms, and correction for attenuation, the reconstructed images (256 x 256 pixels) were corrected for deadtime and isotope decay. Three large regions of interest representing 4 to 5 cm^3 each were drawn on the images of the ^{38}K study. These 3 regions were then copied on all $H_2^{15}O$ dynamic images to construct the corresponding tissue and blood pool time-activity curves. When copied, each region of interest was checked for appropriate location around the blood pool image and to correspond to the myocardial wall activity of the normalized subtraction image. Myocardial perfusion was calculated from $H_2^{15}O$ tomographic data by fitting arterial impute function and tissue time-activity curves to a single-tissue-compartment tracer kinetic model for $H_2^{15}O$ studies. The method has been validated in experimental animals by different groups[4-7].

Relative myocardial perfusion reserve [8] of the anterior segment was defined as the ratio of the maximum achievable absolute flow in the anterior region (depending on the stenotic left anterior descending coronary artery) to the maximum achievable absolute flow in the lateral region (depending on the normal left circumflex coronary artery). Because in this particular group of patients, the left circumflex coronary artery was normal, myocardial relative perfusion reserve defined in this way and assessed by PET, can be considered as equivalent to myocardial fractional flow reserve, defined as the ratio of maximum stenotic to normal maximum flow in the left anterior descending coronary artery dependent myocardium, as will be discussed extensively later.

8.1.3 Quantitative coronary angiography.

The stenosed coronary segment was quantitatively analyzed with the automated coronary analysis program (ACA), implemented on a biplane Optimus 200 radiographic equipment (Philips Medical systems BV, Best, The Netherlands). These algorithms have been described in detail elsewhere[9]. From these geometric data, percent diameter stenosis (DS), area stenosis (AS), minimal obstruction area, and stenosis flow reserve were averaged from at least two orthogonal or nearly orthogonal projections[10].

8.1.4 Pressure measurements.

Catheterization protocol. Central aortic pressure, femoral pressure and distal coronary pressure were recorded through an 7F guiding catheter, the side arm of a femoral introduction sheath, and a 0.015-in. fluid-filled pressure monitoring guide wire, respectively (a sensor-tipped pressure wire was not available yet at the time of this study). The details of this procedure have been described in chapter 5.

Central venous pressure was recorded through a high-fidelity manometer advanced into the right atrium. Maximum vasodilation was induced by a 4-minute intravenous infusion of adenosine (140μg/kg/min).

Calculation of fractional flow reserve and coronary resistance. Myocardial fractional flow reserve (FFR_{myo}) and coronary fractional flow reserve (FFR_{cor}) were calculated as explained in chapter 4 by:

$$FFR_{myo} = (P_d - P_v)/(P_a - P_v)$$

$$FFR_{cor} = (P_d - P_w)/(P_a - P_w)$$

where P_a is the mean aortic pressure, P_d is the mean distal coronary pressure, P_v is the mean right atrial pressure and P_w is the mean coronary wedge pressure during balloon coronary occlusion. An example is shown in figure 8.1. Myocardial vascular resistance in the stenotic territory (R_s) and the normal contra-lateral territory (R_n) were calculated as follows:

$$R_s = (P_d - P_v)/Q_s$$

$$R_n = (P_d - P_v)/Q_n$$

since, in the normal epicardial vessel $P_d = P_a$

$$R_n = (P_a - P_v)/Q_n$$

where Q_s is the myocardial flow in the stenotic area, and Q_n is the myocardial flow in the normal area.

8.2   Rationale for validating pressure-derived fractional flow reserve by PET measurements of relative flow reserve.

Myocardial fractional flow reserve is the ratio of maximum achievable flow in the stenotic myocardial region to the maximum achievable flow in that same region, in the hypothetical case where the epicardial vessel were normal. In contrast, the relative flow reserve is the maximum achievable flow in the stenotic myocardial area divided by the maximum achievable flow in a contra-lateral area dependent on a normal epicardial coronary artery. Figure 8.2

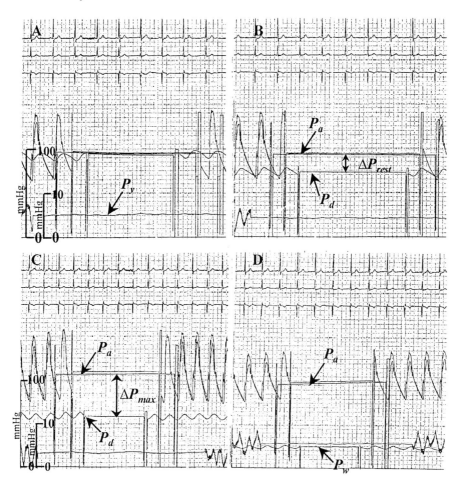

Figure 8.1 *Example of simultaneous pressure recordings in the femoral artery, the coronary ostium, the distal left anterior descending coronary artery and the right atrium. Panel A: The wire is advanced to the tip of the guiding catheter to verify the equality of the mean pressure signals. Panel B: The wire is advanced across the stenosis. At rest the mean translesional pressure gradient is 20 mmHg. Panel C: During adenosine-induced maximum hyperemia, transstenotic pressure gradient increases to 53 mmHg. Panel D: During balloon coronary occlusion the mean distal coronary pressure decreases to 22 mmHg. Mean right atrial pressure remains unchanged in the three conditions (3 to 5 mmHg). Myocardial fractional flow reserve equals 57-3/106-3 = 0.52; coronary fractional flow reserve equals 56-22/106-22 = 0.40. P_a = mean aortic pressure as measured by the guiding catheter at the coronary ostium; P_v = mean right atrial pressure; P_w = mean distal coronary pressure during balloon coronary occlusion; P_d = mean distal coronary pressure as measured by the pressure guide wire; ΔP_{rest} = transstenotic pressure gradient at rest; ΔP_{max} = transstenotic pressure gradient during maximum hyperemia.*

illustrates the rationale of comparing fractional and relative flow reserve in a model of isolated left anterior descending coronary artery stenosis. In that particular case indeed, both fractional and relative myocardial flow reserve should be identical.

Therefore, validation of the concept of myocardial fractional flow reserve against relative flow reserve as derived from PET is justified providing the four following conditions are fulfilled:

(1) The contralateral arteries (in this particular case the left circumflex and the right coronary arteries) should be devoid of any narrowing, which was confirmed by two experienced angiographers in the present study.

(2) The myocardial vascular resistance in the perfusion territory of the circumflex and the left anterior descending coronary artery should be identical during maximum vasodilation. As shown in figure 8.3, our results confirmed that myocardial resistance in the lateral and anterior myocardial segments decreased to a similar level during adenosine infusion although they were significantly different under baseline conditions.

(3) Relative flow reserve determination and fractional flow reserve calculations should be performed under similar hemodynamic conditions. Although both relative and fractional myocardial flow reserve have been shown to be independent of driving pressure, it seems reasonable in a validation study to perform both measurements under similar hemodynamic conditions[1,8]. The hemodynamic data during PET and catheterization are summarized in table 8.1. During PET, there was no significant difference between mean aortic pressure under baseline conditions and during adenosine induced maximum vasodilation. Similarly, at catheterization, no significant difference was noted between mean aortic pressure at rest and during adenosine infusion. More importantly, during maximum vasodilation, mean aortic pressure did not differ significantly during PET data acquisition and during catheterization. Adenosine infusion induced a significant increase in heart rate both during PET and during catheterization but to a similar degree.

(4) The method used as "gold standard" to assess myocardial perfusion should be highly reliable. The methodology of myocardial perfusion assessment by PET, used in our laboratory, has been validated in dogs against microspheres[7]. The correlation was found to be excellent (r = 0.97, systematic error = 26 ml /min/100g) with flow values ranging from 40 to 680 ml/min/100g.

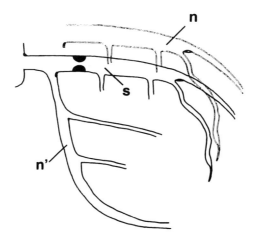

$$RFR = \frac{\textbf{MAX FLOWs}}{\textbf{MAX FLOWn'}}$$

$$FFR = \frac{\textbf{MAX FLOWs}}{\textbf{MAX FLOWn}}$$

In case of ISOLATED coronary artery stenosis

RFR = FFR

(per unit of tissue mass)

Figure 8.2 *Schematic drawing illustrating the rationale of comparing relative and fractional myocardial flow reserve in this particular group of patients. The relative flow reserve (RFR) is the ratio of hyperemic flow in the anterior region (depending on the stenotic left anterior descending coronary artery) to the hyperemic flow in the normal region (depending on the left circumflex coronary artery). The myocardial fractional flow reserve (FFR) is the ratio of hyperemic flow in the anterior region (dependent on the stenotic left anterior descending artery) to hyperemic flow in that same region in the hypothetical case of a normal left anterior descending artery (faint lines). In case of a similar decrease of myocardial resistance during hyperemia in the LAD and the LCX area, the value of both the relative and the fractional myocardial flow reserve should be identical.*
n = hypothetical normal left anterior descending coronary artery; n' = normal left circumflex coronary artery; s = stenotic left anterior descending coronary artery.

Table 8.1 *Hemodynamic data of patients during PET and during catheterization*

		Positron Emission Tomography	Catheterization
MAP	Rest	94 ± 14 mmHg	105 ± 18 mmHg
	Hyperemia	96 ± 13 mmHg	102 ± 13 mmHg
HR	Rest	63 ± 10 bpm	71 ± 13 bpm
	Hyperemia	87 ± 17 bpm	87 ± 15 bpm
RPP	Rest	5955 ± 1379 mmHg.bpm	7579 ± 2465 mmHg.bpm
	Hyperemia	8392 ± 2279 mmHg.bpm	8884 ± 2215 mmHg.bpm
RAP	Rest	NM	5 ± 1 mmHg
	Hyperemia	NM	5 ± 1 mmHg

Abbreviations; bpm: beats per minute; HR: heart rate; MAP: mean aortic pressure; NM: not measured; RAP: mean right atrial pressure; RPP: rate-pressure product. .

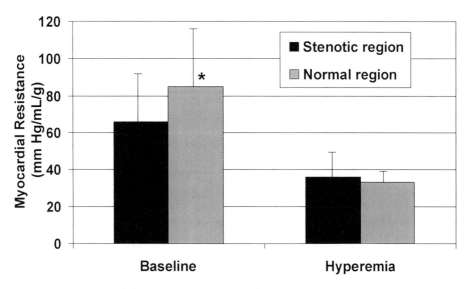

Figure 8.3 *Myocardial resistance at rest and during adenosine-induced hyperemia in the anterior (stenotic) region and in the lateral (normal) region.*

8.3 Feasibility of fractional flow reserve calculation.

All lesions could easily be crossed with the pressure monitoring guide wire and PTCA was performed without need for another guide wire so that this pressure monitoring guide wire adequately fulfilled its dual role as an coronary pressure measurement device and as part of the therapeutic angioplasty system. No complications related to manipulation of the wire were encountered. The additional time needed to perform the measurements is limited to a few minutes and could even be diminished by using a short acting vasodilatory drug as intracoronary papaverine or intracoronary adenosine instead of intravenous adenosine. In this particular study, intravenous adenosine was selected because no intracoronary drugs could be administered during PET. In this validation study, right atrial pressure was monitored invasively throughout the study. Mean right atrial pressure did not change during maximum vasodilation nor during balloon coronary occlusion (table 8.1). Hence, the value of mean right atrial pressure could be estimated clinically or set at an arbitrary value. This would further simplify the procedure since all data needed for fractional flow reserve calculations could be derived from routine coronary angioplasty measurements. Having excluded measurement of right atrial pressure would not have affected the results of this study.

8.4 Myocardial flow by PET versus pressure-derived indexes.

The accuracy of fractional flow reserve calculations from intracoronary pressure measurements as an index of the physiology of a coronary stenosis in humans is shown in figure 7.4. In these patients with an isolated lesion in the left anterior descending coronary artery, a close linear relationship was found between myocardial fractional flow reserve and relative myocardial perfusion reserve as derived from PET over a wide range of stenosis severity (FFR_{myo} ranging from 0.36 to 0.98, mean 0.61 ± 0.17). Theoretically, the presence of the pressure monitoring guide wire (0.015-in. or 0.38 mm) through severe lesions could induce an artifactual increase in transstenotic pressure gradient and hence, an underestimation of the actual myocardial fractional flow reserve. However, this is not supported by our data since no clear deviation from the line of identity was noted in the range of severe stenoses. In patients with normal left ventricular function and very tight coronary lesions, transstenotic pressure gradient depends more on the collateral flow than on the antegrade flow. Therefore, in these tight stenoses, the presence of the guide wire through the lesion will not induce a large overestimation of the actual pressure gradient since, even without guide wire, the pressure gradient is very large. A good correlation was also found between relative myocardial flow reserve by PET and coronary fractional flow reserve by pressure measurements (figure 8.4, right panel). However, the latter relation was best fitted by a quadratic equation showing a clear deviation from the line of identity in the range of severe stenosis. This can be explained as follows: the *myocardial* fractional flow reserve incorporates both the maximum antegrade flow (provided by the epicardial artery) and the maximum flow provided by the collateral circulation under conditions of arteriolar dilatation. In contrast, *coronary* fractional flow reserve only represents the maximum antegrade flow during maximum vasodilation. As a consequence, the difference between *myocardial* and *coronary* fractional flow reserve represents the maximum achievable collateral flow i.e. *collateral* fractional flow reserve. This explains

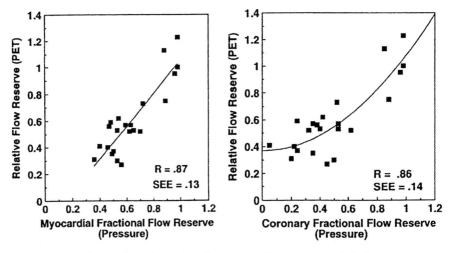

Figure 8.4 *Left panel: relationship between relative myocardial flow reserve as assessed by PET in the anterior region and myocardial fractional flow reserve as calculated from pressure measurements in the distal left anterior descending coronary artery. Right panel: relationship between the relative myocardial flow reserve of the anterior region as determined by PET and the coronary fractional flow reserve of the left anterior descending coronary artery.*

why the fit to the observed values of coronary fractional flow reserve plotted against relative flow reserve values diverged from the line of identity in the range of severe stenoses, when collateral circulation starts to play an increasing role. This issue has been discussed in more detail in paragraph 7.3.2 and is also demonstrated in figure 7.7.

8.5 Myocardial blood flow versus quantitative coronary angiography.

Minimal obstruction area ranged from 0.5 to 2.5 mm^2, diameter stenosis ranged from 22 to 77% (mean 55 ± 14%), area stenosis ranged from 40 to 94% (mean 77 ± 13%) and calculated stenosis flow reserve ranged from 1.03 to 4.6 (mean 2.9 ± 1.1). The correlation between relative flow reserve as derived from PET and angiographic indexes are shown in table 8.2.

Since the length of the lesion and the reference and stenotic diameters can be determined by quantitative coronary angiography, in theory, functional information can be derived from these anatomic data by applying the fluid dynamic equation[10,12,]. The link between the anatomic and functional approach

Table 8.2 *Correlation between relative flow reserve (y) as derived from PET and either pressure-derived indexes or data derived from quantitative coronary angiography (x)*

	Correlation Coefficient	SEE	Equation
Myocardial fractional flow reserve	0.87	0.13	$y=1.22x-0.17$
Coronary fractional flow reserve	0.86	0.14	$y=0.71x^2+0.37$
Resting transstenotic pressure gradient	-0.61	0.22	$y=0.98-0.14\log x$
Hyperemic transstenotic pressure gradient	-0.81	0.14	$y=1.02-0.021x$
Obstruction area	0.66	0.20	$y=0.40+0.14x$
Diameter stenosis	-0.68	0.20	$y=1.28-0.012x$
Area stenosis	-0.70	0.19	$y=1.65-0.014x$
Stenosis flow reserve	0.68	0.20	$y=0.16x+0.14$

has been clearly validated in an animal model instrumented with flow meters where a stenosis was created by external compression of a coronary artery or with precision drilled plastic cylinders placed to create intraluminal stenoses[10,12]. In these instrumented animals, percent area reduction correlated well with absolute and relative coronary flow reserve.

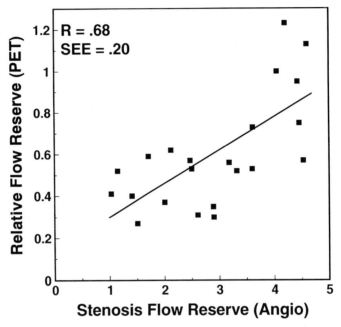

Figure 8.5 *Relationship between relative myocardial flow reserve of the anterior region as assessed by PET and stenosis flow reserve as derived from quantitative coronary angiography of the stenosis in the proximal left anterior descending coronary artery.*

Moreover, it was suggested that arteriographic stenosis flow reserve is a more specific functional measure of stenosis severity than direct measurement of absolute coronary flow reserve by a flow meter because the effects of physiologic variables other than stenosis severity are eliminated[8]. However, as shown in figure 8.5 and in table 8.2 the correlations between indexes derived from quantitative coronary angiography and relative flow reserve (PET) were markedly weaker than the correlation between relative flow reserve (PET) and fractional flow reserve even though the lesions had been selected for their optimal suitability for quantitative coronary angiography.

8.6 Conclusions.

The data presented in this chapter confirm in patients with coronary artery disease that myocardial fractional flow reserve as derived from the ratio of distal coronary pressure to aortic pressure during maximum arteriolar vasodilation corresponds indeed to the fraction of maximum myocardial blood flow preserved despite the presence of the epicardial stenosis and determined by positron emission tomography. Thus, the validity of the concept of myocardial fractional flow reserve was established in conscious humans in the catheterization laboratory. Moreover, the correspondence with PET is much better for FFR than for angiographic indexes and, therefore, pressure-derived fractional flow reserve is a better index of the functional severity of the epicardial lesion than quantitative coronary angiography. Evidence that also in more complex anatomic situations than single vessel disease, coronary and myocardial blood flow can be accurately assessed by coronary pressure measurement, will be provided in paragraph 13.4

References.

1. Pijls NHJ, van Son AM, Kirkeeide RL, De Bruyne B, Gould KL. Experimental basis of determining maximum coronary, myocardial, and collateral blood flow by pressure measurements for assessing functional stenosis severity before and after percutaneous transluminal coronary angioplasty. *Circulation* 1993;87:1354-1367.
2. De Bruyne B, Pijls NHJ, Paulus WJ, Vantrimpont PJ, Sys SU, Heyndrickx GR. Transstenotic coronary pressure gradient measurements in humans: in vitro and in vivo evaluation of a new pressure monitoring angioplasty guide wire. *J Am Coll Cardiol* 1993;22:119-126.
3. Hoffman EJ, Phelps ME, Huang SC, Collard PE, Bidaut LM, Schwab RL, Ricci AR. Dynamic, gated and high resolution imaging with the ECAT III. *IEEE Trans Nucl Sci* 1986;33:452-455.
4. Bergmann SR, Herrerro P, Markham J, Walsh MN: Non-invasive quantitation of myocardial blood flow in human subjects with oxygen-labeled water and positron emission tomography. *J Am Coll Cardiol* 1989;14:639-652.
5. Araujo L, Lammertsma A, Rhodes C, McFalls E, Iida H, Rechavia E, Galassi A, De Silva R, Jones T, Maseri A. Noninvasive quantification of regional myocardial blood flow in coronary artery disease with oxygen-15-labeled carbon dioxide inhalation and positron emission tomography. *Circulation* 1991;83:875-885.
6. Muzik O, Beanlands RSB, Hutchins GD, Mangner TJ, Nguyen N, Schwaiger M. Validation of Nitrogen-13-Ammonia tracer kinetic model for quantification of myocardial blood flow using PET. *J Nucl Med* 1993;34:83-91.

7.   Bol A, Melin LA, Vanoverschelde JL, Baudhuin T, Vogelaers D, De Pauw M, Michel C, Luxen A, Labar D, Cogneau M, Robert A, Heyndrickx GR, Wijns W. Direct comparison of [^{13}N]ammonia and [^{15}O]water estimates of perfusion with quantification of regional myocardial blood flow by microspheres. *Circulation* 1993;87:512-525.
8.   Gould KL, Kirkeeide RL, Buchi M. Coronary flow reserve as a physiological measure of stenosis severity. *J Am Coll Cardiol* 1990;15:459-474.
9.   Reiber JHC, Serruys PW, Kooijman CJ, Wijns W, Slager CJ, Gerbrands JJ, Schuurbiers JCH,   den Boer A, Hugenholtz PG. Assessment of short-, medium- and long-term variations in arterial dimensions from computer-assisted quantification of coronary cineangiograms. *Circulation* 1985;71:280-288.
10. Kirkeeide RL, Gould KL, Parsel L. Assessment of coronary stenosis by myocardial perfusion imaging during pharmacologic coronary vasodilation. VII. Validation of coronary flow reserve as a single integrated functional measure of stenosis severity reflecting all its geometric dimensions. *J Am Coll Cardiol* 1986;7:103-113.
11. De Bruyne B, Sys SU, Heyndrickx GR. Percutaneous transluminal coronary angioplasty catheters versus fluid-filled pressure monitoring guide wires for coronary pressure measurements and correlation with quantitative coronary angiography. *Am J Cardiol* 1993;72:1101-1106.
12. Mancini GBJ, Simon SB, McGillem MJ, LeFree MT, Friedman HZ, Vogel RA. Automated quantitative coronary angiography: morphologic and physiological validation in vivo of a rapid digital angiographic method. *Circulation* 1987;75:452-460.

Chapter 9

INDEPENDENCE OF FRACTIONAL FLOW RESERVE OF HEMODYNAMIC LOADING CONDITIONS

In addition to feasibility and clinical relevance, reproducibility (or absence of variability) is another crucial characteristic of any new diagnostic test. A measurement which is either difficult to obtain, of little clinical relevance, or highly variable, would be clinical nonsense.

The goal of this chapter is to compare the feasibility of distal coronary pressure measurements with other invasive functional indexes and to evaluate the influence of changes in heart rate, blood pressure, and contractility on the calculations of pressure-derived myocardial fractional flow reserve.

9.1   Study design.

The study population consisted of 13 patients scheduled for percutaneous transluminal coronary angioplasty of an isolated lesion in a major epicardial coronary artery (4 left anterior descending coronary arteries, 9 dominant right coronary arteries). Global left ventricular systolic function was normal at rest as assessed by biplane contrast angiography, and wall motion in the territory supplied by the vessel under study was normal. None of the patients had the following conditions that are known to affect resistive vessel function or baseline myocardial blood flow: diabetes mellitus, left ventricular hypertrophy, valvular heart disease as assessed by transthoracic echocardiography, anemia, or previous myocardial infarction.

Patients were brought to the catheterization laboratory in the fasting state. Cardiac medications were not discontinued. A 7.5F introducer sheath was inserted in the right femoral artery and a 7F guiding catheter without side holes was advanced up to the coronary ostium. A 6F bipolar pacemaker lead was advanced into the upper right atrium. After intravenous administration of 10 000 IU of heparin, 3 mg of isosorbide dinitrate was administered through the guiding catheter. This was repeated every 30 minutes during the study protocol to ensure maximum epicardial vasodilation. At least two minutes after nitrates administration, contrast angiograms of the vessel under study were taken in at least 4 different projections.

A 0.014-in Doppler guide wire (Cardiometrics Inc. Mountain View, CA) was advanced distally to the stenosis in a smooth coronary segment and the wire was manipulated until an optimal and stable Doppler flow velocity signal was obtained. The characteristics of this wire and the flow velocity measurements obtained with this system have been validated in vitro and in an animal model using simultaneous electromagnetic flow measurements for comparison[1]. To measure distal coronary pressure, a 0.014-in, fluid-filled pressure monitoring guide wire (Schneider Europe), was advanced distally to the stenosis. The side arm of the introducer sheath, the guiding catheter, and the fluid-filled pressure monitoring wire were connected to three separate pressure transducers (Spectranetics, Statham P23) zeroed at mid-chest level. Femoral pressure (side arm of the sheath), aortic pressure (guiding catheter), distal coronary pressure (pressure monitoring wire), and instantaneous peak flow velocity signal (Doppler guide wire) were recorded on a digital tape. All measurements were taken under resting conditions and during maximum vasodilation induced by an intracoronary bolus of adenosine (12 µg in the right coronary artery and 18 µg in the left coronary artery)[2]. Care was taken not to induce an impairment of flow during maximum hyperemia by the presence of the guiding catheter in the first millimeters of the coronary artery[3]. This can be detected by the occurrence of a pressure difference between the femoral artery and the guiding catheter as illustrated in figure 6.8.

To investigate the effects of hemodynamic changes on the various indexes, both resting and hyperemic pressure and flow velocity measurements were taken under the four following pairs of conditions: (1) twice under reference conditions (without a hemodynamic intervention) at a 3-minute interval; (2) during atrial pacing at 80 and 110 beats per minute (bpm); (3) under basal blood pressure, and during intravenous infusion of nitroprusside (0.5 to 2 µg/kg/min) titrated to reach a decrease in systolic blood pressure of at least 20 mmHg; (4) in basal contractile state, and after a 5-minute intravenous infusion of 10 µg/kg/min of dobutamine to increase contractility. After each intervention, heart rate, mean aortic pressure, coronary blood flow velocity, and distal coronary pressure were allowed to return to their baseline values. Thus, to complete the protocol, both baseline and hyperemic pressure and flow velocity recordings should have been performed 8 times in every patient. In 2 patients, the measurements were performed both before and after angioplasty so that actually 15 stenoses were investigated. However, in

5 patients the spontaneous blood pressure was too low to allow nitroprusside infusion, in 2 patients no pacemaker lead was advanced into the right atrium, and 1 patient did not receive dobutamine. Hence, two pairs of consecutive baseline and hyperemic pressure and flow velocity recordings were obtained without a specific hemodynamic intervention in 15 stenoses; the effect of pacing-induced tachycardia was investigated in 13 stenoses; the effect of changing blood pressure by nitroprusside was studied in 10 stenoses; and the effect of increasing contractility by dobutamine was studied in 14 stenoses.

When pressure and/or flow velocity tracings were considered non-optimal, resting and hyperemic assessments were repeated after verifying proper functioning of the system, and repositioning of the guide wires if needed. If, after three attempts, no satisfactory tracing could be obtained, the measurements were considered non-obtainable. Figure 8.1 and 8.2 illustrate how the various indexes were derived from pressure and flow velocity recordings.

Myocardial fractional flow reserve (FFR$_{myo}$) was calculated as the ratio of mean distal coronary pressure and mean aortic pressure during maximum hyperemia[4,5].

Coronary flow velocity reserve (CFVR) was calculated as the ratio of hyperemic to baseline mean coronary flow velocity[6-8].

The instantaneous hyperemic diastolic velocity pressure slope (IHDVPS) was calculated from the simultaneously recorded aortic pressure and coronary flow velocity signals at peak hyperemia[9-13]. Therefore, the aortic pressure tracing and the instantaneous peak coronary blood flow velocity were digitized with a sample frequency of 125 Hz. The instantaneous relation between coronary flow velocity and coronary pressure during one cardiac cycle was displayed as a velocity-pressure loop by a specially designed software. For each beat, the slope of the diastolic portion of the loop was calculated and expressed in $cm.s^{-1}.mmHg^{-1}$. The diastolic interval of the velocity-pressure loop to be analyzed was selected manually from the maximum diastolic velocity to the onset of rapid decline of coronary flow velocity due to myocardial contraction. The slope values were accepted only when the correlation coefficient of the linear regression between velocity and pressure during the selected diastolic interval was > 0.97, thus eliminating major pressure or velocity tracing artifacts. The values reported in this study are the mean of three consecutive cardiac cycles selected during peak hyperemia.

All lesions under study were analyzed quantitatively during the procedure with a previously validated system operating on digital images[14]. Percent luminal diameter stenosis was calculated with the use of an automatic interpolated technique to measure the reference diameter.

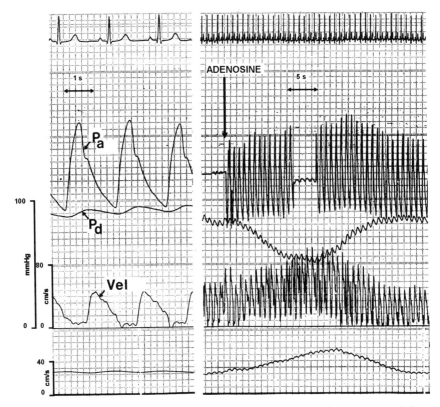

Figure 9.1 *Simultaneous pressure and flow velocity recordings at rest (left) and after injection of intracoronary adenosine (right) in a 69-year-old patient with a 62% diameter stenosis in the mid right coronary artery. Coronary flow velocity reserve (CFVR) can be calculated as the ratio of hyperemic mean coronary flow velocity to resting mean flow velocity and reaches 2.0 in this particular case. Myocardial fractional flow reserve (FFR_{myo}) is calculated as the ratio of mean distal coronary pressure to mean aortic pressure during maximum hyperemia and reaches 0.46 in this case. P_a indicates aortic pressure; P_d mean distal coronary pressure; and vel, Doppler coronary flow velocity.*

9.2 Feasibility of the measurements.

A total of 104 measurements were performed. In all 104 cases myocardial fractional flow reserve could be calculated. In only 4 cases a second bolus of intracoronary adenosine had to be administered to obtain reliable signals and to calculate FFR_{myo}. CFVR could also be calculated in all cases. However, in 15% of cases a second bolus of adenosine had to be administered and in 9% of cases a third bolus of adenosine had be to given to obtain reliable

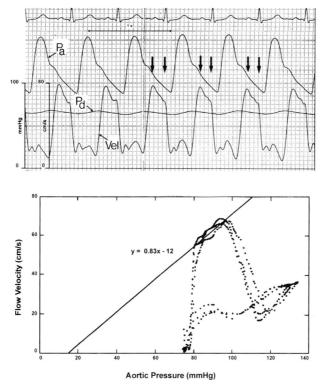

Figure 9.2 *Top: Simultaneous pressure and flow velocity tracings during maximum vasodilation in the same patient as in figure 1. Arrows indicate the start and end point of the segment used for analysis. Bottom: Superimposed instantaneous velocity-pressure loops for the 3 beats indicated with arrows in the top tracing. The instantaneous hyperemic diastolic velocity-pressure slope represents the slope of the linear portion of this loop. P_a indicates aortic pressure; P_d mean distal coronary pressure; and veloc, Doppler coronary flow velocity.*

flow velocity signals in order to calculate CFVR. IHDVPS could only be measured in 79% of the cases. The 26 failures were related to artifacts on the flow velocity tracing precluding the calculation of a satisfactory correlation coefficient of the diastolic velocity-pressure relation.

9.3   Reproducibility under basal hemodynamic conditions.

To study the intrinsic variability of the indexes of flow reserve, two consecutive flow velocity and pressure recordings were performed at a 3-

minute interval without any specific hemodynamic intervention in 15 stenoses. The hemodynamic variables measured at rest and during hyperemia as well as the calculated indexes are given in table 8.1.

Both during the first and the second measurement, mean blood pressure decreased mildly during hyperemia compared with rest. Heart rate did not vary significantly. Resting average peak velocity, mean distal coronary pressure, and translesional pressure gradient were similar during the baseline recordings. Hyperemia induced a similar increase in average peak velocity and translesional pressure gradient and a similar decrease in mean distal coronary pressure. The mean values of FFR_{myo}, CFVR, and IHDVPS, did not change significantly between the two corresponding measurements. The correlation between the first and the second measurement are shown in figure 9.3. The coefficient of variation observed between the first and the second measurement was significantly smaller for FFR_{myo} (4.8% [CI, 3.5% to 7.4%]) than for CFVR (10.5% [CI, 7.7% to 16.2%]). The variation coefficient observed between the first and the second measurements under baseline conditions of IHDVPS (27.7% [CI, 19.9% to 45.8%]) was significantly larger than for both FFR_{myo} and CFVR (figure 9.4).

Table 9.1 *Hemodynamic parameters and calculated indexes during two consecutive recordings (n=15) before any specific hemodynamic intervention was made ("baseline").*

	Baseline 1		Baseline 2	
	Rest	Hyperemia	Rest	Hyperemia
MBP, mmHg	95±1	90±13*	95±14	91±13*
HR, bpm	78±8	79±10	78±7	78±9
MBFV, cm.s^{-1}	17±6	31±17*	18±7	32±17*
P_d, mmHg	83±17	63±19*	82±18	62±17*
ΔP, mmHg	12±11	26±16*	12±11	26±17*
FFR_{myo}	0.70±0.17		0.69±0.17	
CFVR	1.80±0.54		1.72±0.53	
IHDVPS, cm.s^{-1}. mmHg^{-1}	1.01±0.62		1.00±0.70	

*CFVR indicates coronary flow velocity reserve; IHDVPS, instantaneous hyperemic diastolic velocity-pressure slope; HR, heart rate; MBFV, mean blood flow velocity; MBP, mean blood pressure; P_d mean distal coronary pressure; ΔP, translesional pressure gradient; and FFR_{myo}, myocardial fractional flow reserve. *P<.05 hyperemia versus rest.*

9.4   Effects of hemodynamic changes.

9.4.1   Changes in heart rate.

To investigate the effects of heart rate on FFR$_{myo}$, CFVR and IHDVPS these three indexes were obtained in 13 stenoses, first during atrial pacing at 80 bpm and thereafter at 110 bpm. The hemodynamic changes induced by pacing tachycardia and the calculated indexes are summarized in table 9.2.
During atrial pacing at 80 and 110 bpm, blood pressure was significantly lower during hyperemia than at rest. Resting average peak velocity, mean distal coronary pressure, and translesional pressure gradient were similar at 80 and 110 bpm. During hyperemia, average peak velocity and translesional pressure gradient increased and distal coronary pressure decreased to a similar level. The mean values of FFR$_{myo}$ and of IHDVPS at different heart rate were similar. CFVR decreased slightly but significantly from 1.85 ± 0.45 at 80 bpm to 1.66 ± 0.45 at 110 bpm (P < 0.05). The correlation between the various measurements performed at a heart rate of 80 versus 110 bpm is shown in figure 9.3 (second row). The coefficient of variation observed at different heart rate was significantly lower for FFR$_{myo}$ (4.0% [CI, 2.9% to 6.4%])   than for CFVR (14.9% [CI, 10.8% to 24.0%]) and for IHDVPS (29.2% [CI, 20.4% to 51.3%] both P < 0.05; figure 9.4).

9.4.2   Changes in blood pressure.

To study the effects of arterial pressure on FFR$_{myo}$, CFVR, and IHDVPS, these indexes were measured in 10 stenoses at the spontaneous arterial pressure and after intravenous infusion of nitroprusside to obtain a decrease in systolic blood pressure of more than 20 mmHg. The hemodynamic changes induced by nitroprusside infusion and the calculated indexes are summarized in table 9.3.
Systolic blood pressure decreased from 136 ± 12 mmHg before nitroprusside infusion to 100 ± 9 mmHg during nitroprusside infusion (P < .01). No additional effect on blood pressure and heart rate was observed during administration of adenosine. A reflex tachycardia accompanied the nitroprusside-induced decrease in blood pressure. Resting and hyperemic distal coronary pressures were significantly lower during than before nitroprusside infusion. Translesional pressure gradients were similar before and during nitroprusside at rest. Hyperemic translesional gradient was lower during nitroprusside infusion in accordance to the observed decrease of arterial pressure. The mean values of FFR$_{myo}$ and of

IHDVPS remained unaltered before and during nitroprusside. Nitroprusside infusion induced a mild decrease in resting flow velocity and a proportional decrease in hyperemic velocity. As a consequence, CFVR remained unchanged before and during nitroprusside. The correlation between the values of FFR_{myo}, CFVR, and IHDVPS obtained before and during nitroprusside infusion are shown in figure 8.3 (third row). The coefficient of variation observed between the measurements performed before and during infusion of nitroprusside was significantly lower for FFR_{myo} (3.3% [CI, 2.3% to 5.9%]) than for CFVR (13.6% [CI, 9.5% to 23.9%]) and IHDVPS (21.7% [CI, 14.9% to 39.6%]; both $P < .05$; figure 9.4).

Table 9.2 *Hemodynamic parameters and calculated indexes at heart rates of 80 and 110 bpm (n=13)*

	HR 80 bpm		HR 110 bpm	
	Rest	Hyperemia	Rest	Hyperemia
MBP, mmHg	99±9	94±10*	96±11*	88±16*
HR, bpm	81±2	81±2	109±3†	109±3†
MBFV, cm.s^{-1}	17±5	33±14*	18±6	31±14*
P_d mmHg	87±12	65±17*	83±17	60±18*
ΔP, mmHg	12±12	29±12*	14±11	28±16*
FFR_{myo}	0.69±0.16		0.68±0.15	
CFVR	1.85±0.41		1.66±0.45†	
IHDVPS, cm.s^{-1}. mmHg^{-1}	1.10±0.45		1.35±0.72	

CFVR indicates coronary flow velocity reserve; IHDVPS, instantaneous hyperemic diastolic velocity-pressure slope; HR, heart rate; MBFV, mean blood flow velocity; MBP, mean blood pressure; P_d mean distal coronary pressure; ΔP, translesional pressure gradient; and FFR_{myo}, myocardial fractional flow reserve. *P<.05 hyperemia versus rest. †P<.05 HR 110 versus HR 80.

Figure 9.3 (opposite page) *Plots of relation between the pairs of values of myocardial fractional flow reserve (FFR_{myo}), coronary flow velocity reserve (CFVR), and instantaneous hyperemic diastolic velocity pressure slope (IHDVPS). First row: the indexes were measured twice under reference ("baseline") conditions without any specific hemodynamic intervention (BL1 is baseline 1; BL2 is baseline 2). Second row: the indexes were measured at the heart rate of 80 bpm and of 110 bpm. Third row: the indexes were measured before and during infusion of nitroprusside (NIP). Fourth row: the indexes were measured before and during an infusion of dobutamine (DOB). The dotted line represents the line of identity.*

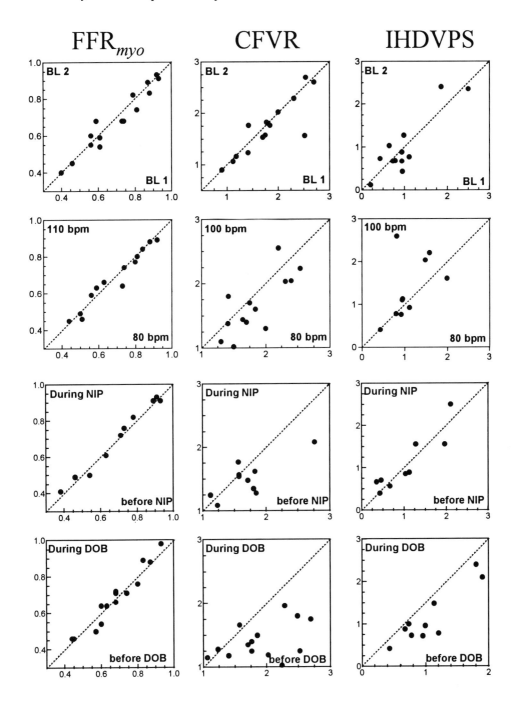

Table 9.3 *Hemodynamic parameters and calculated indexes before and during nitroprusside infusion (n=10)*

	Before Nitroprusside		During Nitroprusside	
	Rest	Hyperemia	Rest	Hyperemia
MBP, mmHg	100±9	98±9	79±6†	78±9†
HR, bpm	78±10	79±11	89±12†	90±10†
MBFV, cm.s^{-1}	21±7	37±16*	17±5†	27±12*†
P_d, mmHg	87±13	67±16*	68±15†	55±13*†
ΔP, mmHg	13±16	30±23*	15±16	23±16*
FFR$_{myo}$	0.70±0.19		0.71±019	
CFVR	1.67±0.44		1.50±0.28	
IHDVPS, cm.s^{-1}. mmHg^{-1}	1.04±0.65		1.08±0.66	

CFVR indicates coronary flow velocity reserve; IHDVPS, instantaneous hyperemic diastolic velocity-pressure slope; HR, heart rate; MBFV, mean blood flow velocity; MBP, mean blood pressure; P_d mean distal coronary pressure; ΔP, translesional pressure gradient; and FFR$_{myo}$, myocardial fractional flow reserve.   *P<.05 hyperemia versus rest. †P<.05 during versus before nitroprusside.

Table 9.4 *Hemodynamic parameters and calculated indexes before and during dobutamine infusion (n=14)*

	Before Dobutamine		During Dobutamine	
	Rest	Hyperemia	Rest	Hyperemia
MBP, mmHg	97±14	93±12*	99±17	95±18*
HR, bpm	78±8	77±9	93±13†	95±12†
MBFV, cm.s^{-1}	20±6	39±17*	26±8†	37±142*
P_d, mmHg	83±19	63±15*	80±22	65±22*
ΔP, mmHg	14±13	29±17*	20±15†	30±17*
FFR$_{myo}$	0.68±0.15		0.68±0.16	
CFVR	1.90±0.50		1.41±0.28†	
IHDVPS, cm.s^{-1}. MmHg^{-1}	1.06±0.48		1.15±0.64	

CFVR indicates coronary flow velocity reserve; IHDVPS, instantaneous hyperemic diastolic velocity-pressure slope; HR, heart rate; MBFV, mean blood flow velocity; MBP, mean blood pressure; P_d mean distal coronary pressure; ΔP, translesional pressure gradient; and FFR$_{myo}$, myocardial fractional flow reserve.   *P<.05 hyperemia versus rest. †P<.05 during versus before dobutamine.

9.4.3 Changes in contractility.

To study the effects of left ventricular contractility on FFR_{myo}, CFVR and IHDVPS, simultaneous pressure and flow velocity tracings were obtained in 14 stenoses before and after a 5-minute intravenous infusion of dobutamine. The hemodynamic changes and the calculated indexes are summarized in table 9.4.

During dobutamine infusion, resting and hyperemic mean blood pressure did not change significantly. Heart rate increased both at rest and during hyperemia. Resting translesional pressure gradient increased during infusion of dobutamine. In contrast, hyperemic distal coronary pressure and translesional pressure gradient did not change significantly. The mean values of FFR_{myo} and IHDVPS did not change significantly during infusion of dobutamine. During dobutamine infusion, a marked increase in resting blood flow velocities was observed, while hyperemic blood flow velocities remained unchanged. As a result, the mean value of CFVR significantly

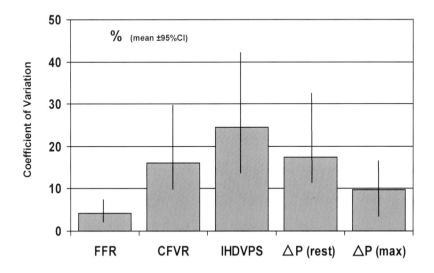

Figure 9.4 *Coefficients of variations for all pairs of measurements of FFR_{myo}, CFVR, IDHVPS, ΔP_{rest}, and ΔP_{max}.*

decreased during dobutamine infusion. The correlation between the individual measurements of FFR$_{myo}$, CFVR, and IHDVPS before and during infusion of dobutamine is shown in figure 9.3 (fourth row). The coefficient of variation observed between the measurements before and during dobutamine infusion was significantly lower for FFR$_{myo}$ (4.4% [3.2% to 6.9%]) than for both CFVR (26.7% [19.5% to 42.1%]) and IHDVPS (17.4% [12.2% to 30.5%]; both P < .05; figure 9.4).

9.5   Reproducibility of translesional pressure gradients.

Figure 9.5 shows the correlation between the values of resting transstenotic pressure gradient and hyperemic transstenotic pressure gradient obtained twice under basal conditions, at a heart rate of 80 versus 110 bpm, before and during infusion of nitroprusside, and before and during dobutamine infusion.   The coefficient of variation of both resting and hyperemic transstenotic pressure gradients are shown in figure 9.4. As expected, ΔP_{max} varied proportionally with aortic pressure, leaving FFR unaffected.

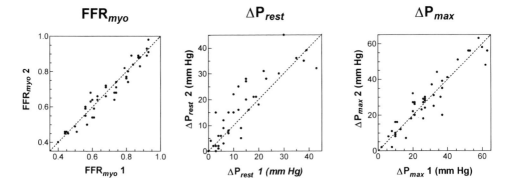

Figure 9.5 *Plots of the relation between all pairs of values of FFR$_{myo}$, ΔP_{rest}, and ΔP_{max}.*

9.6 Comments.

The present data were obtained over a large range of stenosis severity, with special emphasis on lesions of intermediate severity. The latter are usually the most difficult to gauge and therefore may require functional evaluation for clinical decision making. The results of this study demonstrate: (1) that FFR_{myo} is obtainable very easily in all cases and that this pressure-derived measurement is almost independent from the prevailing hemodynamic conditions; (2) that CFVR is easy to determine in most cases, is quite reproducible when hemodynamic conditions remain unchanged, but is highly sensitive to hemodynamic changes; and (3) that IHDVPS can be obtained in only 79% of cases and shows a large variability of the measurements even under baseline conditions.

Several reasons probably explain the high reproducibility of pressure-derived FFR_{myo} irrespective of the prevailing hemodynamic conditions: *first*, FFR_{myo}, like IHDVPS, has the conceptual advantage of relying only on measurements performed during maximum hyperemia. FFR_{myo} is therefore unaffected by changes in resting conditions; *second*, the index incorporates mean arterial pressure, therefore correcting for the changes in driving pressure; *third*, the mean coronary pressure as recorded in the study through tiny pressure monitoring guide wires is an extremely stable signal devoid of artifacts that often obscure the velocity tracings in humans; and *fourth*, distal coronary pressure integrates all possible changes in vessel diameter that could be induced by changes in absolute coronary blood flow [15,16,17].

CFVR has been shown to be quite reproducible, provided the conditions known to affect resting coronary flow remain constant[18,19]. Previous animal and humans studies have demonstrated a significant reduction in coronary flow reserve (and CFVR) under the influence of tachycardia [6,10,18-20], volume loading [10,18], and increased contractility[10]. Two studies conducted in humans did not show a significant change in CFVR accompanying changes in blood pressure because of proportional changes in coronary blood flow velocity so that their ratio remained similar[18,20]. Our data show a decrease in CFVR (albeit not significant) when blood pressure was lowered by nitroprusside. When heart rate was increased by atrial pacing or when contractility was increased under the influence of dobutamine, a significant decrease in CFVR occurred mainly as the result of an increase in resting coronary blood flow velocity. Although a large variability in CFVR measurements accompanied changes in hemodynamic conditions, two serial measurements under baseline conditions were quite reproducible, suggesting that the variability of CFVR measurements cannot be ascribed to technical factors. The hemodynamic dependence of CFVR is chiefly due to the fact that the concept is based on a ratio whose denominator is resting flow velocity, a parameter extremely sensitive to changes in myocardial oxygen consumption. Therefore, in clinical practice, serial measurements of CFVR are often difficult to compare and to interpret because of changes in prevailing myocardial oxygen consumption and secondary changes in basal and/or hyperemic coronary blood flow. Moreover, blood flow velocity is influenced not only by the severity of the epicardial lesion and by its consequences on myocardial resistance, but also by the changes in dimensions of the vessel segment where the flow velocity measurements are taken. However, the data presented above were acquired after administration of intracoronary nitrate so that changes in vessel diameter are unlikely to play a major role in the variability of coronary flow velocity reserve measurements. In addition, flow-induced vasodilation of the epicardial vessel after short lasting hyperemia, is expected to occur only 60 seconds later, at the time when coronary blood flow has already returned to normal[21]. Our results extend data of Di Mario et al, showing a large variability of coronary flow velocity reserve measurements repeated after a 6-month interval[22]. These authors pointed out that this variability can be reduced by normalization for the cross-sectional area at the site of the measurement (coronary flow) and for the aortic pressure at the time of the measurement (flow resistance). Figure 9.6 illustrates some of the mechanisms responsible for the variability of CFVR with changing hemodynamics and makes clear immediately why FFR is not affected by those changes.

IHDVPS is determined by calculating the slope of the linear diastolic segment of the relation between instantaneous aortic pressure and hyperemic coronary flow. During this part of diastole, compressive forces of the ventricle are minimal and coronary flow is exclusively related to the severity of the lesion and to the driving pressure. The steeper the slope, the milder the coronary lesion. To some extent, this index can be compared with the Doppler pressure-half time used to evaluate the severity of mitral valve stenosis. The instantaneous hyperemic flow-versus-hyperemic pressure slope incorporates aortic pressure and showed no significant hemodynamic dependence on left ventricular end-diastolic pressure, heart rate, or contractility in an open chest animal model[10,19]. This concept was recently simplified (IHDVPS) and applied to humans by Di Mario et al[12]. The IHDVPS, also used in this study, differs from the originally proposed index in at least two aspects : *First*, distal flow velocity measurements were used

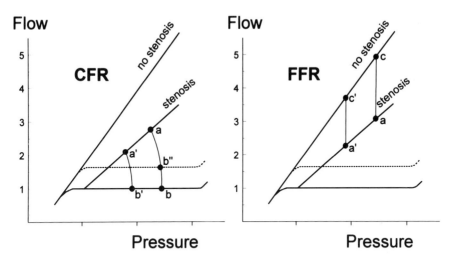

Figure 9.6 *Schematic illustration why coronary flow reserve (CFR) is sensitive to changes in hemodynamic conditions while fractional flow reserve (FFR) remains unaffected by those changes[29]. The coronary pressure-flow relation at maximum hyperemia is indicated both for a normal coronary artery and a coronary stenosis. The resting pressure-flow relation (autoregulatory range) is represented by the solid horizontal line. (Left) CFR is defined as the ratio of hyperemic to resting flow (a/b). It is obvious that with changing blood pressure, the value of CFR changes to a'/b'. Also, when resting flow changes (as with changing heart rate or contractility) CFR changes to a/b". Therefore, no uniform normal value of CFR can be defined. (Right) FFR is defined as the ratio of maximum flow in the presence of a stenosis divided by normal maximum flow (a/c). This ratio remains unaffected by changes in blood pressure (a/c = a'/c') or by variations in resting flow. Its normal value is always 1.0, irrespective of the patient, coronary artery, or prevailing hemodynamic conditions. Therefore, FFR is a more specific measure of functional stenosis severity.*

instead of proximal absolute coronary blood flow normalized for myocardial mass. *Second*, maximum coronary blood flow velocity was used instead of left ventricular high fidelity pressure measurements to detect the diastolic interval of interest for analysis. Although in Di Mario's study inter- and intraobserver reproducibility of IHDVPS was excellent, the latter index could only be obtained in 77% of cases with angiographically proven coronary stenosis. Failed measurements were related to poor quality of the Doppler signal. This is very similar to our findings. Our data demonstrate a large variability of two consecutive values of IHDVPS taken under baseline conditions, while this variability did not seem to increase further with changing hemodynamic conditions. This suggests that technical factors rather than fluctuating hemodynamics are responsible for the observed variability. In addition, at heart rates usually encountered in the catheterization laboratory, the duration of diastole is often too short to reliably calculate the slope of the instantaneous relationship between flow velocity and pressure. These practical pitfalls limit the clinical usefulness of the IHDVPS for evaluation of coronary stenosis severity.

Resting pressure gradient has been shown to poorly correlate with relative flow reserve as assessed by positron emission tomography (see chapter 7, table 7.2)[23]. The data presented in this chapter show a high variability of resting gradient with changing hemodynamic conditions. Both findings are related to the fact that resting pressure gradient depends on baseline coronary blood flow and aortic driving pressure. Therefore the resting pressure gradient cannot be proposed to evaluate lesion severity. In contrast, translesional pressure gradient measured during maximum arteriolar vasodilation is determined by hyperemic flow and is therefore a better index of stenosis severity. However, since even during hyperemia the gradient remains sensitive to changes in blood pressure, hyperemic transstenotic pressure gradient is markedly less reproducible than FFR_{myo}, as demonstrated in figure 9.4 and 9.5.

9.7   Fractional flow reserve and the fluid dynamic equation.

In understanding the pressure independence of FFR, and the variability of other flow indexes, figure 9.7 is helpful, even though it is only a simplified model. Suppose, in the upper panel of that figure, that a patient has a coronary stenosis and that the effect of that stenosis on blood flow is studied at a mean blood pressure of 60 mmHg. Suppose further that the hyperemic gradient across that lesion is 15 mmHg and that P_v equals zero. Thus, P_d will be 45 mmHg and FFR_{myo} equals 0.75.

Suppose now that in this same patient blood pressure is elevated to 120 mmHg. Because of the proportionality between driving pressure and blood flow at maximum vasodilation, this implies that absolute blood flow and blood flow velocity, will also double. Because also resting flow will be affected by the rise of blood pressure, absolute CFR and CFVR will change in an unpredictable way As flow doubles, also ΔP will double and, as a result, distal coronary pressure increases to 90 mmHg.

Therefore, although nothing has changed to the stenosis itself - it still is exactly the same stenosis - blood flow velocity, CF(V)R, and ΔP have all changed significantly and thus none of these indexes can be a complete index of epicardial stenosis severity. FFR_{myo}, however, was 0.75 before the increase of blood pressure and is still 0.75 thereafter, thus reflecting functional stenosis severity itself without dependence on current hemodynamic loading conditions.

The complete explanation is more complex and to understand this, the question should be raised how the pressure-independence of FFR_{myo} relates to the fluid dynamic equation, which states that the pressure drop across a stenosis not only contains a linear but also a quadratic component with respect to flow:

$$\Delta P = fQ + sQ^2$$

where fQ represents the energy loss by friction within the stenosis (which effect can be estimated by Poiseuille's law) and sQ^2 the energy loss by separation effects at the exit of the stenosis (which effect can be estimated by Bernouilli's law). It is argued then, that, if the quadratic component is non-negligible, the increase of flow would result in disproportional increase of ΔP across the lesion[24]. However, since a quadratic component is assumed in the relation between ΔP and Q, in a similar way a quadratic component should be assumed in the relation between driving pressure and flow[25]. It is incorrect to assume a linear relation between P_a and Q and to apply a quadratic term in the relation between ΔP and Q. In other words, if the fluid dynamic equation is applied, it should be applied consistently. In that case, a square root component is present between P_a and Q, and a quadratic component between Q and ΔP. As a result, P_a and ΔP (and thus P_a and P_d) are still linearly related and fractional flow reserve remains unaffected by the change of blood pressure. Therefore, the pressure-independence of FFR is in accordance with the fluid dynamic equation. The correctness of this statement was demonstrated by the results of the present human study, as well as by the animal studies in chapter 7. Looking at figure 7.5 and 7.6, the slope of the regression line in those figures would not have been different if only the circles, squares, or triangles would have been used, representing the 3 different levels of blood pressure and a wide variety of stenosis severity. Some clinical examples to illustrate this, are given in figure 9.8 and 9.9. Besides these theoretical and experimental issues, there are some arguments to be careful in applying the fluid dynamic equation to the intact human circulation. According to that equation and using the coefficients for f and s as presented in earlier studies[26-27], a significant pressure drop of 30-40 mmHg would occur in normal coronary arteries at maximum hyperemia. However, it was demonstrated indisputably in chapter 10, that no decline of pressure occurs along normal coronary arteries in conscious humans. In addition, at the other extremity of the spectrum, in case of total coronary artery occlusion, the fluid dynamic equation is not adequate anymore to describe what happens in the in-vivo circulation because of the role of the collaterals. Myocardial fractional flow reserve still explains the behaviour of the system and even in that case it was demonstrated in dogs that FFR_{myo} (equivalent to fractional collateral flow in that case) is still independent of arterial pressure (figure 7.3 and 7.4).

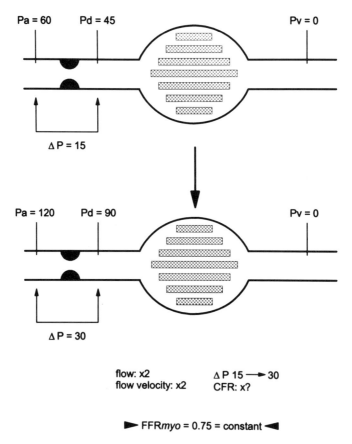

Figure 9.7   *Simplified illustration of the independence of FFR from pressure changes. The complete explanation is more complex and discussed in paragraph 9.7*

Figure 9.8 (next page) *Clinical illustration of the pressure-independence of myocardial fractional flow reserve (FFR$_{myo}$) in a 63-year-old male with an 80% stenosis in the right coronary artery. FFR$_{myo}$ is determined at 2 levels of aortic pressure, with a difference of approximately 35%. As can be observed, FFR$_{myo}$ remains unaffected.*

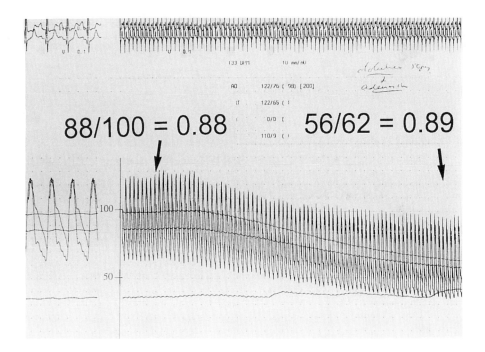

Figure 9.9 *Pressure independency of myocardial fractional flow reserve (FFR$_{myo}$) in a 54-year-old patient with a 50% stenosis in the left circumflex artery. During sustained maximum coronary hyperemia, induced by i.v. adenosine infusion, blood pressure is decreased by i.v. nitroglycerin to 62% of the initial value. It can be clearly observed how ΔP is proportional to P$_a$ and despite this variation of aortic pressure over a large range (from 100 to 62 mmHg), P$_d$ decreases proportionally (from 88 to 56 mmHg) and FFR remains completely unaffected.*

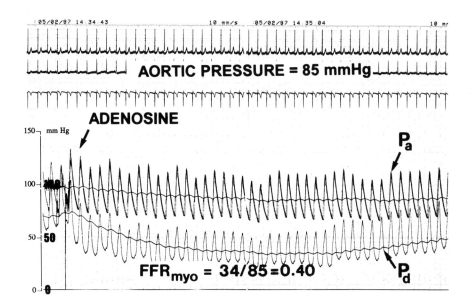

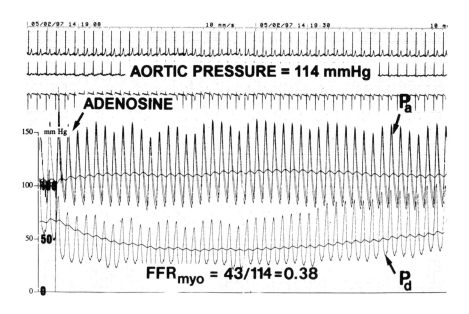

9.8   Clinical implications.

In the present study, lowering blood pressure by nitroprusside infusion was accompanied by a reflex tachycardia. The infusion of dobutamine in addition to an increase in left ventricular contractility also induced an increase in heart rate. Although not specifically monitored in the present study, an increase in heart rate is known to increase left ventricular contractility[28]. Hence, the specific influence of heart rate, blood pressure, and contractility were not really divorced from one another. However, the study protocol closely mimics alterations in hemodynamic parameters that are likely to occur in humans during interventional procedures when changes in heart rate, blood pressure, contractility, and volume loading are closely interrelated and do not fluctuate independently from one another.

The use of intracoronary adenosine to induce maximum hyperemia, may introduce a bias in evaluating the ease of measuring CFVR and IHDVPS. Indeed, if intracoronary papaverine or intravenous adenosine were used, a longer hyperemia would have allowed the manipulation of the Doppler wire during the hyperemic phase. This could have led to a higher success rate in computing IHDVPS.

Temporary changes in heart rate, arterial pressure, and myocardial contractile state are likely to occur in the setting of every diagnostic catheterization and even more so in the setting of interventional cardiology. Prolonged episodes of myocardial ischemia might even limit the return to truly basal hemodynamic conditions and coronary flow. Therefore, methods proposed for gauging the physiological impact of epicardial stenoses or for evaluating the results of an intervention, should provide similar results whatever the prevailing hemodynamic conditions, in order to be interpretable and thus useful for clinical decision-making. In addition, in the era of interventional cardiology, all indexes should be easy, safe, and fast to obtain. Therefore FFR$_{myo}$, by combining the ease and minimal variability, is superior to both CFVR and IHDVPS in providing information on the consequences of an epicardial lesion on the perfusion of the underlying myocardium.

References.

1.   Doucette JW, Corl PD, Payne HM, Flynn AE, Goto M, Nassi M, Segal J. Validation of a Doppler guide wire for intravascular measurement of coronary artery flow velocity. *Circulation* 1992;85:1899-1911.

2.   Wilson RF, Wyche B, Christensen BV, Zimmer S, Laxson DD. Effects of adenosine on human coronary arterial circulation. *Circulation* 1990;82:1595-1606.

3.   De Bruyne B, Stockbroeckx J, Demoor D, Heyndrickx GR, Kern MT. Role of side holes in guiding catheters: observations on coronary pressures and flow. *Cath Cardiovasc Diagn* 1994; 33:145-152.

4.   Pijls NHJ, van Son JAM, Kirkeeide RL, De Bruyne B, Gould KL. Experimental basis of determining maximum coronary, myocardial and collateral blood flow by pressure measurements for assessing functional stenosis severity before and after PTCA. *Circulation* 1993;87:1354-1367.

5.   De Bruyne B, Baudhuin T, Melin JA, Pijls NHJ, Sys SU, Bol A, Paulus WJ, Heyndrickx GR, Wijns W. Coronary flow reserve calculated from pressure measurements in humans. Validation with positron emission tomography. *Circulation* 1994;89:1013-1022.

6.   Gould KL, Lipscomb K, Hamilton GW. Physiological basis for assessing critical coronary stenosis: instantaneous flow response and regional distribution during coronary hyperemia as measures of coronary flow reserve. *Am J Cardiol* 1974;33:87-94.

7.   Hoffman JIE. Maximum coronary flow and the concept of coronary vascular reserve. *Circulation* 1984;70:153-159.

8.   Wilson RF, Laughlin DE, Ackell PH, Chilian WM, Holida MD, Hartley CJ, Armstrong ML, Marcus ML, White CW. Transluminal, subselective measurement of coronary artery blood flow velocity and vasodilator reserve in man. *Circulation* 1985;72:82-92.

9.   Mancini G.B.J., McGillem M.J., DeBoe S.F., Gallangher K.P. The diastolic hyperemic flow vs pressure relation: a new index of coronary stenosis severity and flow reserve. *Circulation* 1989;80:941-950.

10. Mancini GBJ, Cleary RM, DeBoe SF, Moore NB, Gallagher KP. Instantaneous hyperemic flow-vs-pressure slope index. Microsphere validation of an alternative to measures of coronary flow reserve. *Circulation* 1991;84:862-870.

11. Cleary RM, Aron D, Moore NB, De Boe SF, Mancini GBJ. Tachycardia, contractility and volume loading alter conventional indexes of coronary flow reserve, but not the instantaneous hyperemic flow-versus-pressure slope index. *J Am Coll Cardiol* 1992; 20:1261-1269.

12. Di Mario C, Krams R, Gil R, Serruys PW. Slope of the instantaneous hyperemic diastolic coronary flow velocity-pressure relation. A new index for assessment of the physiological significance of coronary stenosis in humans. *Circulation* 1994;90:1215-1224.

13. Kondo M, Azuma A, Yamada H, Kohno H, Kawata K, Tatsukawa H, Ohnishi K, Kohno Yn Asayama J, Nakagawa M. Estimation of coronary flow reserve with the instantaneous flow velocity versus pressure relation: A new index of coronary flow reserve independent of perfusion pressure. *Am Heart J* 1996;132:1127-1134

14. Haase J, Di Mario C, Slager CJ, van der Giessen WJ, den Boer A, de Feyter PJ, Reiber JHC, Verdouw PD, Serruys PW. In vitro validation of on-line and off-line geometric coronary measurement using insertion of stenosis phantoms in porcine coronary arteries. *Cath Cardiovasc Diagn* 1992;27:16-27.

15. Emanuelsson H, Dohnal M, Lamm C, Tenerz. Initial experiences with a miniaturized pressure transducer during coronary angioplasty. *Cath Cardiovasc Diagn* 1991;24:137-143.

16. De Bruyne B, Pijls NHJ, Paulus WJ, Vantrimpont PJ, Sys SU, Heyndrickx GR. Transstenotic coronary pressure gradient measurement in humans: in vitro and in vivo evaluation of a new pressure monitoring angioplasty guide wire. *J Am Coll Cardiol* 1993;22:119-126.

17. Drexler H, Zeiher AM, Wollsläger H, Meinertz T, Just H, Bonzel T. Flow-dependent artery dilatation in humans. *Circulation* 1989;80:466-474.

18. McGinn Al, White CW, Wilson RF. Interstudy variability of coronary flow reserve: influence of heart rate, arterial pressure and ventricular preload. *Circulation* 1990; 1:1319-1330.

19. Cleary RM, Moore NB, De Boe SF, Mancini GBJ. Sensitivity and reproducibility of the instantaneous hyperemic flow-versus-pressure slope index compared to coronary flow reserve for the assessment of stenosis severity. *Am Heart J* 1993;126:57-65.

20. Rossen JD, Winniford MD. Effect of increases in heart rate and arterial pressure on coronary flow reserve in humans. *J Am Coll Cardiol* 1993;21:343-348.

21. Hintze TH, Vatner SF. Reactive dilatation of large coronary arteries in conscious dogs. *Circ Res* 1984;54:50-57.

22. Di Mario C, Gil R, Serruys PW. Long-term reproducibility of coronary flow velocity measurements in patients with coronary artery disease. *Am J Cardiol* 1995;75:1177-1180.

23. Higgins CB, Vatner SF, Franklin D, Braunwald E. Extent of regulation of the heart's contractile state in the conscious dog by alteration in the frequency of contraction. *J Clin Invest* 1973;52:1187-1196.

24. Gewirtz H. Fractional Flow Reserve. *Circulation* 1996;94:2306 (correspondence)

25. Pijls NHJ, Van Gelder B, Van der Voort P, Peels KH, Bracke FALE, Bonnier HJRM, El Gamal MIH. Fractional Flow Reserve. *Circulation* 1996;94:2306-2307 (correspondence)

26. Gould KL. Pressure-flow characteristics of coronary stenoses in unsedated dogs at rest and during coronary vasodilation. *Circ Res* 1978;43:242-253.

27. Sun Y, Most AS, Ohley W, Gewirtz H. Estimation of instantaneous blood flow through a rigid, coronary artery stenosis in anaesthetized domestic swine. *Cardiovasc Res* 1983;17:499-504.

28. De Bruyne B, Baudhuin T, Melin JA, Pijls NHJ, Sys SU, Bol A, Paulus WJ, Heyndrickx GR, Wijns W. Coronary flow reserve calculated from pressure measurements in humans. Validation with positron emission tomography. *Circulation* 1994;89:1013-1022.

29. Pijls NHJ, De Bruyne B. Coronary pressure measurement and fractional flow reserve. *Heart* 1998; 80: 539-542.

Chapter 10

FRACTIONAL FLOW RESERVE IN NORMAL CORONARY ARTERIES

10.1 Introduction.

A major limitation of classical flow reserve indexes such as coronary flow reserve (CFR), blood flow velocity, and absolute flow, is the wide variability of normal values. Normal values of CFR widely vary from patient to patient and strongly depend on the current hemodynamic state (as shown in chapter 9), extent of collaterals (chapter 16), and the technique used to measure that index[1-10]. When CFR is assessed by flow velocity ratios, an additional confounding variable is the sensitivity of the signal to position changes of the wire in the coronary artery, to respiration, coughing, and motion of the patient. Moreover, normal CFR in humans is age-dependent and generally lower in older individuals.

As a result, "normal" values for CFR as presented in literature, vary between 2.3 and 6.0[5-10]. As a consequence of such a large range of normal values, it is illusory to expect a sharply defined cut-off value of CFR separating functionally significant and non-significant stenoses without considerable overlap. In addition, a diminished CFR can be due either to an epicardial obstruction to flow or to microvascular disease, or both, without the possibility to distinguish these different effects. Therefore, despite the valuable physiologic insights provided by CFR, its usefulness for practical decision making in the catheterization laboratory, remains limited and the question whether or not to revascularize a given stenosis will often remain unanswered.

From, the definition of myocardial fractional flow reserve (FFR_{myo}), it is obvious that, at least theoretically, there is one unequivocal normal value of 1.0 for every patient and every coronary artery, irrespective of the current hemodynamic state (figure 10.1)[10,11].Therefore, for FFR_{myo}, it is expected that a well-defined separation exists between stenoses which are or are not associated with inducible ischemia. However, the assumption that no decline of pressure occurs along normal coronary arteries in humans, has never been tested so far and sometimes even been challenged. Because this issue is germane for the clinical applicability of FFR, this chapter validates that no decline of pressure occurs along normal coronary arteries, not even at maximum hyperemia, and as a result that myocardial fractional flow reserve is indeed 1.0 in normal coronary arteries.

Normal Epicardial Artery

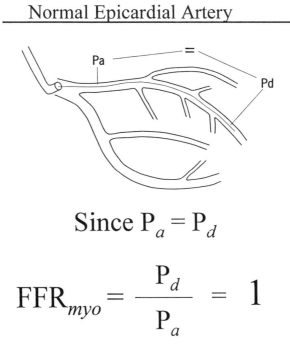

Since $P_a = P_d$

$$FFR_{myo} = \frac{P_d}{P_a} = 1$$

Figure 10.1 *In normal coronary arteries there is no decline of pressure along the epicardial artery not even during maximum hyperemia. Therefore, normal FFR_{myo} is expected to be 1.0 for every patient and every coronary artery, irrespective of the prevailing hemodynamics and myocardial mass.*

10.2 Fractional flow reserve in normal coronary arteries.

Ten patients were investigated (8 men, 2 women; age 44 - 67 years) without cardiovascular risk factors, who had visited the outpatient clinic within the previous year because of atypical chest complaints, and who had a normal coronary angiogram at that time. After informed consent had been obtained, these individuals underwent exercise testing, [201]Thallium scintigraphy, and dobutamine stress echocardiography. After it had been concluded that all these tests were normal, coronary angiography was repeated and FFR_{myo} was determined in all large coronary arteries and side branches.

A 7F guiding catheter was introduced into one femoral artery and after administration of 10.000 U heparin i.v., this catheter was advanced into the coronary artery. Mean aortic pressure (P_a) was monitored by this guiding catheter. Nitroglycerin 0.5 mg SL was administered and angiograms of the target vessels were made as usual.

To measure distal coronary pressure (P_d), an 0.014-in high-fidelity pressure monitoring guide wire was used as described in the previous chapters (Radi Medical, Uppsala, Sweden).

After proper calibration, this wire was introduced into the guiding catheter and advanced to its tip. At that point, equality of pressures registered by the guiding catheter and the pressure guide wire, was verified (figure 10.2, upper panel). The wire was then advanced into the distal third part of all easily accessible large branches. Steady state maximum coronary hyperemia was obtained then by intravenous administration of adenosine (140 µg/kg/min) infused through a femoral venous sheath. From the simultaneous recordings of P_a and P_d at steady state maximum hyperemia, fractional flow reserve of the dependent myocardial bed was calculated by:

$$FFR_{myo} = \frac{P_d}{P_a}$$

The diameter of the respective coronary artery at its proximal part and at the location of the distal pressure measurement, was calculated from the coronary arteriogram by QCA. These values are presented in table 10.1. No complications occurred in any of the patients, and FFR_{myo} could be calculated for 41 different normal coronary arteries and branches as presented in table 10.1 All these values were close to 1.0 (range 0.94 - 1.02) demonstrating that no significant decline of pressure occurs along a normal coronary artery. In all these vessels the distal third of the artery could be reached without problems. Some examples of the pressure recordings in these normal patients, are shown in figures 10.2 and 10.3.

At adenosine-induced hyperemia, there was a decrease of mean aortic pressure of 15 mmHg and an increase in heart rate of 7 bpm (table 10.2). These values are slightly larger than the hemodynamic changes as observed in PTCA patients during i.v. adenosine administration (table 11.2).

Figure 10.2 (opposite page) *Examples of phasic and mean pressure recordings in one of the normal patients. Even at maximum hyperemia, no noticeable decline of pressure occurs along these normal arteries.*

Table 10.1   *Quantitative angiographic diameter and FFR_{myo} in 41 coronary branches in 10 normal individuals. prox $\varnothing$: proximal diameter of the investigated artery; dist $\varnothing$: diameter of the artery at the distal location where P_d was measured. Diag: diagonal branch; MOCX: obtuse marginal branch; PLCX posterolateral branch; RV: right ventricular branch.*

Vessel		prox $\varnothing$	dist $\varnothing$	FFR_{myo}
LAD	(n = 10)	3.6 ± 0.9	2.3 ± 0.5	0.97 ± 0.03
DIAG	(n = 7)	2.2 ± 0.6	1.8 ± 0.5	0.96 ± 0.01
MOCX	(n = 7)	3.4 ± 0.7	2.6 ± 0.2	0.97 ± 0.01
PLCX	(n = 6)	2.7 ± 0.5	2.4 ± 0.2	0.99 ± 0.01
RCA	(n = 10)	3.9 ± 0.7	2.7 ± 0.4	0.98 ± 0.02
RV	(n = 1)	2.1	1.7	0.98
Total	(n = 41)			0.98 ± 0.02

Table 10.2 *Hemodynamic data in normal patients at rest and at adenosine-induced maximum hyperemia.*

	Resting	*Hyperemic*
MAP (mmHg)	96 ± 17	82 ± 12
Heart rate (bpm)	73 ± 12	79 ± 12

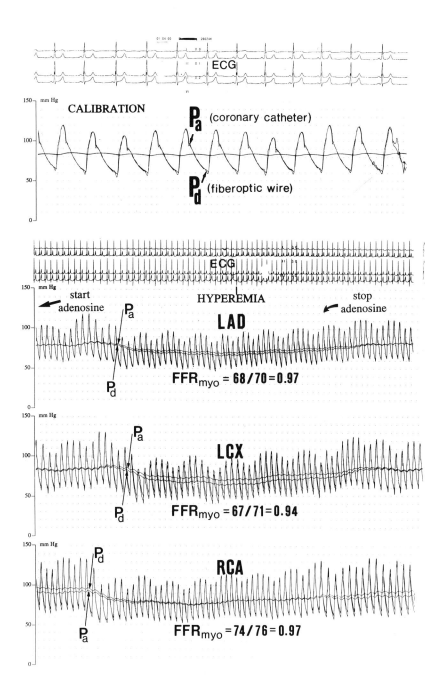

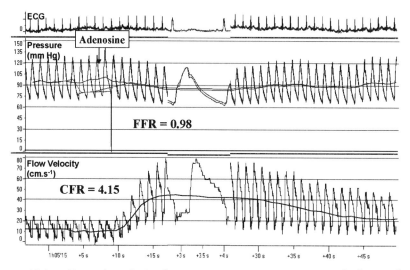

Figure 10.3 *Example of simultaneous coronary pressure and flow velocity measurement in the LAD coronary artery of a 47-year old man with angiographically completely normal coronary arteries. In spite of a 4.1 fold increase in flow velocity after an intracoronary bolus of adenosine, no decrease in pressure is observed in the very distal part of the vessel.*

10.2.1 Clinical Implications

In this study in 41 truly normal coronary arteries, FFR_{myo} equaled 0.98 ± 0.02. Therefore, the range of normal values can be defined as 0.94 - 1.00 which means in fact that no significant decline of pressure occurs along a normal coronary artery, not even at maximum hyperemia. From earlier animal experiments, contradictory data had been obtained with respect to the resistance of epicardial coronary arteries to normal coronary blood flow. Theoretically, using the fluid dynamic equation and estimating friction and separation coefficients, some decline of pressure along normal coronary arteries was predicted[12-14], but animal experiments, using ultrathin wires instead of 3F hypotubes, failed to confirm this[15]. In the present series of 41 normal coronary arteries in conscious humans, FFR_{myo} equaled 0.98 ± 0.02. For the first time, therefore, it has been indisputably demonstrated that no noticeable decline of pressure occurs along normal coronary arteries in conscious humans and thus that normal human coronary arteries do not provide noticeable resistance to blood flow[11]. The clinical implications of

Table 10.3 *FFR$_{myo}$ of truly normal coronary arteries in normal persons (group A), and apparently normal contralateral coronary arteries in patients with remote coronary artery disease (group B).*

	Group A	Group B
# persons	10	50
# vessels	41	90
FFR$_{myo}$	0.98 ± 0.02	0.90 ± 0.08

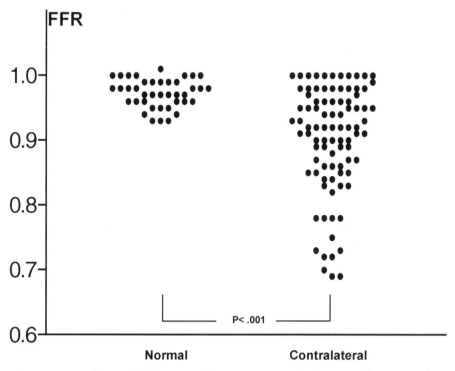

Figure 10.4 *Values of FFR$_{myo}$ in 41 coronary arteries in normal persons (true normal values, left) and 90 apparently normal contralateral arteries in patients with remote coronary artery disease (right).*

these observations are important: not only a unique reference value is provided to which pathologic values can be compared, but also the way is open to confirm presence or absence of normalization of epicardial conductance after coronary interventions. This may be important particularly after stent implantation as will be discussed in chapter 14.

10.3 FFR$_{myo}$ in apparently normal contralateral coronary arteries in patients with remote coronary artery disease.

In the search for normal values for different physiologic parameters of the coronary circulation, it is frequent that data from apparently normal contralateral coronary arteries are used, obtained in patients with a coronary stenosis in the ipsilateral coronary artery. A problem in doing so is that one can never be sure that such an apparently normal contralateral vessel, is truly normal indeed. Therefore, FFR$_{myo}$ was determined in 90 apparently normal contralateral coronary arteries in 50 patients who underwent single-vessel PTCA and had a normal left ventricular function.

As will be clear from table 10.3, FFR$_{myo}$ of the apparently normal contralateral arteries in patients with coronary disease in another vessel, was slightly, but significantly lower. More importantly, the scatter of these values was quite large, with lowest values as low as 0.69. Moreover 54% of the values were outside the normal range (figure 10.4). In general, therefore, caution should be taken in defining normal values of physiologic parameters from measurements in apparently normal contralateral arteries, because some degree of "hidden" , angiographically inapparent disease in

Figure 10.5 (opposite page) *Example of coronary pressure measurement during hyperemia after implantation of a stent in the mid-LAD. The stented segment is indicated by the black line. When the sensor is in the distal LAD (indicated by the arrow in panel A), calculated FFR equals 0.74. However, FFR calculated just distal (panel B) and just proximal to the stent (panel C), are identical, indicating that there is no pressure drop across the stent, that the conductance of the stented segment is normal, and that the stent is well deployed. When the sensor is further pulled back, to the left main (panel D), FFR is almost equal to 1.0. The difference in FFR between the distal part of the vessel and the stented segment, and between the stented segment and the left main, indicates diffuse disease distal and proximal to the stented segment. Note: especially in a case like this patient, the use of intravenous instead of intracoronary adenosine is helpful because a pressure pull-back recording at sustained hyperemia can be made.*

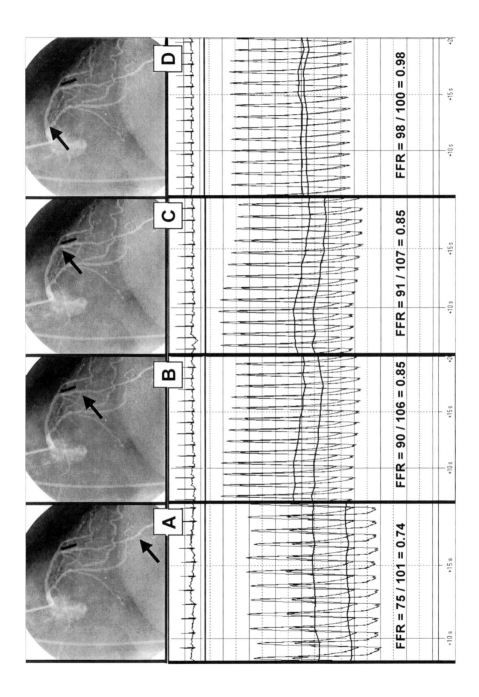

those vessels is not uncommon. This observation justifies the study in normal persons as described in this chapter.

At last, these observations indicate that for the evaluation of the conductance of a dilated or stented coronary segment, the pressure measurements should be performed immediately proximal and immediately distal to the treated segment. When the sensor is positioned several centimeters distal to the segment under study, the pressure gradient which may happen to exist during hyperemia reflects the conductance of both the treated segment and the remainder of the atherosclerotic vessel. If, after stent implantation, FFR is still below 0.90, a slow pull-back of the pressure sensor during intravenous adenosine-induced maximal hyperemia is the easiest way to unmask the actual location of the abnormal resistance and to differentiate between suboptimal stent deployment and abnormal

conductance of the more distal or proximal part of the vessel. When intracoronary vasodilators are preferred, a hyperemic pressure measurement should first be obtained immediately distal to the stent and thereafter just proximal to the stented segment. If the two values of FFR are identical or very close to each other, one can state that the conductance of the stented segment is normal (figure 10.5). Also, in case of irregular or diffusely diseased vessels, the pull-back curve of the pressure sensor under maximum hyperemia is the best way to quantify and localize abnormal residual resistance, both during a diagnostic procedure or after a coronary intervention.

References.

1. Hoffmann JIE: Maximal coronary flow and the concept of coronary vascular reserve. *Circulation* 1984; 70: 153-159.
2. Nissen SE, Gurley JC: Assessment of the functional significance of coronary stenosis: Is digital angiography the answer ? *Circulation* 1990; 81: 1431-1435.
3. Kirkeeide RL, Gould KL, Parsel L: Assessment of coronary stenoses by myocardial perfusion during pharmacologic coronary vasodilation: VIII. Validation of coronary flow reserve as a single integrated functional measure of stenosis severity reflecting all its geometric dimensions. *J Am Coll Cardiol* 1986; 7: 103-113.
4. Gould KL, Kirkeeide RL, Buchi M: Coronary flow reserve as a physiologic measure of stenosis severity. *J Am Coll Cardiol* 1990; 15: 459-74.
5. Hongo M, Nakatsuka T, Watanabe N, Takenaka H, Tanaka M, Kinoshita O, Okubo S, Sekiguchi M: Effects of heart rate on phasic coronary blood flow pattern and flow reserve in patients with normal coronary arteries: A study with an intravascular Doppler catheter and spectral analysis. *Am Heart J* 1994; 127: 545-551.

6. Zijlstra F, Reiber JHC, Juilliere Y, Serruys PW: Normalization of coronary flow reserve by percutaneous transluminal coronary angioplasty. *Am J Cardiol* 1988; 61: 55-63.

7. Kern MJ, Deligonul U, Tatineni S, Serota H, Aguirre FV, Hilton TC: Intravenous adenosine continous infusion and low dose bolus administration for determination of coronary vasodilatory reserve in patients with and without coronary artery disease. *J Am Coll Cardiol* 1991; 18: 718-729.

8. Wilson RF: Assessment of the human coronary circulation using a Doppler catheter. *Am J Cardiol* 1991; 67: 44D-56D.

9. McGinn AL, White CW, Wilson RF: Interstudy variability of coronary flow reserve. Influence of heart rate, arterial pressure, and ventricular preload. *Circulation* 1990; 81: 1319-1330.

10. De Bruyne B, Bartunek J, Sys SU, Pijls NHJ, Heyndrickx GR, Wijns W. Simultaneous coronary pressure and flow velocity measurements in humans. Feasibility, reproducibility, and hemodynamic dependence of coronary flow velocity reserve, hyperemic flow versus pressure slope index, and fractional flow reserve. *Circulation* 1996; 94: 1842-1849.

11. Pijls NHJ, Van Gelder B, Van der Voort P, Peels K, Bracke FALE, Bonnier JJRM, El Gamal MIH. Fractional Flow Reserve: a useful index to evaluate the influence of an epicardial coronary stenosis on myocardial blood flow. *Circulation* 1995; 92: 3183-3193.

12. Gould KL. Pressure-flow characteristics of coronary stenoses in unsedated dogs at rest and during coronary vasodilation. *Circ Res* 1978; 43: 242-253.

13. Folts JD, Gallagher K, Rowe GG: Hemodynamic effects of controlled degrees of coronary artery stenosis in short-term and long-term studies in dogs. *J Thorac Cardiov Surg.* 1977; 73: 722-727.

14. Young DF, Cholvin NR, Roth AC: Flow in the major branches of the left coronary artery during experimental coronary insufficiency in the unanesthetized dog. *Circ Res* 1975; 735-743.

15. Pijls NHJ, Van Son J, Kirkeeide RL, De Bruyne B, Gould KL. Experimental basis of determining maximum coronary, myocardial, and collateral blood flow by pressure measurements for assessing functional stenosis severity before and after PTCA. *Circulation 1993; 87: 1354-1367.*

Chapter 11

FRACTIONAL FLOW RESERVE TO DISTINGUISH SIGNIFICANT STENOSIS: USE AT DIAGNOSTIC CATHERIZATION
Cut-off values to detect reversible ischemia

11.1 Rationale for cut-off values of invasive indexes.

The ultimate goal of every diagnostic method should be to facilitate clinical decision-making and to enable evaluation of the results of therapeutic interventions. This is especially true with respect to physiologic investigations in the catheterization laboratory. A number of studies establishing the value of coronary pressure measurement and FFR to distinguish between functionally significant and non-significant stenoses, is presented in this chapter.

Coronary arteriography remains one of the cornerstones of diagnosis in patients with coronary artery disease and will remain necessary to define the presence, location, and extent of disease as well as the anatomic possibilities for revascularization. Nevertheless, it has been well recognized that the functional significance of an arteriographic lesion cannot be determined from the angiogram alone.

In most patients with coronary artery disease, the decision to perform a revascularization procedure should be based not only on coronary anatomy, but also on the functional severity of a lesion. Ideally, such information should be obtained before cardiac catheterization, by non-invasive tests such as exercise testing, Thallium scintigraphy, or stress-echocardiography. In clinical practice, however, many patients enter the catheterization room without previously documented objective proof of reversible ischemia by non-invasive tests. Such tests may have been inconclusive, negative, or simply not performed. Moreover, in case of multivessel disease it is often not possible to predict by non-invasive testing which lesion is the culprit one and should be dilated, and which is not. In other patients, estimation of angiographic stenosis severity can be difficult because of overprojection and other shortcomings of the imaging technique.

Therefore, much research has been devoted by many investigators for decades to develop physiologic indexes, which can be obtained "on the spot" in the catheterization laboratory and enable on-line decision-making with respect to revascularization of a particular lesion. For that purpose, a sharp discriminating value of such an index with minimal overlap between "significant" and "non-significant" values is mandatory.

As outlined in chapter 9 and 10, neither absolute flow nor coronary flow (velocity) reserve fulfill that condition. Due to the variability of normal values, the hemodynamic dependence, and the failure to account for collateral flow, the clinical usefulness of these indexes is clouded by a wide gray zone between values which are or are not associated with inducible ischemia. Moreover, because coronary flow (velocity) reserve does not distinguish between epicardial and microvascular disease, further scatter is introduced (figure 11.1).

Because FFR_{myo} has one unique and unequivocal normal value of 1.0 irrespective of the patient and artery under study (chapter 10), because that index is not influenced by the prevailing hemodynamic conditions (chapter 9), and because it takes into account collateral blood flow (chapter 16), theoretically it is likely that a well-defined cut-off point of FFR_{myo} exists, discriminating lesions which are or are not associated with inducible ischemia, with minimal overlap. Furthermore, because in normal subjects no myocardial ischemia can be provoked[1], not even during exhaustive exercise, it is likely that such a cut-off point will be lower than 1.0.

In this chapter, several independent studies are presented to establish such a cut-off value. As will be shown, that value is approximately 0.75 with minimal overlap. Therefore, from a practical point of view it can be stated that, when the clinical significance of a particular coronary lesion is uncertain, a value of FFR_{myo} of ≤ 0.75 justifies revascularization (which, in the case of PTCA, can be performed "on-the-spot"), whereas a value of FFR_{myo} of > 0.75 mostly excludes reversible ischemia and indicates that an intervention is generally not appropriate. Some special anatomic or physiologic situations, such as sequential stenoses within one vessel, previous subendocardial infarction, and left ventricular hypertrophy, will be discussed separately (chapter 13).

In the first study in 60 patients the results of regular exercise testing were correlated to FFR_{myo}, measured at subsequent coronary arteriography.

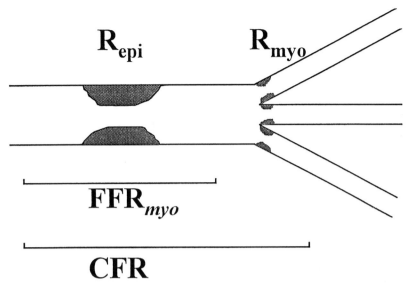

Figure 11.1 *Absolute Coronary Flow Reserve (CFR) is an index of the serial resistances of an epicardial stenosis and microvascular disease, and does not distinguish between these two entities. Fractional flow reserve (FFR) is a specific index of epicardial stenosis but does not account for microvascular disease.*

In that study, it was found that in no patient with $FFR_{myo} > 0.72$, reversible ischemia was inducible by exercise testing. Although known confounding factors influencing the exercise test results were avoided, in this study false negative exercise tests must have been present in 10-15% of the patients, according to the well-known limited sensitivity of well performed exercise tests even in a selected study population[2,3]. This may explain why in a few patients in that study population, FFR-values less than 0.72 were observed in the presence of negative exercise tests. False positive tests in that study were less likely because positive tests were followed by revascularization, followed in turn by a repeated exercise test which had returned to negative in all but one patient. *Therefore, that first study, presented in paragraph 11.2, has established the lower threshold value of* FFR_{myo} *, associated with normal stress-testing or the absence of inducible ischemia.*

In the second study, performed in a subsequent cohort of 60 PTCA patients, false positive and false negative exercise tests were completely excluded (paragraph 11.3). That study was restricted to patients with single vessel disease and a clearly positive exercise test before PTCA which returned to normal after PTCA. In that specific study population, a value of FFR_{myo} of

0.74 was found to discriminate best between stenoses which are or are not associated with reversible ischemia. The separation was almost complete and overlap minimal, with only 2 exceptions out of 60 patients. *Therefore, this study has established the upper threshold value of FFR$_{myo}$, associated with inducible ischemia.*

A third study comparing dobutamine echocardiography with FFR values in patients with one-vessel coronary artery disease confirmed that a threshold value of 0.75 accurately discriminates lesions associated with dobutamine-induced wall motion abnormalities from those which are not (paragraph 11.4).

Having established with these studies that the cut-off point should be close to 0.75, a final prospective and more general study was performed during diagnostic catheterization in patients with intermediate anatomic lesions in whom a definite diagnosis with respect to inducible ischemia could not be established by regular tests. In this study, a unique gold standard of inducible ischemia was composed of all presently used non-invasive tests. It was shown that the diagnostic accuracy of that gold standard was almost 100% and FFR$_{myo}$ was compared to that gold standard. In that study, the diagnostic accuracy of FFR$_{myo}$ for correct identification of reversible ischemia was proven to be approximately 95% with a sensitivity of 90% and a specificity of 100%. That final study in diagnostic catheterization is presented in chapter 12. The 3 other studies are presented below.

11.2   Relation between FFR$_{myo}$ and exercise-induced myocardial ischemia. Part I: Lower threshold value of FFR$_{myo}$, not associated with inducible ischemia.

11.2.1 Study design.

Sixty patients with normal left ventricular function and an isolated lesion in a major coronary artery were studied. All patients underwent a maximal bicycle exercise test and, within the following 6 hours, intracoronary pressure measurements to determine resting and hyperemic translesional pressure gradient and myocardial fractional flow reserve as described in chapter 5.

To minimize as much as possible the occurrence of false positive exercise ECG's, the following inclusion criteria were applied: 1. No history of myocardial infarction or the presence of abnormal wall motion as assessed by a biplane left ventricular angiogram; 2. A normal resting ECG; 3. No electrolytes abnormalities; 4. No left ventricular hypertrophy or mitral valve prolapse as assessed by echocardiography.

To minimize as much as possible the occurrence of false negative results at stress ECG, the patients were selected only if:
1. They were physically able to perform a maximal bicycle stress test. In the absence of obvious signs of myocardial ischemia, a heart rate of at least 85% of the maximal predicted heart rate was required; 2. The reference diameter of the lesion to be assessed was > 2.6 mm in order to avoid a too small myocardial region at risk of ischemia; 3. All cardiac medication had been stopped at least 36 hours before the stress test and replaced by aspirin. Despite this selection, one should realize that statistically 10-15% of this population will still have false negative exercise tests.

11.2.2 Values of FFR$_{myo}$ not associated with ST depression during exercise.

In the study population as a whole, FFR$_{myo}$ varied from 0.28 to 0.98 (mean ± SD: 0.60 ± 0.18), ΔP_{max} from 5 to 88 mmHg (mean ± SD: 37 ± 19 mmHg), and ΔP_{rest}, from 0 to 73 mmHg (mean ± SD: 23 ± 21 mmHg).
Figure 11.2 shows the values of FFR$_{myo}$ and the transstenotic pressure gradient according to the results of the exercise ECG. Not surprisingly, FFR$_{myo}$ was significantly lower (0.50 ± 0.12% versus 0.77 ± 0.13%, P < .01) and both ΔP_{max} and ΔP_{rest} were significantly higher (47 ± 14 versus 20 ± 13 mmHg and 31 ± 20 versus 11 ± 14 mmHg, respectively; both P < .01) in patients with a positive exercise ECG compared to patients with a negative exercise ECG.
There was some overlap between the values of myocardial fractional flow reserve associated with a normal and abnormal stress test and with an abnormal test. However, of major importance for clinical decision-making in the catheterization laboratory, is that the value of FFR$_{myo}$ above which the exercise ECG was uniformly normal, is 0.72 (100% sensitivity level of 0.72). The values of ΔP_{max} and of ΔP_{rest} below which the exercise ECG were uniformly normal were 21 mmHg and 2 mmHg respectively, with considerably more overlap. From figure 11.2, it can be observed that the hyperemic pressure gradient has some value for discriminating patients with

inducible ischemia at exercise testing, but the resting pressure gradient has not. At last, because in a population as in this study, false negative exercise tests will still be present in 10-15% of the patients, this could explain the 7 negative exercise tests (12%) in patients with FFR_{myo} below 0.72.

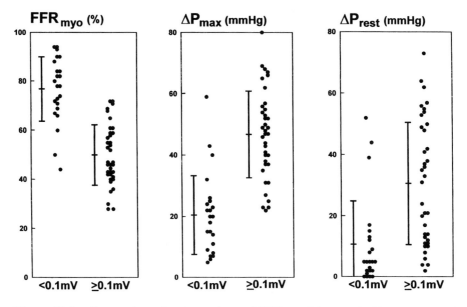

Figure 11.2. *Scatterplots showing values of FFR_{myo}, ΔP_{max}, and ΔP_{rest} associated with normal and abnormal exercise ECG (< 0.1 mV and ≥ 0.1 mV, respectively).*

11.2.3 FFR_{myo} versus the magnitude of ST depression during ischemia.

It has been demonstrated in animal studies that ST-segment abnormalities at exercise occur only when myocardial flow is reduced by at least 25-30% and that generally a correlation exists between the ST-segment changes and both the magnitude of the flow deprivation and the intramyocardial oxygen tension [4-9]. A similar relation has been reported between myocardial blood flow and the endocardial electrocardiogram[10]. A linear relation has been reported between the magnitude of ST depression and the severity of myocardial flow deprivation[11].

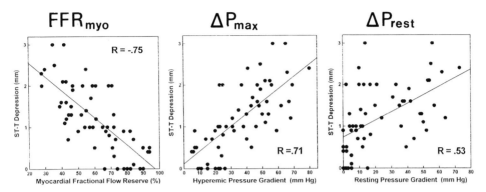

Figure 11.3 *Scatterplots showing the relation between FFR$_{myo}$, ΔP$_{max}$, and ΔP$_{rest}$ and the magnitude of ST depression (vertical axis) during peak exercise.*

Also in the present study, a correlation was observed between ST-segment depression and pressure-derived indexes (figure 11.3). FFR$_{myo}$ correlated well with the magnitude of ST-segment depression during peak exercise (y = 0.032x+3.15 ; r = - 0.75, SEE = 0.53 ; P < .01). Also ΔP$_{max}$ correlated well with the magnitude of ST-segment depression on the exercise ECG (y = 0.030x+0.11 ; r = .71, SEE = 0.56 ; P < .01). However, the correlation between ΔP$_{rest}$ and the extent of ST-segment depression (y = 0.020x+0.74 ; r = .53, SEE = 0.67 ; P < .01) was significantly weaker (P < .001 versus both FFR$_{myo}$ and ΔP$_{max}$).

Among the patients who developed significant ST-segment depression during exercise, weak but significant correlations were observed between heart rate at the initial occurrence of 0.1 mV ST-segment depression and FFR$_{myo}$ (r = 0.39, P < .05), ΔP$_{max}$(r = -0.36, P < .05), and ΔP$_{rest}$ (r = -.041, P < .05). These findings suggest that the intensity of ischemia (rather than the extent of ischemia in terms of area at risk) within a given vascular bed plays a major role in producing the clinical range of ST-segment depression. At last, the percent correct classification of the exercise ECG as a function of the different pressure-derived indexes, is shown in figure 11.4.

11.2.4 Diagnostic importance of hyperemic versus resting measurements.

Figure 11.2 shows a larger overlap between positive and negative exercise ECG as predicted by the ΔP_{rest} than by the ΔP_{max} or FFR_{myo}. As illustrated in figure 11.4, the discriminating power of FFR_{myo} and ΔP_{max} (both obtained at maximum vasodilation) in predicting the results of the exercise ECG was significantly larger than that of ΔP_{rest}: 88%, 84%, and 74%, respectively. These results emphasize the importance of hyperemic measurements to evaluate the functional repercussions of a coronary stenosis on the underlying myocardium. Under normal circumstances, myocardial resistance and blood flow are fit to meet the metabolic demands of the myocardium by coronary autoregulation. At rest, the coronary vascular system behaves as a low-flow, high-resistance system in which flow is determined by the peripheral resistance. During maximal exercise or during pharmacological vasodilation, peripheral resistances in normal individuals decrease by a factor four to five. In the case of epicardial narrowing and increase in epicardial resistance, peripheral myocardial resistance decreases and flow is determined by resistances in series: the resistance of the coronary stenosis and the resistance of the myocardial vascular bed. At rest, the proximal stenosis has to be severe before its resistance exceeds that of the resting myocardial vascular bed. Resting blood flow will not be hampered by the

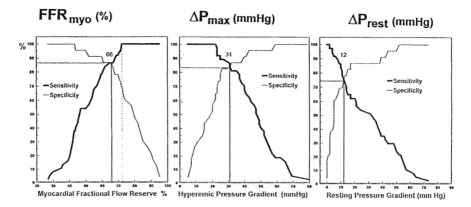

Figure 11.4 *Graphs showing percent correct classification of an abnormal exercise ECG (sensitivity, %) and percent correct classification of a normal exercise ECG (specificity, %) as a function of the different pressure-derived indexes.*

narrowing until the lesion reaches approximately an 80% diameter stenosis[12,13]. In contrast, during maximal vasodilation, the peripheral myocardial resistances are minimal and hyperemic flow is determined mainly by the severity of the narrowing. Accordingly, measurements performed under conditions of resting flow are less sensitive measures of stenosis severity. Since translesional pressure gradient is highly dependent on blood flow, ΔP_{rest} is expected to correlate less closely with indexes of exercise-induced ischemia than ΔP_{max} and FFR_{myo}, which are both obtained under conditions of minimal myocardial resistance (conditions that are also supposed to prevail during maximum exercise). In addition, from a clinical point of view, making functional measurements of stenosis severity from ΔP_{max} rather than ΔP_{rest} is intuitively reasonable, since the functional capacity and the complaints of patients with ischemic heart disease are determined mainly by maximum achievable myocardial blood flow rather than by resting flow.

11.2.5 Methodologic limitations.

It is extremely difficult to establish the value of any new diagnostic index when the test to which that index is compared, has a limited accuracy in itself, as is the case for exercise testing in a general population as in this study. As a consequence, this study allows only to conclude that inducible ischemia is unlikely above a FFR_{myo} of 0.72. It does not prove the converse, i.e. that inducible ischemia will uniformly be present below that value. To establish also this converse issue, it was necessary to design a study population in such a way, that false positive and false negative exercise tests were completely excluded. Testing of FFR_{myo} in such a population, is described below.

Table 11.1 *Matrix describing myocardial fractional flow reserve (FFR$_{myo}$), coronary fractional flow reserve (FFR$_{cor}$), and fractional collateral blood flow (Q$_c$/Q^N) before and after PTCA and at balloon occlusion in the patient of figure 11.5. The values in such a matrix are independent of loading conditions.*

	Before PTCA	At occlusion	After PTCA
FFR$_{myo}$	0.50	0.18	0.97
FFR$_{cor}$	0.39	0.00	0.96
Q$_c$/Q^N	0.11	0.18	0.01

11.3 Relation between FFR$_{myo}$ and exercise-induced myocardial ischemia. Part II: Upper threshold value of FFR$_{myo}$ associated with inducible ischemia.

11.3.1 Study design.

The study population in this second study consisted of another 60 consecutive patients (41 men, 19 women, age 57 ± 8 years, range 39 - 74 years) accepted for elective PTCA with stable angina pectoris, single vessel coronary disease (LAD: 39; LCX: 8; RCA: 13), normal left ventricular function, and a clearly positive exercise test < 24 hours before PTCA. Exercise testing in these patients was performed on a bicycle ergometer starting with a workload of 20 W that was increased by 20 W every minute. The test was considered positive when ST-depression of ≥ 1 mm occurred 80 msec after the J-point in at least 2 adjacent leads.

At the PTCA, fractional flow reserve (FFR) was determined before and after balloon dilatation according to the protocol described below. After successful PTCA, all medication was stopped except nifidepine 20 mg b.i.d. which was stopped 48 h later, and aspirin 80 mg daily which was continued. The exercise test was then repeated 5-7 days after the PTCA. *Only if this second exercise test was completely normal, the pre-PTCA value of FFR was considered to be compatible with inducible ischemia and the post-PTCA value was not.* If the second exercise test was still positive, coronary arteriography, including determination of FFR, was repeated within 10 days to confirm or exclude early restenosis.

11.3.2 Coronary pressure measurements.

At cardiac catheterization, arterial pressure (P$_a$) was measured by a 6-8F guiding catheter, and venous pressure (P$_v$) was measured by a 6F multipurpose catheter in the right atrium. As P$_v$ was close to zero in all patients, not having measured P$_v$ would not have affected the results of this study.

Coronary pressure measurements during maximum hyperemia were performed immediately before and 10 minutes after PTCA and the fractional flow reserve of the coronary artery and its dependent myocardium was calculated as outlined in chapter 4 by:

$$FFR_{cor} = \frac{P_d - P_w}{P_a - P_w}$$

and

$$FFR_{myo} = \frac{P_d - P_v}{P_a - P_v} \approx \frac{P_d}{P_a}$$

where P_a, P_v, and P_d represent mean arterial pressure, central venous pressure, and distal coronary pressure, all measured at maximum coronary hyperemia; and where P_w represents coronary wedge pressure during balloon occlusion.

The difference between FFR_{myo} and FFR_{cor} represents the contribution of collateral flow to total myocardial perfusion and is called fractional collateral flow[15-18]. The calculated values of FFR_{myo}, FFR_{cor}, and fractional collateral blood flow of the patient in figure 11.5, are summarized in table 11.1.

11.3.3 Procedural and clinical results.

No complications occurred due to the specific study protocol in any of the patients. In all patients, excellent pressure signals were obtained before and after PTCA. In 7 patients, no reliable coronary wedge pressure could be recorded during balloon inflation.

In one patient, a large dissection with occlusion of the proximal left anterior descending artery occurred after the second balloon inflation and emergency bypass surgery was necessary. In another patient, no satisfactory angiographic result could be obtained despite many inflations. Because of recurrent angina at rest 2 days later, bypass surgery was performed and no post-PTCA exercise test was available. Therefore, in our group of 60 PTCA patients fulfilling the primary inclusion criteria, an angiographically successful result was obtained in 58 patients and 56 patients had a normal exercise test 5-7 days after the PTCA. Therefore, based upon Bayesian considerations, it can be stated that inducible ischemia had been present in these 56 patients before PTCA and absent thereafter[19,20]. This means that the FFR_{myo} values in those patients before and after PTCA represent the "normal" and "abnormal" range of FFR_{myo}, i.e. values which are or are not

Figure 11.5 (opposite page) *Simultaneous phasic and mean recordings of arterial (P$_a$), distal coronary (P$_d$) and central venous pressure (P$_v$) before, during, and after PTCA of a LAD stenosis in a 59-year-old lady. For the sake of clarity, P$_v$ is not displayed in the panels B to F. P$_a$ is measured by the 7F guiding catheter and P$_d$ by a pressure guide wire with the sensor at 3 cm from the floppy tip. A: Before introducing the pressure guide wire into the coronary artery, the tip of the pressure wire is at a location close to the tip of the guiding catheter and equality of P$_a$ and P$_d$ at that point is verified. B: The pressure wire is advanced into the coronary artery and crosses the stenosis (#). C: After start of i.v. adenosine infusion, steady state hyperemic pressure curves are obtained, enabling calculation of myocardial fractional flow reserve (FFR$_{myo}$) before PTCA. D: The balloon is advanced into the stenosis and inflated. E: The balloon is deflated and withdrawn. The wire remains in the distal coronary artery. Note the large artificial gradient merely caused by the presence of the deflated balloon at the site of the stenosis. F: After i.v. adenosine infusion has been started again, steady state hyperemic pressure curves are obtained, enabling calculation of FFR$_{myo}$ after PTCA. G: At the end of the procedure, the pressure wire is withdrawn to the tip of the guiding catheter, and it is verified that no drift has occurred during the procedure.*

associated with inducible ischemia (figure 11.6). In the remaining 2 patients, the exercise test after 5-7 days was still positive and coronary arteriography was repeated subsequently. In both of them, the angiographic result was still satisfactory and FFR$_{myo}$, being 0.94 and 0.76 at the end of the initial PTCA-procedure, was 0.84 and 0.82 at the repeated angiography. For that reason, the pre-PTCA values of FFR$_{myo}$ in these 2 patients cannot be claimed to be associated with inducible ischemia, which is indicated in figure 11.6 by hatching these 2 points.

The hemodynamic data during catheterization and PTCA are summarized in table 11.2. In all patients steady state hyperemia was achieved within 2 minutes of starting the adenosine infusion. In a few patients, some prolongation of the PR-interval occurred but no second degree AV-block was observed. In the majority of the patients, the adenosine infusion was accompanied by some chest pain or a burning sensation in the neck. During infusion, a small decrease of mean arterial pressure and increase of heart rate was observed compared to baseline, as shown in table 11.2.

The maximum hyperemic transstenotic gradients before and after PTCA are presented in figure 11.6. The highest hyperemic gradient after successful PTCA was 24 mmHg. The lowest hyperemic gradient before PTCA and associated with inducible ischemia was 19 mmHg. This indicates that the gradient itself, when measured at maximum hyperemia with an adequately thin wire, is also a useful parameter, especially if blood pressure is normal.

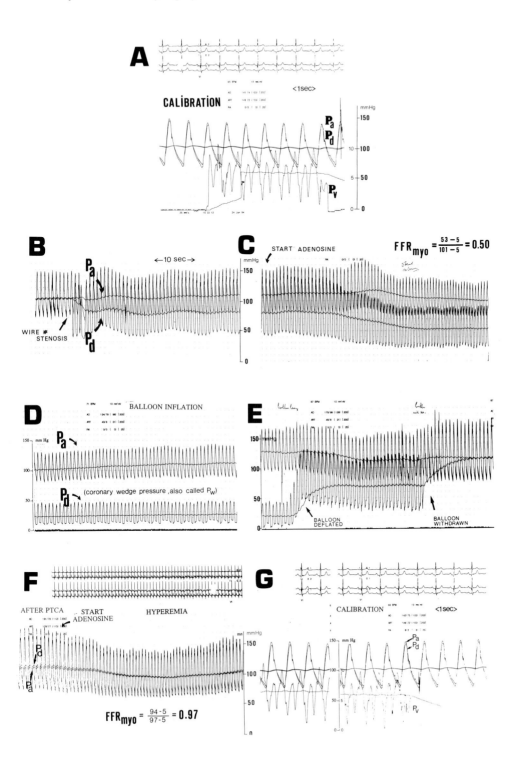

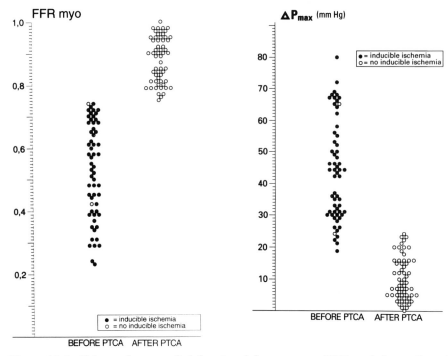

Figure 11.6 *Values of myocardial fractional flow reserve (FFR$_{myo}$, left panel) and maximum hyperemic transstenotic pressure gradient (ΔP$_{max}$, right panel) before and after PTCA. Those values associated with proven ischemia, are indicated by solid points and those values not associated with ischemia are indicated by open points. As explained in the text, in 2 patients doubt existed regarding inducible ischemia before PTCA. These patients are indicated by hatched points.*

11.3.4 Myocardial fractional flow reserve (FFR$_{myo}$).

In all patients, FFR$_{myo}$ before PTCA was ≤ 0.74. In other words, exercise-induced ischemia at exercise testing was always accompanied by FFR$_{myo}$ ≤ 0.74. Therefore, 0.74 can be considered in this study as the upper threshold of FFR$_{myo}$ associated with inducible ischemia. After successful PTCA (as assessed by the reversal of the positive exercise test result to negative), FFR$_{myo}$ was always > 0.74 (figure 11.6). Therefore, it can be stated that well-defined ranges of FFR$_{myo}$, associated with inducible ischemia or not, can be distinguished with minimal overlap. As a result, the accuracy of FFR$_{myo}$ to indicate or exclude inducible ischemia (i.e., to indicate or exclude a functionally significant coronary stenosis) was close to 100% in this study population.

11.3.5 Coronary fractional flow reserve (FFR$_{cor}$) and fractional collateral flow.

To assess the relative contribution of arterial and collateral flows to myocardial blood flow, P$_w$ must be known[15]. Therefore, the separate contributions of collateral and coronary flow to myocardial flow could be obtained in those 53 patients in whom P$_w$ was measured. The results for the specific patient shown in figure 11.5, are presented in table 11.1, while table 11.3 summarizes the results for all 53 patients.

The pressure-derived fractional collateral blood flow was 15 ± 8% (range 2 - 35%) before and 4 ± 3% (range 0 - 12%) after PTCA. From the differences in FFR$_{myo}$ and FFR$_{cor}$ in these tables, it is apparent that without knowing the contribution of collateral flow to myocardial flow, classical coronary flow indexes may overestimate the physiologic impact of the stenosis.

11.3.6 Discussion and clinical implications.

As validated in chapter 10, normal FFR$_{myo}$ equals 1. Therefore, because in healthy subjects no myocardial ischemia is inducible, not even during exhaustive exercise, the value of FFR$_{myo}$ below which ischemia may be inducible is likely to be less than 1.0. To find that cut-off value and thus define ranges of values of FFR$_{myo}$ that are associated with inducible ischemia or not, it was necessary to have at our disposal a test which unequivocally discriminates between the presence and absence of inducible ischemia.

To achieve that goal, we selected a particular group of patients with stable angina, single vessel disease, normal LV function and a positive exercise test before PTCA that reversed to negative after angiographically successful PTCA. In such a population, false negative and false positive tests are excluded and both the positive predictive value of a positive exercise test before PTCA and the negative predictive value of a negative exercise test after PTCA, are nearly 100%[19,20]. Therefore, in this particular group of patients, the exercise test could be used as a completely reliable standard to indicate or exclude inducible ischemia and to assess ranges of FFR$_{myo}$ indicating or excluding significant coronary artery disease. As shown in figure 11.6, there was only minimal overlap between "normal" and "pathologic" values and the cut-off point was 0.74. This value is very close to the value of 0.72 found in the earlier study presented in paragraph 11.2.

It should be noted in this context that in most patients FFR$_{myo}$ after successful PTCA, although obviously sufficient to prevent inducible ischemia, did not completely return to values as encountered in normal coronary arteries (table 11.3, in comparison to table 10.1). Further data and discussion about FFR_{myo} values after coronary interventions, will be presented in chapter 14.

No adverse reactions were observed during adenosine infusion except some chest discomfort, due to its physiologic action.

The results of this study would not have been different if P_v would not have been measured. For clinical practice, therefore, measurement of P_v can be omitted, as long as conditions associated with markedly increased central venous pressure are absent. Some numerical examples on this issue, are presented in chapter 16.

A last qualification in this context is that the reaction of a diseased coronary artery after pharmacologic vasodilation can be different from exercise induced stress (paragraph 13.5). In the latter case, arteriolar vasodilation can be accompanied by paradoxical constriction at the site of the stenosis, provoked by sympathetic nerve stimulation[21]. Whatever the role of such a mechanism may be, in most patients exercise induced ST-depression before PTCA was associated with $FFR_{myo} \leq 0.74$ and absence of ST-depression after PTCA with $FFR_{myo} > 0.74$ in this selected study population.

Table 11.2 *Hemodynamic data in the study population of paragraph 11.3 (n = 60) at rest and at adenosine induced maximum hyperemia. HR: heart rate (bpm); MAP: mean arterial pressure (mmHG); ΔP: transstenotic pressure gradient (mmHg). RAP: mean right atrial pressure (mmHg).*

	Before PTCA	After PTCA
MAP_{rest}	101 ± 15	97 ± 17
$MAP_{hyperemia}$	93 ± 16	86 ± 15
ΔP_{rest}	26 ± 13	6 ± 4
$\Delta P_{hyperemia}$	44 ± 16	10 ± 7
HR_{rest}	68 ± 14	67 ± 12
$HR_{hyperemia}$	74 ± 18	73 ± 15
RAP_{rest}	2 ± 3	2 ± 2
$RAP_{hyperemia}$	3 ± 3	3 ± 2

Table 11.3 *Mean values ± 1 SD of myocardial fractional flow reserve (FFR$_{myo}$), coronary fractional flow reserve (FFR$_{cor}$), and fractional collateral flow (Q$_c$/Q^N) before and after successful PTCA and at balloon occlusion in the patients of paragraph 11.3 (n = 53). Those 7 patients in whom P$_w$ at balloon occlusion could not be reliably measured and in whom only FFR$_{myo}$ is available, have been omitted.*

	Before PTCA	At occlusion	After PTCA
FFR$_{myo}$	0.53 ± 0.15	0.23 ± 0.10	0.88 ± 0.07
FFR$_{cor}$	0.38 ± 0.19	-	0.83 ± 0.12
Q$_c$/Q^N	0.15 ± 0.08	0.23 ± 0.10	0.04 ± 0.03

The clinical implications of this study may be important both in diagnostic and interventional catheterization. In diagnostic catheterization, the significance of an epicardial coronary lesion in terms of inducibility of ischemia can be better assessed. In patients with an intermediate stenosis in one of the large epicardial coronary arteries, this technique can be particularly helpful in deciding on revascularization if ambiguity exists with respect to the functional significance of that stenosis, as further discussed and applied in chapter 13.

In interventional cardiology, great concern exists about the large number of patients undergoing PTCA without prior objective evidence of ischemia at exercise test, thallium scintigraphy, or other tests[22]. Realizing that the prevalence of coronary artery stenosis in an arbitrary population of asymptomatic 60-year-old males is at least 20%[23], it is not unlikely that in a number of patients with negative non-invasive tests but accepted for PTCA on anatomic grounds, the coronary lesion found at angiography is coincidental and the PTCA is performed unnecessarily. By measuring FFR$_{myo}$ before PTCA, these cases can be better identified and unnecessary PTCA's may be avoided. Recently, a large prospective randomized multicenter study has been completed (DEFER Study), where a coronary intervention was either performed or deferred in patients who were referred for PTCA without documented ischemia and who had a stenosis with a FFR$_{myo}$ of $\geq$ 0.75. This study indicated the safety of deferring PTCA in stenosis with FFR > 0.75; and confirmed the appropriateness of performing PTCA in stenosis with FFR < 0.75. This study is discussed in more detail in chapter 15. The outcome of this and similar studies warrants physiologic measurements "on the spot" before performing a coronary intervention of a stenosis without prior documented ischemia.

In conclusion, myocardial fractional flow reserve (FFR_{myo}) is a lesion-specific index which reflects the effect of the epicardial stenosis on maximum myocardial perfusion. In this study, in patients with single vessel disease and normal left ventricular function, a value of FFR_{myo} of 0.74 discriminated accurately between lesions associated with inducible ischemia or not. Therefore, FFR_{myo} is a reliable index to assess the functional significance of an epicardial coronary artery stenosis and especially useful for clinical decisions in the catheterization laboratory with respect to the question if an intervention is appropriate or not.

11.4 Comparison of dobutamine echocardiography and fractional flow reserve.

From the two preceding studies it appears that the FFR value of approximately 0.75 is optimal to distinguish stenoses which are associated with exercise-induced reversible myocardial ischemia from those which are not. Dobutamine echocardiography is another established and widely applied method for the detection and risk stratification of coronary artery disease[24-29]. To further validate the clinical usefulness of FFR as a surrogate for non-invasive stress testing this pressure-derived index was compared to the results of dobutamine echocardiography[30].

11.4.1 Methods.

Seventy-five patients with isolated single-vessel coronary artery disease and normal left ventricular function were selected. The lesion was located in the left anterior descending coronary artery in 38 patients, in the right coronary artery in 32, and in the left circumflex coronary artery in 5 of them. All patients underwent dobutamine stress testing within 6 hours before catheterization. Administration of beta-adrenergic blocking agents and calcium channel blocking agents was stopped 36 hours before the test and patients were given molsidomine, 4 mg three times daily. Dobutamine echocardiography was performed according to McNeill et al[31]. Dobutamine was infused starting at the dosages of 10 μg/kg/min and increased by 10 μg/kg/min every 3 minutes up to the dosage of 40 μg/kg/min. In case of inadequate increase in heart rate, a bolus of 1.0 mg of atropine was injected during the last minute of the test. A two-dimensional echocardiogram was monitored throughout the procedure in 4 standard views and analysed according to a 16-segment model[32]. Segmental wall motion were graded as follows: 1 = normal response to dobutamine (i.e. a progressive and synchronous increase in systolic contraction); 2 = hypokinesia (i.e. a reduction of systolic wall thickening and inward motion during dobutamine infusion as compared to the previous stage); 3 = akinesia (i.e. a lack of wall thickening or inward motion during dobutamine infusion); 4 = dyskinesia (i.e. an outward motion during dobutamine infusion). Coronary pressure measurements and calculation of fractional flow reserve were performed as described in chapter 5. Quantitative coronary angiography was performed and minimal luminal diameter, diameter stenosis and area stenosis were calculated from two views.

Thirty-seven patients had both dobutamine and exercise stress testing. The results of these non-invasive tests were compared side by side to the value of FFR.

11.4.2 Results.

The individual data of FFR of patients with (n = 42) and without (n = 33) dobutamine-induced wall motion abnormalities are shown in the left panel of figure 11.7. FFR was significantly lower in patients with a positive than in patients with a negative dobutamine stress test result (0.47 ± 0.12 versus 0.77 ± 0.15, P < 0.001), although a large overlap of the individual data was observed between the two groups. Sensitivity, specificity, positive and negative predictive values of dobutamine echocardiography for predicting a FFR ≤ 0.75 were 76%, 97%, 98% and 61%, respectively (table 11.4). The most severe degree of dyssynergy correlated markedly better with FFR (figure 11.7, right panel) than with the angiographic indices of stenoses severity (figure 11.8, right panels). Likewise, wall motion score index during dobutamine infusion correlated better with FFR than with the angiographic diameter stenosis (table 11.5).

Patients with false negative results on dobutamine echocardiography (FFR ≤ 0.75 and negative dobutamine echocardiographic findings) reached similar levels of heart rate, blood pressure and rate-pressure product during dobutamine infusion as those of patients with true positive dobutamine echocardiographic results (FFR ≤ 0.75 and positive dobutamine echocardiographics findings) (153 ± 9 vs 158 ± 13 bpm, 154±16 vs 153 ± 29 mmHg and 20,189 ± 3801 vs 19,738 ± 3,153 bpm mmHg, respectively, all P = NS). Furthermore, the incidence of submaximal stress test (heart rate < 85% of maximal age-predicted heart rate) was similar between patients with true negative (FFR ≥ 0.75 and negative dobutamine echocardiography) and patients with false negative echocardiography (46% [6 of 13] vs 45% [9 of 20], P = NS).

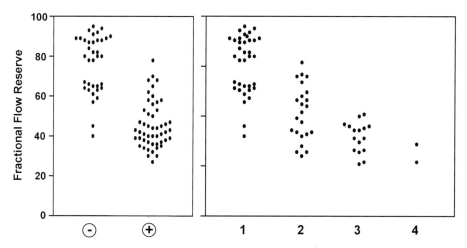

Figure 11.7 *Relation between FFR and dobutamine echocardiography (ECHO). The left panel shows the individual values of FFR in patients with positive (+) and negative (-) dobutamine stress test results. The right panel shows the relation between the most severe dyssynergy during peak dobutamine infusion and the value of FFR. r_s = Spearman rank correlation coefficient.*

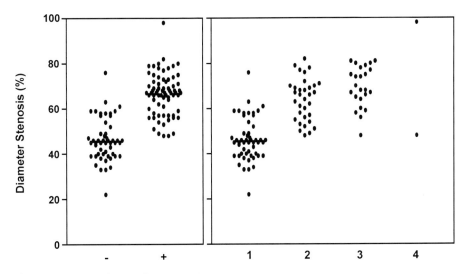

Figure 11.8 *Relation between the percent diameter stenosis and dobutamine echocardiography (ECHO). Left panel, individual angiographic values in patients with a positive (+) and a negative (-) dobutamine stress test result. Right panel, relation between the most severe dyssynergy during peak dobutamine infusion and diameter stenosis (1 = normokinesia; 2 = hypokinesia; 3 = akinesia; 4 = dyskinesia). r_s = Spearman rank correlation coefficient.*

11.4.3 Discussion.

These results indicate that, in patients with isolated single-vessel coronary artery disease and normal left ventricular function, values of FFR larger than 0.75 virtually exclude dobutamine-induced wall motion abnormalities. In only one out of the 42 patients with abnormal dobutamine echocardiographic findings, FFR was larger than 0.75. In addition, the magnitude of dobutamine-induced wall motion abnormalities correlated significantly better with FFR than with angiographic indexes of stenosis geometry. In contrast, in 39% of patients without dobutamine-induced wall motion abnormalities, FFR was lower than 0.75 suggesting a large proportion of false negative dobutamine stress tests. Therefore, the present results reinforce the FFR value of 0.75 as the lower threshold associated with a normal dobutamine stress test.

Table 11.4 *Sensitivity, specificity, positive and negative predictive values of dobutamine echocardiography according to angiographic indices and FFR.*

	Sensitivity (%)	Specificity (%)	PPV (%)	NPV (%)	Accuracy (%)
MLD ≤ 1 mm	83	61	58	85	72
MLD ≤ 1.5 mm	71	100	100	46	73
DS ≥ 50%	80	88	92	63	78
FFR_{myo} ≤ 0.75	76	97	98	61	80

DS: diameter stenosis; FFR_{myo}: myocardial fractional flow reserve; MLD: minimal lumen diameter; NPV: negative predictive value; PPV: positive predictive value.

Table 11.5 *Spearman rank correlation coefficients (r_s) and 95% confidence intervals (CI) between the degree of dyssynergy during peak dobutamine infusion and angiographic and functional indices of stenosis severity. Abbreviations: see table 11.4.*

	R_s	Lower CI	Upper CI
MLD	- 0.60	- 0.73	- 0.42
% DS	0.68	0.53	0.78
% AS	0.68	0.54	0.79
FFR_{myo}	- 0.77	- 0.84	- 0.65

11.5 Practical use of the cut-off value of 0.75 in diagnostic catheterization.

In the studies presented in this chapter, the values of 0.72 and 0.74 turned out to be a lower threshold for absence of inducible ischemia and an upper threshold for presence of inducible ischemia, respectively. These values are very close, indicating that there is only a narrow grey zone of overlap between values of FFR_{myo} associated with inducible ischemia or not.

In the next chapter, FFR_{myo} for on-line clinical decision-making is further validated and tested against a unique gold standard, composed of all presently used non-invasive diagnostic tests. In that prospective study, a value of 0.75 as cut-off point had an accuracy of 93% for correct identification of inducible ischemia. Therefore, despite the fact that a number of pathologic conditions have not been fully explored yet, from these studies we believe that a cut-off value of FFR_{myo} of 0.75 can be generally recommended to answer the clinical question whether a particular stenosis can be held responsible for reversible ischemia and if the patient can be helped by revascularization of that artery. Because, measurement of FFR_{myo} can be quickly and easily performed during diagnostic catheterization, on-line decisions can be made. This is especially useful in case of intermediate lesions, difficult coronary anatomy or overprojection, multiple lesions when it is not clear which stenosis is culprit and which is not, negative or unclear results of non-invasive tests, and other situations where doubt is present regarding if a particular stenosis is responsible for ischemia or not. Also after incomplete myocardial infarction, this cut-off value seems to remain useful (paragraph 13.1). Microvascular disease can lead to overestimation of FFR_{myo}, but does not affect the clinical applicability of FFR_{myo} in the interventional laboratory (paragraph 13.2). The conclusions so far can be summarized as follows:

In conclusion:

♦ *at diagnostic catheterization, generally a FFR_{myo} < 0.75 indicates that the stenosis is capable of inducing reversible ischemia. Revascularization of the lesion can be considered. FFR_{myo} > 0.75 generally indicates that revascularization is not warranted.*

♦ *values of FFR_{myo} which are useful to evaluate the results of coronary interventions, are further discussed in chapter 14.*

♦ *the use of FFR_{myo} in some specific pathologic conditions is discussed in chapter 13.*

The threshold value of 0.75 is further corroborated in chapter 12. The only real limitation for applying FFR to detect significant stenosis, is left ventricular hypertrophy as will be discussed in paragraph 13.3. Finally, exercise-induced spasm can be a confounding factor but it can mostly be treated by adequate drug therapy.

11.6 The cut-off value of 0.75 in a physiologic perspective.

As already noted, in healthy people it is generally impossible to provoke myocardial ischemia, not even during exhaustive exercise. Maximum workload is determined by limitations of the musculo-skeletal system and not by cardiorespiratory limitations[1]. Therefore, in the physiologic situation it is obvious that there must be some reserve in maximum achievable coronary blood flow. This implies that the expected value of FFR_{myo} below which ischemia can be provoked, must be lower than 1.0.

From the studies in this and in the following chapter, it can be concluded that when maximum achievable myocardial blood flow decreases to a value of less than 75% of its normal value, myocardial ischemia can generally be induced, irrespective of the person or the artery under study and - within certain limits - irrespective of the current hemodynamic conditions.

When a coronary stenosis develops, maximum achievable blood flow will gradually decrease[12,13,34,35]. For concentric stenoses in animal experiments, this decrease in maximum blood flow starts at a diameter stenosis of approximately 50%. In irregular atherosclerotic lesions in human coronary arteries, the anatomic variability is much larger. Anyhow, as soon as the stenosis has become severe enough to reduce maximum flow to less than 75% of its initial, normal value (equivalent to a reduction of FFR_{myo} to less than 0.75), the patient will develop myocardial ischemia if sufficiently stressed. With further narrowing, maximum flow becomes more and more compromised and the ischemic threshold is further decreased.

The lowest values of FFR_{myo} observed in patients with stable angina pectoris, are in the range of 0.25 - 0.30. Below that value, generally resting ischemia will be present with the clinical image of unstable angina or angina at rest[17,18]. In fact, this is completely in accordance with many earlier studies[12,36,37], indicating that resting blood flow in a normal human myocardium is approximately 25-30% of maximum achievable blood flow and that normal absolute coronary flow reserve (CFR) in humans under standard conditions is approximately 3-5, although with considerable scatter as understandable from chapter 10.1.

It is also interesting in this respect that in a number of earlier studies to determine absolute CFR by videodensitometry, positron emission tomography, or by Doppler velocimetry, the cut-off points between significant and non-significant lesions were found at values of approximately 70 - 75% of the normal reference values for those techniques, although the scatter was much larger than for FFR$_{myo}$ [25,38-41].

References.

1. Guyton AC. The coronary circulation and ischemic heart disease, in: *Textbook of medical Physiology.* Saunders Company, Philadelphia 1986, pp 295-304.

2. Wilson RF, Marcus ML, Christensen BV. Accuracy of exercise electrocardiography in detecting physiologically significant coronary arterial lesions. *Circulation* 1991; 83: 412-421.

3. ECS working group on exercise physiology, physiopathology, and electrocardiography. Guidelined for cardiac exercise testing. *Eur Heart J* 1993; 14: 969-988.

4. Becker RC, Alpert JS. Electrocardiographic ST segment depression in coronary heart disease. *Am Heart J* 1988; 115: 862-868.

5. Mirvis DM, Gordey RL. Electrocardiographic effects of myocardial ischemia induced by atrial pacing in dogs with coronary stenosis, I: repolarization changes with progressive left circumflex arterial narrowing. *J Am Coll Cardiol* 1983; 1: 1090-1098.

6. Smith HJ, Singh BN, Norris RM, John MB, Hurley PJ. Changes in myocardial blood flow and ST-segment elevation following coronary artery occlusion in dogs. *Circ Res* 1975; 36: 697-705.

7. Khuri SF, Flaherty JT, O'Riordan JB, Pitt B, Brawley RK, Donahoo JS, Gott VL. Changes in intramyocardial ST segment voltage and gas tensions with regional myocardial ischemia in the dog. *Circ Res* 1975; 37: 455-463.

8. Angell CS, Lakatta EG, Weisfeldt ML, Shock NW. Relationship of intramyocardial oxygen tension and epicardial ST segment changes following acute coronary artery ligation: effects of coronary perfusion pressure. *Cardiovasc Res* 1975; 9: 12-18.

9. Heng MK, Singh BN, Norris RM, John MB, Elliott R. Relationship between epicardial ST segment elevation and myocardial ischemic damage after experimental coronary artery occlusion in dogs. *J Clin Invest* 1976; 58: 1317-1326.

10. Ruffi R, Lovelace DE, Mueller TM, Knoebel SB, Zipes DP. Relationship between changes in bipolar electrograms and regional myocardial blood flow during acute coronary artery occlusion in the dog. *Circ Res* 1979; 45: 764-770.

11. Mirvis DM, Ramanathan KB, Wilson JL. Regional blood flow correlates of ST segment depression in tachycardia-induced myocardial ischemia. *Circulation* 1986; 73: 365-373.

12. Gould KL, Lipscomb K, Hamilton GW. Physiologic basis for assessing critical coronary stenosis. Instantaneous flow response and regional distribution during coronary hyperemia as measures of coronary flow reserve. *Am J Cardiol* 1974; 33: 87-94.

13. Uren NG, Melin JA, De Bruyne B, Wijns W, Baudhuin T, Camici PG: Relation between myocardial blood flow and the severity of coronary artery stenosis. *N Engl J Med* 1994; 330: 1782-1788.

14. Wilson RF, Wyche K, Christensen BV, Zimmer S, Laxson DD: Effects of adenosine on human coronary arterial circulation. *Circulation* 1990; 82: 1595-1606.

15. Pijls NHJ, Van Son JAM, Kirkeeide RL, De Bruyne B, Gould KL. Experimental basis of determining maximum coronary, myocardial, and collateral blood flow by pressure measurements for assessing function stenosis severity before and after percutaneous transluminal coronary angioplasty. *Circulation* 1993; 87: 1354-67.

16. De Bruyne B, Baudhuin T, Melin JA, Pijls NHJ, SYS SU, Bol A, Paulus WJ, Heyndrickx GR, Wijns W. Coronary flow reserve calculated from pressure measurements in man. Validation with positron emission tomography. *Circulation* 1994; 89: 1013-1022.

17. De Bruyne B, Bartunek J, Sys SU, Heyndrickx GR. Relation between myocardial fractional flow reserve calculated from coronary pressure measurements and exercise-induced myocardial ischemia. *Circulation* 1995; 92: 39-46.

18. Pijls NHJ, Van Gelder B, Van der Voort P, Peels K, Bracke FALE, Bonnier JJRM, El Gamal MIH. Fractional Flow Reserve; a useful index to evaluate the influence of an epicardial coronary stenosis on myocardial blood flow. *Circulation* 1995; 92: 3183-3193.

19. Hamilton GW, Trobaugh GB, Ritchie JL, Gould KL, DeRouen A, Williams DL: Myocardial imaging with [201]thallium: An analysis of clinical usefulness base on Bayes' theorem. *Semin Nucl Med* 1978; 8: 358-364.

20. Melin JA, Piret LJ, Vanbutsele RJM, Rousseau MF, Cosyns J, Brasseur LA, Beckers C, and Detry JMR. Diagnostic value of exercise electrocardiography and thallium myocardial scintigraphy in patients without previous myocardial infarction: a Bayesian approach. *Circulation* 1981; 63: 1019-1024.

21. Nabel EG, Ganz JB, Alexander RW, Selwyn AP: Dilation of normal and constriction of atherosclerotic coronary arteries caused by the cold pressor test. *Circulation* 1988; 77: 43-52.

22. Topol EJ, Ellis SG, Cosgrove DM, Bates ER, Muller DWM, Schork NJ, Schork MA, Loop FD: Analysis of coronary angioplasty practice in the United States with an insurance-claims data base. *Circulation* 1993; 87: 1489-1497.

23. Chaitman BR, Bourassa MG, Davis K, Rogers WJ, Tyras DH, Berger R, Kenedy JW, Fisher L, Judkins MP, Mock MB, Killip T: Angiographic prevalence of high-risk coronary artery disease in patient subsets. *Circulation* 1981; 64: 360-367.

24. Berthe C, Pierard LA, HIERnaux M, Trotteur G, Lempereur P, Carlier J, Kulbertus HE, Predicting the extent and location of coronary artery disease in acute myocardial infarction by echocardiography during dobutamine infusion. *Am J Cardiol* 1986; 58: 1167-1172.

25. Sawada SG, Segar DS, Ryan T, Brown SE, Dohan AM, Williams R, Fineberg NS, Armstrong WF, Feigenbaum H. Echocardiographic detection of coronary artery disease during dobutamine infusion. *Circulation* 1991; 83: 1605-1614.

26. Cohen JL, Greene TO, Ottenweller J, Binenbaum SZ, Wilchfort SD, Kim CS. Dobutamine digital echocardiography for detecting coronary artery disease. *Am J Cardiol* 1991; 67: 1311-1318.

27. Mazeika PK, Nadazdin A, Oakley CM. Dobutamine stress echocardiography for detection and assessment of coronary artery disease. *J Am Coll Cardiol* 1992; 19: 1203-1211.

28. Marwick T, D'Hondt AM, Baudhuin T, Willemart B, Wijns W, Detry JM, Melin J. Optimal use of dobutamine stress for the detection and evaluation of coronary artery disease: combination with echocardiography or scintigraphy, or both? *J Am Coll Cardiol* 1993; 22: 159-167.

29. Marwick T, Willemart B, D'Hondt AM, Baudhuin T, Wijns W, Detry JM, Melin J. Selection of the optimal nonexercise stress for the evaluation of ischemic regional myocardial dysfunction and malperfusion. *Circulation* 1993; 87: 345-354.

30. Bartunek J, Marwick TH, Rodrigues ACT, Vincent M, Van Schuerbeeck E, Sys SU, De Bruyne B. Dobutamine-induced wall motion abnormalities: correlations with myocardial fractional flow reserve and quantitative coronary angiography. *JACC* 1996; 27: 1429-1436.

31. McNeill AJ, Fioretti PM, El-Said EM, Salustri A, Forster T, Roelandt JRTC. Enhanced sensitivity for detection of coronary artery disease by addition of atropine to dobutamine stress echocardiography. *Am J Cardiol* 1992; 70: 41-46.

32. Bourdillon PD, Broderick TM, Sawada SG, Armstrong WF, Ryan T, Dillin JC, Fineberg NS, Feigenbaum H. Regional wall motion index for infarct and noninfarct regions after reperfusion in acute myocardial infarction: comparison with global wall motion index. *J Am Soc Echo* 1989; 2: 298-407.

33. Bartunek J, Van Schuerbeeck E, De Bruyne B. Comparison of exercise electrocardiography and dobutamine echocardiography with invasively assessed myocardial fractional flow reserve in evaluation of severity of coronary arterial narrowing. *Am J Cardiol* 1997: 79: 478-481.

34. Wilson RF, White CW: Intracoronary papaverine: An ideal coronary vasodilator for studies of the coronary circulation in conscious humans. *Circulation* 1986; 73: 444-451.

35. Wilson RF: Assessment of the human coronary circulation using a Doppler catheter. *Am J Cardiol* 1991; 67: 44D-56D.

36. White CW, Wright CB, Doty DB, Hiratza LF, Eastham CL, Harrison DG, Marcus ML: Does visual interpretation of the coronary arteriogram predict the physiological importance of a coronary stenosis ? *N Engl J Med* 1984; 310: 819-824.

37. Gould KL: Functional measures of coronary stenosis severity at cardiac catheterization. *J Am Coll Cardiol* 1990; 16: 198-9.

38. Zijlstra F, Reiber JHC, Juillière Y, Serruys PW: Normalization of coronary flow reserve by percutaneous trasnluminal coronary angioplasty. *Am J Cardiol* 1988; 61: 55-63

39. Kern MJ, Deligonul U, Tatineni S, Serota H, Aguirre FV, Hilton TC: Intravenous adenosine continuous infusion and low dose bolus administration for determination of coronary vasodilatory reserve in patients with and without coronary artery disease. *J Am Coll Cardiol* 1991; 18: 718-729.

40. McGinn AL, White CW, Wilson RF: Interstudy variability of coronary flow reserve. Influence of heart rate, arterial pressure, and ventricular preload. *Circulation* 1990; 81: 1319-1330.

41. Pijls NHJ, Aengevaeren WRM, Uyen GJH, Hoevelaken A, Pijnenburg T, Van Leeuwen K, Van der Werf T. The concept of maximal flow ratio for immediate evaluation of PTCA-results by videodensitometry. *Circulation* 1991; 83: 854-865.

Chapter 12

FRACTIONAL FLOW RESERVE TO ASSESS INTERMEDIATE STENOSIS

Comparison to non-invasive tests

As outlined in the previous chapters, myocardial fractional flow reserve (FFR_{myo}) is a lesion-specific index of the functional severity of a coronary stenosis, calculated from pressure measurements during coronary arteriography[1-8]. It has been shown in chapter 11 that a value of 0.75 distinguishes lesions, associated with reversible ischemia or not, with minimal overlap. In this chapter the usefulness of fractional flow reserve is investigated for clinical decision-making in patients with intermediate coronary stenosis, and compared to an ischemic standard composed by all presently used non-invasive tests: exercise testing, thallium scintigraphy, and dobutamine stress-echocardiography.

12.1 The limited accuracy of non-invasive tests to identify inducible ischemia.

Clinical decision-making remains challenging in patients with chest pain and an intermediate stenosis at coronary angiography. Often, many diagnostic tests are repeatedly performed without convincing either the physician or the patient that the complaints are truly of ischemic origin or not. In a considerable number of such patients, a coronary intervention is performed without clear evidence that the lesion is responsible for the complaints.[1,2]

If FFR_{myo} is an accurate index for identifying inducible ischemia in this difficult subset of patients, it can be generally proposed as a lesion-specific invasive alternative for determining if a particular stenosis can be held responsible for inducible ischemia and to support decisions for coronary revascularization when other objective proof of reversible myocardial ischemia is lacking or when non-invasive tests are inconclusive or have not been performed[9,10]. Accordingly, the purpose of the present study was to investigate the usefulness of myocardial fractional flow reserve for clinical decision-making during diagnostic coronary angiography in patients with an ambiguous clinical presentation, contradictory or inconclusive non-invasive test results, and an angiographically intermediate stenosis in one large coronary artery; and to compare the clinical value of FFR_{myo} to exercise testing, thallium scintigraphy, and stress-echocardiography. Because the accuracy of all these non-invasive tests, if performed alone, is limited, especially in this difficult subset of patients, at first a unique gold standard for inducible ischemia was composed of all the non-invasive tests together and FFR_{myo} was compared to that gold standard.

12.2 Design of the study.

12.2.1 Study population.

The study population consisted of 45 consecutive patients (28 male, 17 female; age 54 ± 8 yrs, range 36-74 yrs) with the following characteristics: 1) chest pain; 2) an angiographically intermediate stenosis in the proximal part of one major coronary artery; 3) normal left ventricular function; 4) all study patients were referred for a second opinion because of conflicting data between the clinical presentation, previous non-invasive tests, and previous coronary arteriography regarding the certainty that the chest pain could be attributed to reversible ischemia caused by that intermediate stenosis.

In fact, most of these patients underwent many diagnostic tests in the previous year without reaching a clear diagnosis as to whether their chest pain could really be attributed to reversible myocardial ischemia. In table 12.1 previous diagnostic tests and treatments in our study population, are summarized.

The study protocol was approved by the Institutional Review Board and informed consent was obtained from all participants for all tests.

12.2.2 Outlines of the study protocol.

All medications were stopped for 7 days, except aspirin 80 mg once daily. Thereafter, and within 48 hours, bicycle exercise testing, thallium scintigraphy, dobutamine stress-echocardiography, and coronary arteriography with intracoronary pressure measurements and calculation of myocardial fractional flow reserve were performed in all patients. The clinical decision to perform a revascularization (percutaneous transluminal coronary angioplasty or bypass surgery) was based upon a value of $FFR_{myo} <$ 0.75, based upon earlier study results as presented in chapter 11. In those patients in whom revascularization was performed, all positive non-invasive tests were repeated within 6 weeks after the revascularization.

Table 12.1 *Number of previous diagnostic tests and treatments performed in the study population because of the chest pain up to the present study. Despite all these tests, no definite diagnosis had been made (i.e.: it was not established whether the chest pain was due to inducible myocardial ischemia or not).*
The extra costs made are calculated for the period starting after the first angiography until the start of the present study and do not include any drug treatment. These costs had been saved if fractional flow reserve had been determined at the first coronary angiography.

◆ regular exercise testing	2.7 (range: 0 - 8)
◆ thallium[201] scintigraphy or MIBI-spect	1.8 (range: 1 - 4)
◆ coronary angiography	2.1 (range: 1 - 7)
◆ number of tested drugs	4.6 (range: 2 - 9)
◆ hospital admissions (not related to diagnostic angiography)	0.9 (range: 0 - 6)
◆ duration of complaints (months)	5.6 (range: 2 - 14)
◆ average extra costs made per patient (USD)	9417

12.2.3 Exercise testing and thallium scintigraphy.

Upright bicycle exercise testing was performed starting with a workload of 20 W that was increased by 20 W every minute. A 12-lead-electrocardiogram was continuously recorded. The test was considered positive when horizontal or downsloping ST-depression $\geq$ 0.1 mV was present 80 ms after the J-point in 2 adjacent leads. At peak exercise, 73

MBq thallium[201]-chloride was administered in a large antecubital vein, exercise was maintained for one more minute, and planar imaging was performed subsequently in the 3 standard views[11]. After 3 hours, re-injection of 37 MBq thallium[201]-chloride was performed and redistribution images were obtained[12]. All thallium scintigrams were evaluated independently by visual analysis of the analogue images by two experienced reviewers blinded to all other data.

12.2.4 Dobutamine stress echocardiography.

Dobutamine stress echocardiography was performed, using a quad-screen comparison technique of identical views[13,14]. Intravenous dobutamine infusion was started at a rate of 10 μg/kg/min and increased by 10 μg/kg/min every 3 minutes until wall motion abnormalities occurred or to a maximum of 50 μg/kg/min. In patients who did not achieve 90% of age-adjusted maximum heart rate and had no objective signs of ischemia, 1 mg of atropine was administered intravenously while dobutamine infusion was continued[15]. The occurrence of wall motion abnormalities was evaluated off-line as previously described[16,17] by two independent echocardiographers blinded to all other data.

12.2.5 Pressure measurements and calculation of FFR_{myo}.

At catheterization, a 6-8F guiding catheter was introduced into one femoral artery and advanced into the ostium of the coronary artery. A pressure guide wire (Radi Medical Systems, Uppsala, Sweden) was zeroed, calibrated, advanced through the catheter, introduced into the coronary artery, and positioned distal to the stenosis as described in chapter 5. Intravenous adenosine was then infused (140 μg/kg/min) to induce maximum coronary blood flow, corresponding to minimal distal coronary pressure[18-25]. When a steady state hyperemia was achieved, myocardial fractional flow reserve was calculated as the ratio between mean distal intracoronary pressure from the wire and mean arterial pressure from the guiding catheter as described in chapter 4 and 5.

12.2.6 On-line clinical decision making, based upon FFR_{myo}.

If FFR_{myo} was ≥ 0.75, no intervention was performed. If FFR_{myo} was < 0.75, revascularization was recommended. In case of a lesion suitable for coronary angioplasty, this procedure was performed during the same session and repeat measurements of fractional flow reserve were performed 15 minutes after successful angioplasty. If the lesion was not suitable for coronary angioplasty, bypass surgery was performed within 4 weeks.

12.3 Definition of a gold standard of inducible ischemia by combination of the non-invasive tests.

Notwithstanding the excellent sensitivity and specificity of thallium exercise testing and stress-echocardiography in patients with an angiographic significant coronary stenosis, it is well known that the accuracy of these tests decreases in patients with atypical complaints or with only moderate angiographic lesions[12,17,26-29]. It is thus difficult to establish the value of any new parameter for diagnosis of the functional severity of coronary artery disease, because no single unequivocal or "gold" standard exists, a consideration especially true in the difficult population selected for this study.

To overcome this problem we compared the value of the new invasive index FFR_{myo} *to an ischemic ("gold") standard composed of a combination of all presently used non-invasive indexes as follows:*

First, it was postulated that functionally significant disease (corresponding with inducible myocardial ischemia) was present *if and only if* at least one of the non-invasive tests yielded a clearly positive result *and* reverted to negative after successful coronary angioplasty or bypass surgery.

Second, it was postulated that no functionally significant stenosis (and therefore no inducible ischemia) was present *if and only if* all non-invasive tests could be exhaustively performed and yielded negative results.

In the only remaining situation, i.e. one or more positive non-invasive tests but not followed by revascularization because FFR_{myo} exceeded 0.75, no ischemic standard was present and the positive test would be indeterminate by definition. However, to avoid any overvaluation of the new index, those patients were considered as false negatives for the fractional flow reserve index.

As will be discussed in paragraph 12.5.2, the use of such an ischemic or "gold" standard, composed of the sequentially performed different non-invasive tests, provides a diagnostic accuracy of almost 100% according to sequential Bayesian considerations[30-35]. Myocardial fractional flow reserve ≥ 0.75 *or* < 0.75, *was compared to that standard.*

12.4 Results.

12.4.1 Procedural and clinical results.

Patient characteristics, results of non-invasive tests, and angiographic data are shown in table 12.2. There was no difference in percent stenosis or minimal luminal diameter between the patients with FFR_{myo} < or ≥ 0.75.

Exercise testing and thallium scintigraphy could be performed in all patients. In 4 patients, stress-echocardiographic images were poor and not interpretable.

Coronary pressure recordings and myocardial fractional flow reserve were obtained in all patients. An example is shown in figure 12.1. Also the patient in figure 4.4 and 4.5 belongs to this study population.

FFR_{myo} was ≥ 0.75 in 24 patients and, accordingly, no revascularization was performed in any of them. FFR_{myo} was < 0.75 in 21 patients. In 20 of these 21 patients, coronary angioplasty (n=13) or bypass surgery (n=7) was performed whereafter all previously positive tests were repeated and all reverted to negative. In one patient with FFR_{myo} of 0.40 and a proximal left anterior descending artery stenosis, revascularization was recommended but refused.

In those patients undergoing coronary angioplasty, measurement of FFR_{myo} was repeated 15 minutes after the procedure and always increased to a value > 0.75 (0.87 ± 0.06, range 0.77 - 0.96) in agreement with the reverted non-invasive tests.

12.4.2 Comparison of myocardial fractional flow reserve to the ischemic gold standard.

The relation between myocardial fractional flow reserve and the results of the non-invasive tests is presented in figure 12.2. In all patients with FFR_{myo} < 0.75 (n = 21), signs of myocardial ischemia could be induced by at least one non-invasive test. Because all positive tests in this group were repeated after revascularization and reverted to negative, a non-invasive standard of inducible ischemia as defined in the methods section was present and there was concordance between "inducible ischemia according to FFR_{myo}" and "inducible ischemia according to the ischemic standard" in all these patients. In 21 of the 24 patients with FFR_{myo} ≥ 0.75, all non-invasive tests were negative. Therefore, concordance between "no inducible ischemia according to FFR_{myo}" and "no inducible ischemia according to the ischemic standard" was present in those 21 cases.

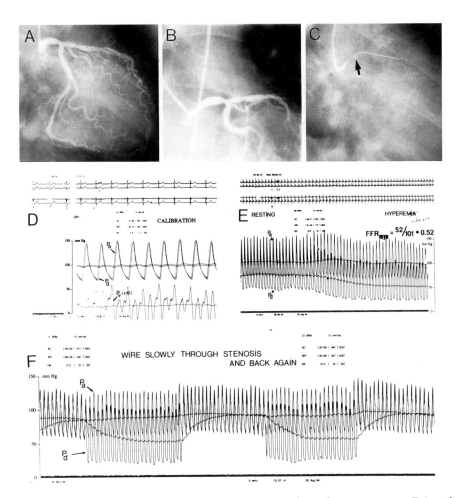

Figure 12.1 *Angiogram of the left coronary artery and simultaneous aortic (P_a) and transstenotic pressure (P_d) recordings in a 65-year-old lady with an intermediate stenosis in the left main and left anterior descending coronary artery (panel A and B). At first, the pressure recordings in panel D were obtained with the pressure sensor located at the tip of the coronary catheter to verify that 2 equal pressures are obtained at that location. Subsequently in panel E, the pressure wire has crossed the left main stenosis and a rather large resting gradient of 22 mmHg is found, which further increases after intravenous infusion of adenosine. At steady state maximum hyperemia, Pa equals 101 mmHg and P_d equals 52 mmHg, resulting in a myocardial fractional flow reserve (FFR_{myo}) of 0.52, indicating a significant stenosis from a functional point of view. In panel C and F, it is demonstrated how the wire is slowly advanced across the stenosis and withdrawn again, showing exactly and reproducibly the site and functional severity of the stenosis. The sensor is indicated by the arrow.*

Table 12.2 *Patient characteristics, non-invasive test data, and quantitative angiographic parameters.*

		FFR$_{myo}$ ≥ 0.75	FFR$_{myo}$ < 0.75
Male/female	:	13/11	15/6
Age (years)	:	55 ± 9	54 ± 8
LM/LAD/LCX/RCA*	:	1 / 10 / 4 / 9	1 / 14 / 2 / 4
Reference diam (mm)	:	3.31 ± 0.67	3.10 ± 0.63
diam stenosis (percent)	:	44 ± 9	41 ± 8
Minimal luminal diam (mm)	:	1.94 ± 0.47	1.78 ± 0.41
Heart rate at exercise/Thallium	:	146 ± 18	162 ± 19 **
% of age-adjusted heart rate	:	95 ± 12	104 ± 12
# posit. exercise tests	:	2	16
# posit. Thallium scans	:	1	12
Heart rate at stress echo	:	149 ± 11	147 ± 13
% of age-adjusted heart rate	:	98 ± 7	95 ± 8
# posit. stress echo	:	0	10
TREATMENT	:	All medical	Medical : 1
			PTCA : 13
			Bypass surg.: 7

* LM, LAD, LCX, and RCA denote left main, left anterior descending, left circumflex, and right coronary artery, respectively.
** P = 0.033 versus FFR$_{myo}$ ≥ 0.75 (Student's unpaired t-testing)

Of the remaining 3 patients, two had a positive regular exercise test and one had positive thallium scintigraphy. Therefore, according to definition, these 3 patients had to be considered false negatives for the fractional flow reserve method, because inducible ischemia could have been present despite FFR$_{myo}$ ≥ 0.75. Even then, sensitivity, specificity, positive and negative predictive value, and accuracy of FFR$_{myo}$ was 88, 100, 100, 88, and 93 percent, respectively (table 12.3).

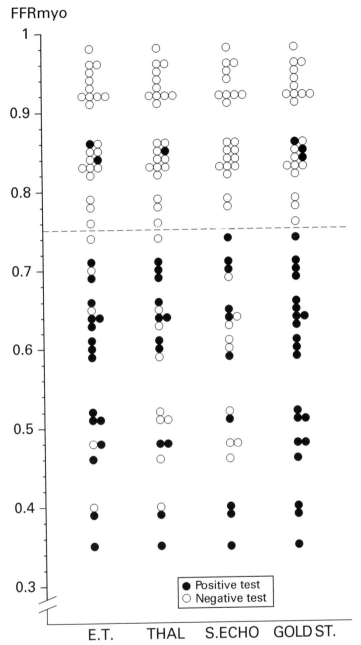

Figure 12.2 *Relation between myocardial fractional flow reserve (FFR$_{myo}$) and the results of the non-invasive tests. Every line represents the different test results in one individual patient. Positive test results are indicated by solid points and negative test results by open points. E.T.: regular exercise test; THAL: thallium[201] scintigraphy; S.ECHO: dobutamine stress-echocardiography; GOLD ST: gold standard of reversible ischemia, composed of all non-invasive tests.*

12.4.3 Follow-up of the patients with $FFR_{myo} \geq 0.75$.

The results of the tests were explained to all patients and in those patients with $FFR_{myo} \geq 0.75$, it was explicitly stated that the ischemic-like complaints were not due to a flow-limiting fixed coronary artery stenosis and that mechanical revascularization was not warranted. Seventeen of these patients were treated by aspirin only, and 7 of them by the combination of aspirin and a calcium-antagonist. At a follow-up visit 4 weeks later, the functional class of these patients according to the CCS-classification had decreased from 2.8 to 1.3. After a follow-up of 14 ± 5 months (range 5-21 months), no ischemic events occurred in this patient group, no revascularization was necessary, and 17 were completely asymptomatic. In the meantime, a similar favorable outcome has been confirmed in large prospective series of patients in whom intervention was deferred based upon FFR > 0.75[35-38]. Those studies are further discussed in chapter 15.

12.5   Discussion.

12.5.1 The reliability of FFR_{myo} for clinical decision-making.

The present study suggests that myocardial fractional flow reserve is a reliable index on which to base decisions for revascularization in this difficult subset of patients with chest pain and an intermediate coronary stenosis. Its accuracy in indicating or excluding reversible ischemia is equivalent to that of the exercise-electrocardiogram, thallium scintigraphy, and dobutamine stress-echocardiography together, and superior to any of these tests if performed alone[36].

Decision making based upon FFR_{myo} resulted in excellent clinical outcome in those patients in whom unnecessary revascularization was avoided.

In most patients with coronary artery disease, the decision to perform revascularization should be based not only on coronary anatomy but also on additional information on the functional significance of a lesion and lesion-related inducible ischemia[39-41]. This is especially true in patients with intermediate narrowings on the coronary angiogram. If, in the presence of such an intermediate lesion, ischemia can be clearly demonstrated by exercise or pharmacologic stress tests, revascularization is appropriate when medical therapy fails[40-41]. However, in some patients, the non-invasive tests are not conclusive, confounded by conditions interfering with reliable test interpretation, not available, or simply not performed. Moreover, the sensitivity of both exercise-thallium scintigraphy and stress-echocardio-

Table 12.3 *Comparison between inducible ischemia according to myocardial fractional flow reserve (FFR$_{myo}$) and according to the non-invasive gold standard. The "+" and "-" signs indicate the presence or absence of inducible ischemia.*

	Gold standard +	Gold standard -
FFR$_{myo}$ < 0.75	21	0
FFR$_{myo}$ ≥ 0.75	3	21

graphy in these patients is limited. When chest pain persists in spite of repeatedly negative test results, confusion often arises about the actual significance of such an angiographically intermediate lesion[1,2].

Therefore, it would be clinically helpful to have an index which can be easily obtained at diagnostic coronary angiography and clearly indicates if the stenosis under consideration is responsible for reversible ischemia. If equivalent or superior to the best non-invasive test, such an index could be a surrogate for stress testing and used for on-line clinical decision-making regarding revascularization when other objective evidence of reversible ischemia is lacking. Conversely, such an index can also be used to avoid unnecessary coronary interventions.

Myocardial fractional flow reserve is such an invasive, lesion-specific index of the effect of an epicardial coronary artery stenosis on maximum myocardial perfusion[5-10]. As outlined in chapter 11, in previous studies in selected series of patients undergoing percutaneous transluminal coronary angioplasty, a FFR$_{myo}$ value of approximately 0.75 distinguished lesions associated with inducible ischemia or not with minimal overlap[9,10].

The present study extends those previous observations to the clinical application of FFR$_{myo}$ in the diagnostic setting. The usefulness of FFR$_{myo}$ at diagnostic angiography in patients considered as difficult from a diagnostic point of view, was tested against a gold standard combined by all currently available non-invasive tests. If FFR$_{myo}$ is a useful tool in this difficult patient subset, this index may be used more generally as a lesion-specific invasive alternative to stress tests to determine if a particular stenosis can be responsible for reversible ischemia. The clinical follow-up and reverted test results after revascularization, support this position.

12.5.2 Methodological considerations for the composite ischemic standard.

Because in a patient population such as in this study the accuracy of every individual non-invasive test is limited, the main methodologic problem was how to create an ischemic "gold" standard which incorporated the information from all non-invasive tests together and to which FFR_{myo} could be compared.

The combined standard in this study as described in paragraph 12.3, is unique among studies assessing ischemia. The basis for its acceptance is as follows: It is assumed that any positive test result, in general, could be a true positive or false positive result, depending on the characteristics of the test and the patient population[32,35]. However, if that same positive test reverts to negative after a successful intervention, it can be assumed that the positive test result before the intervention was a true positive and that the negative result thereafter is a true negative[30-35].

In other words, it is not the positive or negative test in itself, but the reversal of the result after the intervention which justifies the a posteriori conclusion that the test was true positive before and true negative after the intervention.

In the patients in whom FFR_{myo} was less than 0.75 and in whom coronary angioplasty or bypass surgery was performed consequently, a total of 38 positive exercise ECG's, thallium tests and dobutamine stress-echocardiograms were encountered (figure 12.2). All these tests were repeated and reversed to normal after revascularization. Therefore, a gold standard for inducible ischemia was present in all those patients with FFR_{myo} < 0.75. Similarly, exclusion of inducible ischemia was assumed to be present if all non-invasive tests could be exhaustively performed without any evidence of ischemia. In all patients fulfilling that condition, FFR_{myo} was ≥ 0.75. The assumption of absence of inducible ischemia in the case of sequentially negative results at the different tests has been described and defended earlier[30,33].

It is interesting to note that reversal of one test from positive to negative after revascularization, not only indicates that this particular test was true positive before and true negative after the intervention; but also indicates that other tests which were negative in that patient before the revascularization, must have been false negative. This emphasizes the limited sensitivity of regular non-invasive tests in the assessment of intermediate stenosis, if performed alone.

12.5.3 Clinical implications.

This study indicates that FFR$_{myo}$, obtained at coronary arteriography, is an excellent index to confirm whether or not an angiograhically intermediate stenosis is functionally significant and can be held responsible for reversible ischemia. A value of 0.75 discriminates between functionally significant and non-significant stenosis. The accuracy of FFR$_{myo}$ for this purpose is approximately 95% compared to a gold standard integrating the combined information provided by all presently used non-invasive tests. In fact, FFR < 0.75 *always* indicates inducible ischemia (specificity ≈ 100%), whereas FFR > 0.75 generally excludes ischemia related to that epicardial stenosis with a few exceptions (sensitivity ≈ 90%).Therefore, myocardial fractional flow reserve is an ideal index for clinical decision-making regarding revascularization of a particular stenosis when other objective evidence of reversible ischemia is lacking.

References.

1. Topol EJ, Ellis SG, Cosgrove DM. Analysis of coronary angioplasty practice in the United States with an insurance-claims data base. *Circulation* 1993; 87: 1489-97.
2. Kern MJ, Donohue TJ, Aguirre FV. Clinical outcome of deferring angioplasty in patients with normal translesional pressure-flow velocity measurements. *J Am Coll Cardiol* 1995; 25: 178-87.
3. Kirkeeide RL, Gould KL, Parsel L. Assessment of coronary stenoses by myocardial perfusion imaging during pharmocologic coronary vasodilation. VIII. Validation of coronary flow reserve as a single integrated functional measure of stenosis severity reflecting all its geometric dimensions. *J Am Coll Cardiol* 1986; 7: 103-13.
4. Gould KL, Kirkeeide RL, Buchi M. Coronary flow reserve as a physiologic measure of stenosis severity. *J Am Coll Cardiol* 1990; 15: 459-74.
5. Pijls NHJ, Van Son JAM, Kirkeeide RL, De Bruyne B, Gould KL. Experimental basis of determining maximum coronary, myocardial, and collateral blood flow by pressure measurements for assessing functiona l stenosis severity before and after percutaneous transluminal coronary angioplasty. *Circulation* 1993; 87: 1354-67.
6. De Bruyne B, Baudhuin T, Melin JA, Pijls NHJ, Sys SU, Bol A, Paulus WJ, Heyndrickx GR, Wijns W. Coronary flow reserve calculated from pressure measurements in man. Validation with positron emission tomography. *Circulation* 1994; 89: 1013-22.
7. De Bruyne B, Paulus WJ, Pijls NHJ. Rationale and application of coronary transstenotic pressure gradient measurements. *Cathet Cardiovasc Diagn* 1994; 33: 250-61.
8. Pijls NHJ, Bech GJW, El Gamal MIH, Bonnier HJRM, De Bruyne B, Van Gelder B, Michels HR, Koolen JJ. Quantification of recruitable coronary collateral blood flow in conscious humans and its potential to predict future ischemic events. *J Am Coll Cardiol* 1995; 25: 1522-28.

9. Pijls NHJ, Van Gelder B, Van der Voort P, Peels KH, Bracke FALE, Bonnier HJRM, El Gamal MIH. Fractional Flow Reserve: A useful ideal index to evaluate the influence of a coronary stenosis on myocardial blood flow. *Circulation* 1995; 92: 3183-93.

10. De Bruyne B, Bartunek J, Sys SA, Heyndrickx GR. Relation between myocardial fractional flow reserve calculated from coronary pressure measurement and exercise-induced myocardial ischemia. *Circulation* 1995; 92: 39-46

11. Ritchie JL, Bateman TM, Bonow RO. Guidelines for clinical use of radionuclide imaging. *Circulation* 1995; 91: 1278-1303.

12. Dilsizian V, Rocco TP, Freedman NMT. Enhanced detection of ischemic but viable myocardium by the reinjection of thallium after stress-redistribution imaging. *N Engl J Med* 1990; 323: 141-6.

13. Salustri A, Fioretti PR, Pozzoli MMA, McNeill AJ, Roelandt JR. Dobutamine stress echocardiography; its role in the diagnosis of coronary artery disease. *Eur Hear t J* 1992; 13: 70-7.

14. Sawada SG, Segar DS, Ryan T. Echocardiographic detection of coronary artery disease during dobutamine infusion. *Circulation* 1991; 83: 1605-14.

15. McNeill AJ, Fioretti PR, El-Said EM, Salustri A, De Feyter PJ, Roelandt JR. Enhanced sensitivity for detection of coronary artery disease by addition of atropine to dobutamine stress echocardiography. *Am J Cardiol* 1992; 70: 41-6.

16. N Engl J Bourdillon PDV, Broderick TM, Sawada SG, Armstrong WF, Ryan T, Dillon JC, Fineberg NS, Feigenbaum H. Regional wall motion index for infarct and non infarct regions after reperfusion in acute myocardial infarction: comparison with global wall motion index. *J Am Soc Echo* 1989; 2: 398-407.

17. Marwick T, Willemart B, D'Hondt A-M. Selection of the optimal nonexercise stress for the evaluation of ischemic regional myocardial dysfunction and malperfusion. *Circulation* 1993; 87: 345-54.

18. Emanuelsson H, Dohnal M, Lamm C, Tenerz L. Initial experiences with a miniaturized pressure transducer during coronary angioplasty. *Cathet Cardiovasc Diagn* 1991; 24: 137-43.

19. Lamm C, Dohnal M, Serruys PW, Emanuelsson H. High fidelity translesional pressure gradients during percutaneous transluminal coronary angioplasty: correlation with quantitative coronary angiography. *Am Heart J* 1993; 126: 66-75.

20. Serruys PW, Di Mario C, Meneveau N. Intracoronary pressure and flow velocity with sensor-tip guide wires: A new methodologic approach for assessment of coronary hemodynamics before and after coronary interventions. *Am J Cardiol* 1993; 71: 41D-53D.

21. Wilson RF, Wijche K, Christensen BV, Zimmer S, Laxson DD. Effects of adenosine on human coronary arterial circulation. *Circulation* 1990; 82: 1595-1606.

22. Kern MJ, Deligonul U, Tatineni S, Serota H, Aguirre FV, Hilton TC: Intravenous adenosine continuous infusion and low dose bolus administration for determination of coronary vasodilatory reserve in patients with and without coronary artery disease. *J Am Coll Cardiol* 1991; 18: 718-29.

23. Uren NG, Melin JA, De Bruyne B, Wijns W, Baudhuin T, Camici PG. Relation between myocardial blood flow and the severity of coronary artery stenosis. *N Engl J Med* 1994 330: 1782-8.

24. Redberg RF, Sobol Y, Chou TM, Malloy M, Kumar S, Botvinick E, Kane J. Adenosine-induced coronary vasodilation during transesophageal Doppler echocardiography. *Circulation* 1995; 92: 190-6.

25. Van der Voort P, Van Hagen E, Hendrix G, Van Gelder B, Bech GJW, Pijls NHJ. Comparison of intavenous adenosine to intracoronary papaverine for calculation of pressure-derived fractional flow reserve. *Cathet cardiov Diagn* 1996; 39:120—125.

26. Marwick T, D'Hondt A, Baudhuin T. Optimal use of dobutamine stress test for the detection and evaluation of coronary artery disease: combination with echocardiography, scintigraphy or both ? *J Am Coll Cardiol* 1993; 22: 159-67.

27. Picano E, Parodi O, Lattanzi F. Assessment of anatomic and physiological severity of single-vessel coronary artery lesions by dipyridamole echocardiography. *Circulation* 1994; 89: 753-61.

28. Gould KL. Positron emission tomography compared to other imaging modalities, in: Gould KL (ed), Coronary Artery Stenosis. *Elsevier* 1991: pp 197-207.

29. Detrano R, Janosi A, Lyons KP, Marcondes G, Abbassi N, Froelicher VF. Factors affecting sensitivity and specificity of a diagnostic test: the exercise thallium scintigram. *Am J Medic* 1988; 84: 699-710.

30. Fryback DG. Bayes' theorem and conditional nonindependence of data in medical diagnosis. *Comput Biomed Res* 1978; 11: 423-32.

31. Hamilton GW, Trobaugh GB, Ritchie JL, Gould KL, DeRouen A, Williams DL. Myocardial imaging with [201]thallium: An analysis of clinical usefulness based on Bayes' theorem. *Semin Nucl Med* 1978; 8: 358-64.

32. Melin JA, Piret LJ, Vanbutsele RJM. Diagnostic value of exercise electrocardiography and thallium myocardial scintigraphy in patients without previous myocardial infarction: a Bayesian approach. *Circulation* 1981; 63: 1019-24.

33. Weintraub WS, Madeira SW, Bodenheimer MM. Critical analysis of the application of Bayes' theorem to sequential testing in the noninvasive diagnosis of coronary artery disease. *Am J Cardiol* 1984; 54: 43-9.

34. Detrano R, Leatherman J, Salcedo EE, Bayesian analysis versus discriminant function analysis: Their relative utility in the diagnosis of coronary disease. *Circulation* 1986; 73: 970-7.

35. Patterson RE, Horowitz SF. Importance of epidemiology and biostatistics in deciding clinical strategies for using diagnostic tests: A simplified approach using examples from coronary artery disease. *J Am Coll Cardiol* 1989; 13: 1653-65.

36. Pijls NHJ, De Bruyne B, Peels K, Van der Voort PH, Bonnier HJRM, Bartunek J, Koolen JJ. Measurement of fractional flow reserve to assess the functional severity of coronary-artery stenoses, *N Engl J Med* 1996; 334: 1703-1708.

37. Bech GJW, De Bruyne B, Bonnier HJRM, Bartunek J, Wijns W, Peels K, Heyndrickx GR, Koolen JJ, Pijls NHJ. Long-term follow-up after deferral of PTCA of intermediate stenosis on the basis of coronary pressure measurement. *J Am Coll Cardiol* 1998; 31: 841-847.

38. Bech GJW, De Bruyne B, Pijls NHJ. Comparison of deferral versus performance of PTCA based upon fractional flow reserve: the DEFER study. *J Am. Coll Cardiol* 1999; 33: 89A.

39. Klocke FJ, Cognition in the era of technology: "Seeing the shades of gray". *J Am Coll Cardiol* 1990; 16: 763-9.

40. Ryan TJ, Faxon DP, Gunnar RM. Guidelines for percutaneous transluminal coronary angioplasty. *Circulation* 1988; 78: 780-9.

41. Kirklin JW, Akins CW, Blackstone EH, et al. ACC/AHA guidelines and indications for coronary artery bypass graft surgery. *Circulation* 1991; 83: 1125-73.

Chapter 13

FFR IN SOME SPECIFIC CONDITIONS

An essential prerequisite for the calculation of FFR from aortic and coronary pressure is to obtain the measurements under conditions of maximum hyperemia. Only in this situation it can be assumed that the resistance of the vascular bed is minimal and therefore equal to the resistance in the same vascular bed but not depending on an epicardial stenosis. This condition has been demonstrated in animals (chapter 7) and in humans (chapter 8). Only when the resistance of the vascular bed depending on an epicardial stenosis equals the resistance of the same vascular bed but without stenosis, these resistances can be cancelled in the calculation of FFR[2]. It has been shown in animals and in humans, in the physiological range of aortic pressure, that the relation between myocardial flow and driving pressure is linear during maximum microvascular vasodilation[3-4]. This implies that, during maximum hyperemia, the ratio of two myocardial flows (which corresponds to the definition of FFR) equals the ratio of their respective driving pressures. The key point with respect to FFR is not the slope but the linearity of the pressure-flow relation under conditions of maximum vasodilation. When maximum hyperemia is not achieved the relation between hyperemic flow and driving pressure is curvilinear, and thus, the ratio of these ('non-hyperemic') flows does *not* equal the ratio of their respective driving pressures.

In several commonly encountered pathologic conditions, it is not obvious whether minimal microvascular resistance and/or whether maximum transstenotic flow can be achieved by pharmacological vasodilation. Therefore, the relation between the value of pressure-derived FFR during pharmacologic vasodilation and the occurrence of myocardial ischemia should be further established. These conditions are discussed in the following paragraphs and include previous myocardial infarction, resistance vessel dysfunction, left ventricular hypertrophy, the presence of diffuse atherosclerosis, serial stenoses within the same artery, and stress-induced paradoxical vasoconstriction.

13.1 FFR*myo* after myocardial infarction.

A considerable proportion of patients undergoing coronary angiography or angioplasty, have experienced a prior myocardial infarction. It is generally accepted that post-infarction residual stress-induced reversible ischemia warrants some revascularization procedure as these patients may benefit from revascularization of the infarct artery[5,6]. However, noninvasive evaluation of the presence of residual myocardial ischemia in a partially infarcted territory is clouded by a high percentage of false negative and false positive results. Whether the FFR value of 0.75 is valid as a cut-off point to detect (or exclude) reversible ischemia after (incomplete) myocardial infarction, was unknown so far.

Basal myocardial flow per gram of perfusable tissue is lower in infarcted regions than in regions remote from the infarction[7,8]. In addition, hyperemic flow is lower in infarcted territories, not only one week but also 6 months after myocardial infarction[8]. For similar degree of stenosis Claeys et al. also found coronary flow velocity reserve to be lower in regions with than in regions without prior myocardial infarction, both before and after angioplasty[9]. The mechanisms responsible for these reduced basal and hyperemic flows remain largely speculative and include the decreased oxygen consumption in the residual (partially necrotic) myocardium, inappropriate constriction of both the epicardial and the resistance vessels distal to the site of coronary thrombosis, "stunning" of the resistive vessels and partial obliteration of the microvasculature. Therefore, with respect to pressure-derived FFR, there are two main differences between a region with and a region without prior myocardial infarction: (1) the myocardial mass depending on the stenosis is smaller although the reference diameter of the infarct vessel has not changed; (2) Resistive vessel dysfunction may blunt the maximal hyperemic response.

Nevertheless, on theoretical grounds, it seems logical to postulate that, in patients with a prior myocardial infarction, a similar cut-off value could be proposed as in patients without prior infarction. The explanation for that phenomenon is as follows (figure 13.1): let us assume that incomplete myocardial infarction has occurred in a particular distribution and that the infarct artery is still patent but stenotic to a similar degree as before the infarct. Part of the distal myocardium is still viable and part of it is necrotic, with partial or complete obliteration of the microvasculature[10]. Maximum blood flow to that distribution is lower than it was before the infarction. Consequently, the hyperemic gradient across the residual stenosis is smaller and the FFR higher than before the infarction. Therefore, at the first glance, the occurrence of a myocardial infarction has led to an underestimation of

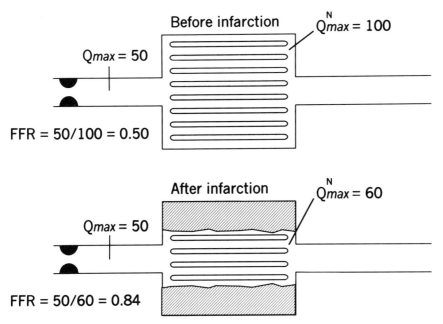

Figure 13.1 *After myocardial infarction, the amount of viable myocardium distal to the stenosis is smaller than before. Therefore, in the hypothetical case the lesion severity has remained unchanged, the functional severity of the stenosis has decreased because of the decrease of viable tissue to be supplied.* Q_{max} *, maximum achievable blood flow in the coronary artery;* Q^N_{max} *, normal maximum blood flow to the vital myocardium, supplied by that artery.*

the lesion by pressure measurements. However, FFR_{myo} of the *vital* myocardium supplied by the residual lesion, can be defined as maximum flow in the presence of that (residual) lesion, divided by maximum flow without that residual lesion, *the latter being only determined by the vital tissue and not by the necrotic tissue.* With respect to residual ischemia and FFR_{myo} associated with the residual lesion, actual maximum flow has to be related to maximum flow in the absence of the epicardial lesion (which is "normal" maximum flow for the viable compartment). Stated another way - even though this is a simplification - after myocardial infarction the distal myocardium could be divided into two compartments: the "vital" compartment and the "scar". Just as is the case for residual myocardial ischemia, FFR_{myo} of the residual stenosis is determined by the relation between stenosis severity and viable myocardial mass. Therefore, it seems logical to postulate that the value of FFR above which residual ischemia will not occur and below which ischemia will occur, remains similar.

This also means that a lesion, which was functionally significant before incomplete infarction, is not necessarily significant thereafter, even when lesion severity remained unchanged. A numerical example will illustrate this point: a 75% stenosis in a vessel with a diameter of 3 mm, has more functional importance in case of a large distribution area than in case of a smaller myocardial territory to be supplied. Because after incomplete myocardial infarction, the distribution area of the infarct-related artery decreases, an anatomically unchanged stenosis becomes less significant. Stated another way: two anatomically completely identical lesions may have a different FFR_{myo} if the depending myocardial distribution is different. This further emphasizes the necessity of functional assessment of coronary stenoses in addition to angiographic studies. This is also illustrated in figure 13.1 where FFR_{myo} increases from 0.50 to 0.84 after 50% of the distal perfusion area has been "removed" by becoming a scar.

This also explains why in a number of patients after partial or incomplete myocardial infarction, no residual ischemia can be induced anymore, not even if there is an anatomically equally severe residual stenosis.

It may be anticipated that, if in the presence of a severe stenosis in an infarct-related artery only a small pressure gradient can be provoked across the lesion, this is indicative for severe myocardial damage and only little viable myocardium. Even in such case, the high FFR indicates that PTCA does not make much sense, as beautifully demonstrated in case 14 of chapter 17. On the other hand, if a considerable gradient can be provoked in such case, this indicates viable myocardium and mostly justifies an intervention (chapter 17, case 15).

Of course, these theoretical considerations need further validation. To validate this theoretical model and to determine whether the FFR value of 0.75 might also be applied in patients with a prior myocardial infarction, the presence of residual ischemia by MIBI-Spect was compared to FFR measurements. Preliminary data are reported in the next paragraph.

13.1.1 Methods.

Twenty-seven patients were studied at least 5 days after myocardial infarction. Twenty-five of them had isolated one-vessel disease. Two patients had also an angiographically significant stenosis in another epicardial artery. In all patients, only the infarct related vessel had to be dilated. Within three days before catheterization, all patients underwent a

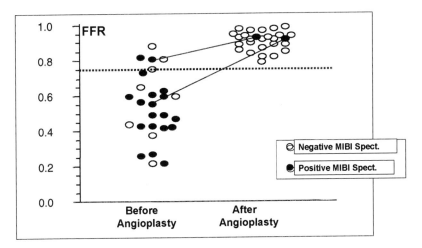

Figure 13.2 *Individual data of FFR in relation to the results of the MIBI Spect before and after successful coronary angioplasty. The black dots indicate a positive MIBI Spect for reversible flow maldistribution in the territory of the infarct vessel. The open circles indicate negative MIBI Spect examinations.*

MIBI-Spect scintigram at rest and after intravenous administration of 140 μg/kg/min of adenosine. The MIBI Spect examination was repeated both at rest and after adenosine within 2 weeks after successful angioplasty. Before and after angioplasty, FFR was measured and diameter stenosis was assessed by quantitative coronary angiography. The analysis of the MIBI-Spect nuclear scan was done without knowledge of the FFR and the angiographic data. A MIBI-Spect scan was considered positive for reversible myocardial ischemia only if, on top of a fixed perfusion defect, a reversible perfusion defect was observed in the area of the infarct vessel.

13.1.2 Results.

All patients underwent PTCA as initially planned, the operator being blinded to the scintigraphic data. In 23 out of 27 patients a stent was implanted. The angiographic diameter stenosis ranged from 54 to 91% (mean 68 ± 10%) before angioplasty and from 2 to 28% (mean 19 ± 7%) after angioplasty. FFR ranged from 0.24 to 0.87 (mean 0.54 ± 0.18) before angioplasty and from 0.82 to 0.99 (mean 0.91 ± 0.04) after angioplasty. The individual FFR data in relation to the results of the MIBI Spect before and after angioplasty are shown in figure 13.2. MIBI-spect scans showed reversible flow maldistribution in 19 out of 27 patients (70%) before angioplasty. Seventeen of them could be considered truly positive as they normalized after angioplasty. In two patients the MIBI Spect scan was positive before angioplasty and remained positive after angioplasty. The FFR of the latter patients was 0.55 and 0.80, respectively. In 8 patients the MIBI Spect scan did not show any signs of flow maldistribution neither before nor after angioplasty.

More importantly, of all positive scans, 17/21 were associated with FFR < 0.75 and of all negative scans, 28/33 were associated with FFR ≥ 0.75, corresponding with a sensitivity of 81%, specificity of 85%, positive predictive value of 77% and a negative predictive value of 87%. When only true positive MIBI-scans were considered, the negative predictive value of FFR increased to 96%. Although these numbers are somewhat lower than in patients without previous infarction, these data suggest that, after the (sub-) acute phase of myocardial infarction has been passed, FFR is a reliable index to decide if the residual stenosis in the infarct-related artery should be dilated or not, and its predictive value in that respect is similar to that of nuclear SPECT-imaging after previous myocardial infarction.

13.1.3 Discussion.

These preliminary results indicate that the FFR value of more than 0.75 remains useful to exclude the occurrence of residual flow maldistribution at adenosine MIBI-Spect nuclear scans in patients after a prior myocardial infarction. The likelihood of residual ischemia in a patient with prior myocardial infarction is indeed very low if FFR is larger than 0.75. It should be noted, however, that FFR < 0.75 in a patient with previous infarction, only indicates reversible ischemia in 77% of the patients.

In summary, in patients with prior myocardial infarction, a FFR value larger than 0.75 reliably excludes the presence of reversible myocardial ischemia, (specificity 85%, negative predictive value 87%) while a FFR value less than 0.75 often, but not always, indicates residual ischemia (sensitivity 81%, positive predictive value 77%). These data have to be confirmed in a larger series of patients.

No data are presently available concerning the influence of the *extent* of myocardial viability after infarction on FFR. Nevertheless, it might be speculated that in patients with a large akinetic area soon after myocardial infarction, the occurrence of a considerable increase in transstenotic pressure gradient during hyperemia might be indicative of viable myocardium and, hence, of potential recovery of contractile function after revascularization. An example of such patient is presented in chapter 17, case 15.

13.2 FFR$_{myo}$ in the presence of microvascular disease.

The presence of resistive vessel dysfunction develops with aging as well as in many pathologic conditions including coronary atherosclerosis. Therefore, some degree of resistive vessel dysfunction is almost invariably present in patients with atherosclerotic epicardial stenosis. It can be assumed that hyperemic flow in these patients is not as high as it was when these patients were younger. This is corroborated by the finding that in patients with atherosclerosis but angiographically normal vessels and in older individuals coronary flow (velocity) reserve is significantly lower than in younger individuals without atherosclerosis[11,12]. Resistive vessel dysfunction implies that the slope of the hyperemic pressure-flow relation is lower than without resistive vessel dysfunction. However, even in the presence of resistive vessel dysfunction the definition of FFR still holds. In that case FFR is also defined as the ratio of maximum hyperemic flow in the stenotic area to maximum hyperemic flow in that same region if the epicardial vessel were normal. If the epicardial artery and the distal microvasculature are considered as two resistances in series, a decrease in hyperemic flow (velocity) or in flow reserve indicates that somewhere in that system an abnormal resistance to flow is present: epicardial, microvascular, or both. Flow (velocity) measurements, therefore, are not be able to distinguish between these two components. In contrast, the decreased hyperemic epicardial coronary pressure, expressed by FFR$_{myo}$,is an indication of the extent of the obstruction caused by the epicardial lesion. *From an interventionalist's viewpoint, FFR still exactly determines to what extent a successful angioplasty (i.e. the reestablishment of the epicardial conductance) will increase maximal myocardial flow whether or not resistive vessel dysfunction is present.* Therefore, from a pathophysiologic point of view, pressure-derived FFR$_{myo}$ and Doppler velocimetry are complementary by providing information as to what extent the epicardial stenosis and the microvascular disease contribute to the occurrence of myocardial ischemia. However, to make a clinical decision whether a patient can be helped by revascularization of an epicardial lesion, FFR_{myo} is the index of choice. Conversely, to determine whether ischemia may occur in a patients without epicardial stenosis, coronary flow (velocity) reserve is the index of choice. An example to illustrate this is presented in chapter 17, case 13.

Further insights in the interpretation of simultaneously determined FFR and CFR in case of microvascular disease, have to be obtained but require determination of both indexes by one single wire, which is anticipated for the near future (paragraph 5.2.2).

13.3 FFR in case of left ventricular hypertrophy.

In left ventricular hypertrophy (LVH), growth of the vascular bed is not proportional to increase of muscle mass[13,14]. Therefore, the normal flow reserve of the myocardial vascular bed will be reduced as LVH develops. As a result, the cut-off value of 0.75 will probably not be valid anymore and become higher with more severe LVH since it is well known that in severe LVH, myocardial ischemia can be present, even if the epicardial coronary arteries are completely normal[15].

No experimental or clinical studies are available so far on the relation between FFR and ischemia in patients with LVH. On theoretical grounds the cut-off value of FFR_{myo} below which ischemia can be induced, will be higher than 0.75 depending on the extent of LVH. When FFR is below 0.75, as a matter of fact reversible myocardial ischemia will be inducible but a higher value does not necessarily exclude ischemia.

For the time being, therefore, it is recommended to be careful in the interpretation of FFR_{myo} in case of LVH.

13.4 Multiple stenoses within one coronary artery.

Coronary atherosclerosis is commonly diffuse and coronary arteriograms frequently demonstrate one or more consecutive stenoses or plaques along the same epicardial artery. It would be desirable to determine functional severity of each of these lesions separately. So far, no invasive or non-invasive method allows to predict the individual contribution of several lesions within one artery to the decrease of myocardial perfusion. As will be shown in this paragraph, coronary pressure measurements enable to determine not only the reduction in maximum blood flow produced by the sum of all the stenoses, but also the exact contribution of each stenosis separately to the reduction of maximum myocardial blood flow.

In case of two consecutive stenoses, the fluid dynamic interaction between the stenoses alters their relative severity and complicates determining FFR for each stenosis separately from the simple ratio of P_d/P_a for a single stenosis. Consequently, for stenoses in series, FFR determined by this simple ratio for a single stenosis may not predict to what extent a proximal lesion will influence myocardial flow after complete relief of the distal stenosis and vice versa.

Therefore, theoretical equations were developed for two serial stenoses to predict the FFR of each stenosis separately as if hypothetically the other stenosis were absent. An animal model of sequential stenoses was used to validate these theoretical equations. In addition these equations were validated in patients with multiple lesions within one coronary artery.

13.4.1 Definitions and mathematical model.

The equations for predicting FFR of each of two sequential stenoses, as if the other stenosis were removed, will be derived mathematically from the initially measured pressures P_a, P_m, P_d and P_w as illustrated in figure 13.3. The terminology is consistent with the original paper on the concept of fractional flow reserve[2]: P_a, P_m, P_d and P_w indicate mean aortic pressure, coronary pressure between both stenoses, coronary pressure distal to the second stenosis, and coronary wedge pressure (distal coronary pressure during total coronary occlusion) at that particular P_a, all measured at maximum coronary hyperemia before any intervention. For simplicity, it is assumed that the resistances of the microvasculature bed are minimal and that the central venous pressure (P_v)is close to zero.

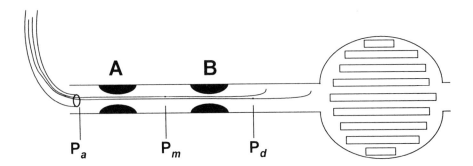

Figure 13.3 *Schematic representation of the experimental setting. An epicardial vessel (with two stenoses A and B, induced by pneumatic occluders) and its depending myocardial bed are shown. P_a, arterial pressure, i.e. the pressure recorded proximal to stenosis A by the guiding catheter; P_m, pressure in between stenosis A and stenosis B, recorded by a pressure-monitoring 0.014-in. guide wire; P_d, pressure distal to stenosis B measured by a second pressure-monitoring guide wire.*

Apparent FFR (FFR$_{app}$): at a first glance, the apparent FFR of stenoses A and B (FFR(A)$_{app}$ and FFR(B)$_{app}$) can be calculated by dividing the pressure distal to stenosis A or B by the pressure proximal to the stenosis A or B, respectively:

$$FFR(A)_{app} = P_m / P_a$$

$$FFR(B)_{app} = P_d / P_m$$

Predicted FFR (FFR$_{pred}$): fluid dynamic theory suggests, however, that the FFR of the proximal stenosis A is influenced by the presence of stenosis B and, vice versa, that the FFR of stenosis B is influenced by the presence of stenosis A since hyperemic flow through one stenosis is limited by the presence of the other stenosis. As described in details elsewhere (16), the predicted FFR of the proximal stenosis (A) and of the distal stenosis (B) as in the hypothetical case that the other stenosis were absent can be calculated by the following equations:

$$FFR(A)_{pred} = \frac{P_d - (P_m / P_a) P_w}{P_a - P_m + P_d - P_w}$$

$$FFR(B)_{pred} = 1 - \frac{(P_a - P_w)(P_m - P_d)}{P_a (P_m - P_w)}$$

Actual or true FFR (FFR_{true}): When stenosis B is actually physically absent, the true FFR of stenosis A is called $FFR(A)_{true}$ and when stenosis A is actually physically absent, the true FFR of stenosis B is called $FFR(B)_{true}$. These indexes can be calculated as follows:

$$FFR(A)_{true} = P_m'/P_a' = P_d'/P_a'$$

$$FFR(B)_{true} = P_d'/P_m' = P_d'/P_a'$$

where P_a', P_m', and P_d' are the hyperemic pressures measured at the corresponding locations after complete removal of one stenosis (see also figure 13.7). To validate the theoretical basis of FFR_{pred}, its calculated values were compared to both FFR_{app} and FFR_{true}. This in vivo validation was performed both in animals and in humans and is presented below.

13.4.2 Animal validation.

In five mongrel dogs, two stenoses were created by pneumatic occluders in the left circumflex coronary artery. During steady state hyperemia (IV adenosine, 140 to 300 µg/kg/min) phasic and mean pressures were recorded by the guiding catheter (P_a) and by two pressure wires (P_m, coronary pressure between both occluders; and P_d ,coronary pressure distally to the distal occluder). Several degrees of proximal and distal stenoses were induced while the other stenosis was left constant. To investigate the influence of a stenosis B on a given stenosis A, 71 combinations of a fixed stenosis A and a variable stenosis B were obtained. For each of these combinations, FFR(A)$_{app}$ and FFR(A)$_{pred}$ were compared to FFR(A)$_{true}$ by linear regression analysis. To investigate the influence of a stenosis A on a given stenosis B, 84 combinations of a fixed stenosis B and a variable stenosis A were created (figure 13.4). For each of these combinations FFR(B)$_{app}$ and FFR(B)$_{pred}$ were compared to FFR(B)$_{true}$ by linear regression analysis.

13.4.3 Human validation.

Thirty-two patients referred for an angioplasty of a native coronary artery with at least 2 stenoses of at least 50% by visual estimation and at least 2 cm apart were investigated. A pressure guidewire (PressureWire XT, Radi Medical Systems, Uppsala, Sweden) was advanced to the distal part of the coronary artery to be treated. Under steady state maximum hyperemia the wire was slowly pulled back from the distal to the proximal part of the coronary artery to identify P_a, P_m and P_d. (figure 13.6). As illustrated in figure 13.7, the proximal stenosis was dilated first in 19 patients and the distal stenosis was dilated first in 13 patients. P_w was measured during balloon inflation. To calculate FFR$_{true}$ a second pull-back pressure recording was performed after PTCA/stenting of one lesion to measure again the hyperemic pressure at the different locations as described above.

Figure 13.4 (opposite page) *Example of hyperemic pressure tracings obtained in dog n°4. The upper panel shows the influence of a varying distal stenosis (B) on a fixed proximal stenosis (A). The lower panel shows the influence of a varying proximal stenosis A on a fixed distal stenosis B. In both examples the predicted fractional flow reserve (FFR_{pred}) remains very close the true value of fractional flow reserve (FFR_{true}) while the apparent value of fractional flow reserve (FFR_{app}) progressively diverges from FFR_{true} as the second stenosis is getting tighter.*

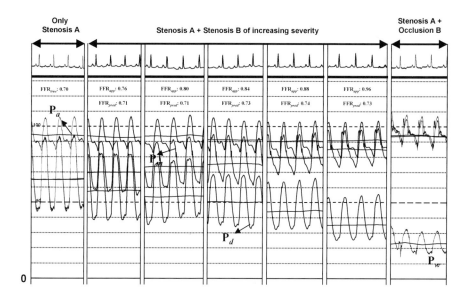

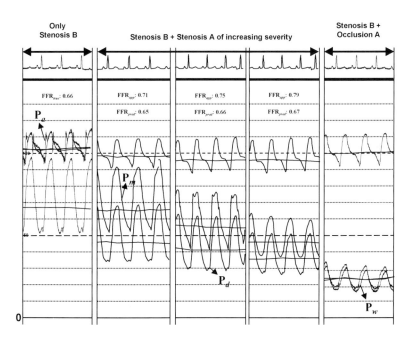

At last, a hyperemic pressure pull-back recording was made after complete removal of both stenoses. Finally, the pressure wire was completely pulled back into the guiding catheter and it was verified that no drift had occurred during the procedure. Some examples of patients in this study are shown in chapter 17, case 18 and 19. Indeed, FFR_{app} progressively overestimated FFR_{true} as expected, whereas FFR_{pred} was close to FFR_{true} in almost every case.

The correlation of FFR_{app} and FFR_{pred} vs FFR_{true} are shown in figure 13.8.

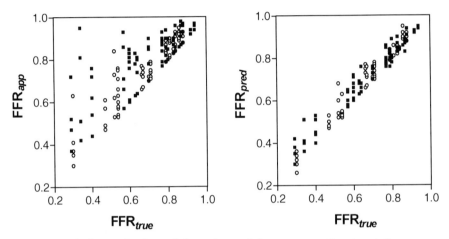

Figure 13.5 *Left panel, plots of the values of the apparent fractional flow reserve (FFR$_{app}$) versus the true fractional flow reserve (FFR$_{true}$). Right panel, plots of the values of the predicted fractional flow reserve (FFR$_{pred}$) versus FFR$_{true}$. The squares represent the FFR values for a fixed stenosis A and a varying stenosis B, the open circles represent the FFR values for a fixed stenosis B and a varying stenosis A.*

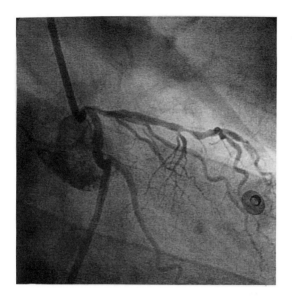

pressure wire pulled back from distal LAD to ostium of LCA during sustained hyperemia

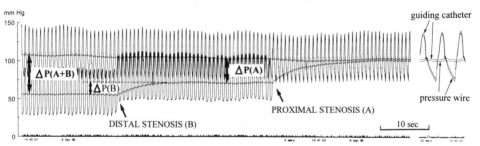

Figure 13.6 *Example of coronary pressure measurement in case of two stenoses within one artery. During sustained maximum coronary hyperemia, the pressure wire is pulled back slowly from the distal coronary artery to the tip of the guiding catheter. Phasic and mean aortic pressure is measured by the guiding catheter, and phasic and mean coronary pressure is measured by the pressure wire. When the pressure sensor crosses either of the stenoses, a discrete pressure gradient is registered (arrows). Both the location and the severity of the different stenoses can be exactly determined by such a hyperemic pull-back curve.*

Figure 13.7 *(opposite page) Representation of the sequence of treatment in the patients in this study with two stenoses in one coronary artery, and definition of pressures. P_a, P_m, and P_d represent mean aortic pressure, coronary pressure in between both stenoses, and coronary pressure distal to the second stenosis, all measured during steady-state maximum coronary hyperemia. The pressures obtained at similar locations after PTCA of one lesion, are indicated by the superfix'. If the proximal stenosis is treated first, in case of an optimal result P_m' will equal P_a' ; if the distal stenosis is treated first, in case of an optimal result P_d' will equal P_m' . The true values FFR $(A)_{true}$ and FFR $(B)_{true}$ as measured after complete elimination of stenosis B and A, were compared to the predicted values FFR $(A)_{pred}$ and FFR $(B)_{pre}$ as predicted from the initial pressures according to equations presented in paragraph 13.4.1.*

13.4.4 Comments.

For serial epicardial stenoses, the classical equation of FFR (P_d /P_a) remains valid for determining the cumulative hemodynamic consequences of the sum of both stenoses. However, the present study confirms that this simple ratio cannot be applied to predict the FFR for each stenosis separately as if the other were removed. In contrast, the individual FFR of each stenosis separately can be predicted by different equations from P_a, P_m, P_d and P_w recorded during maximum hyperemia. The data also suggest that FFR calculated as the P_d/P_a ratio for the stenosis has a greater error in the presence of a second distal stenosis than in the presence of a second proximal lesion.

The importance of maximum transstenotic flow. Pressure-derived FFR is defined as the ratio of hyperemic flow in a stenotic territory expressed as a fraction of what it would be in the hypothetical case the epicardial stenosis were absent. This ratio of two flows can be derived, during maximum hyperemia from the ratio of their respective driving pressures. It has been shown in animals and in humans that, in the range of physiological coronary driving pressure during maximal vascular bed dilation, a linear relation exists between pressure and flow[17,18]. Therefore, during maximum hyperemia, the ratio of two flows equals the ratio of their respective driving pressure. An essential prerequisite for the calculation of pressure-derived FFR is the achievement of maximum transstenotic flow. When only one discrete stenosis is present, pharmacologically-induced maximum vasodilation of the microvasculature will correspond to maximum

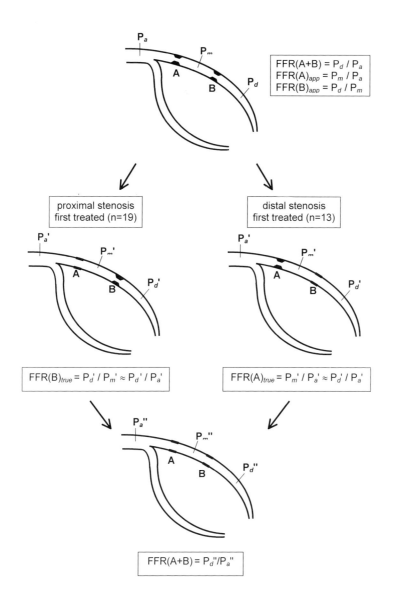

transstenotic flow for a given lesion in a given patient. For that reason FFR tells us exactly to what extent hyperemic flow is limited by the presence of an epicardial stenosis and, conversely, to what extent hyperemic flow will increase after restoring the conductance of the epicardial vessel.

In contrast, when a second stenosis is present along the same epicardial vessel without intervening branches, flow through one stenosis will be submaximal due to another flow limiting stenosis even during maximum vasodilation of the microvasculature. Hence, hyperemic transstenotic gradient will be smaller across any of the two stenoses due to flow being limited by the other stenosis. FFR calculated as the simple ratio of the pressures distal and proximal to each individual stenosis will be smaller than for the same stenosis alone without the more severe second stenosis. It is clear, therefore, that both stenoses influence each other to an extent which is difficult to predict. Nevertheless, as shown in the animal and human studies in this paragraph, coronary pressure still enables accurate prediction of the hemodynamic impact of both stenoses.

Importance of collateral flow. In patients with chronic significant epicardial stenoses, collateral circulation frequently develops. The growth of this collateral circulation depends on the hemodynamic severity of the epicardial stenosis, among other factors. Therefore, in patients with severe coronary artery disease, myocardial perfusion may depend both on antegrade flow through the stenotic epicardial artery and on collateral flow. A more than twofold increase of myocardial perfusion can be provided solely by collaterals in some patients[17]. Myocardial FFR takes into account the contribution of collateral circulation to hyperemic myocardial flow since the distal coronary pressure is determined by aortic pressure and by the extent of collateral circulation in case of isolated epicardial stenosis. Measurements of P_w obtained during coronary occlusion enable determination of the separate contribution of antegrade flow and of collateral flow to total hyperemic myocardial perfusion[2]. In case of multiple stenoses along the same coronary artery, collateral flow will influence both P_w and P_m (the pressure in between the two stenoses). Therefore, the value of P_w cannot be neglected and was therefore incorporated into the equations[16]. The extent to which collateral flow will influence P_m depends on the severity of the second stenosis.

Limitations. When one stenosis is very tight, so that the pressure distal to that stenosis is very close to P_w, very small inaccuracies in measuring P_w might induce large errors in FFR_{pred}. However, this limitation is somewhat academic since a very tight stenosis with a severe pressure gradient will be dilated anyway and the second stenosis evaluated after treatment of the first stenosis.

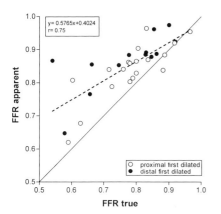
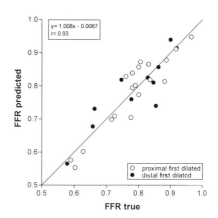

Figure 13.8 *Influence of the presence of one stenosis within a coronary artery on the hemodynamic effect of the other. FFR$_{app}$ indicates the apparent value of fractional flow reserve associated with one stenosis before elimination of the other stenosis, FFR$_{true}$ indicates the measured value of that respective stenosis after elimination of the other stenosis, and FFR$_{pred}$ the predicted value on the basis of the initially measured pressures. The closed points indicate the patients in whom the proximal stenosis was treated first, the open points the patients in whom the distal stenosis was treated first.*

In the left panel, it can be observed how, with increasing severity of one stenosis, the underestimation of the hemodynamic severity of the other stenosis becomes more pronounced. The drawn line is the line of identity and the dashed line the regression line. In the right panel, the regression line coincides with the line of identity.

Moreover, for the two stenoses equations to be applicable, there should be no major arterial branch in between the two stenoses being investigated. If there is an arterial branch between the two stenoses, the non-stenotic low resistance branch increases flow through the first stenosis thereby causing a greater pressure drop across the first stenosis than would occur without the intervening arterial branch. With a lower pressure between the stenoses, flow through the distal stenosis would be reduced in the presence of an arterial branch compared to that without the side branch. Thus the side branch between the stenoses would divert a "steal" flow away from the second stenosis so that the flow through the second stenosis would not be maximal. The pressure gradient across the second stenosis would therefore be less than it would have been in the absence of the side branch. Since the flow through the second stenosis would be reduced in the presence of a side branch, removal of the distal stenosis would result in only limited increased flow capacity through the first stenosis.

With several serial stenoses and intervening branches, this phenomenon of "branch steal"[18] cumulatively along the length of a branching coronary artery may cause a fall in flow at the apex to below normal resting flow after creating maximum hyperemia with resulting ischemia. In diffuse coronary artery disease, this phenomenon is seen as a longitudinal base to apex perfusion gradient on dipyridamole PET perfusion imaging.

Clinical implications. The *first clinical implication* of this study is showing the usefulness of coronary pressure measurement - and especially the pull-back curve at sustained hyperemia - to evaluate the individual hemodynamic effects of different stenoses within one coronary artery. This is important to select the most appropriate lesion(s) for PTCA and to evaluate the separate results of PTCA or stenting at the different locations. Coronary pressure measurement is unique in this way. To our best knowledge, there is no other invasive or non-invasive method to assess the separate hemodynamic effects of different stenoses within one vessel.

The *second implication* is the awareness that the presence of one stenosis in a coronary artery will influence the apparent hemodynamic significance of the other, and that treating one lesion will unmask the true severity of the second one. As shown in this study, it is possible to calculate this effect quantitatively by measuring pressures at the relevant sites within the artery. This also means that the former clinical precept that coronary hemodynamics are determined by the most severe lesion in a coronary artery, is not correct. After stenting, a marked hyperemic gradient is often observed within the artery and one should realize that this does not always indicate suboptimum stent deployment but may also be due to a more proximal or distal stenosis which seemed to be insignificant by angiography before the intervention but has been unmasked by the increased maximum achievable flow due to restoration of the conductance of the stented segment[19]. The awareness that in case of several complex lesions within one coronary artery, the hemodynamic effect of an apparently less severe stenosis may become more pronounced after PTCA of the other, may also influence the decision to aim for bypass surgery instead of multiple PTCA in borderline cases.

A *third important implication* for everyday PTCA practice, is the risk of underestimating functional stenosis severity when large guiding catheters (8F or 9F) are used. In fact, such a guiding catheter often induces an artificial stenosis at the ostium, proximal to the target lesion. When that target lesion is physiologically evaluated, underestimation of its CFR or overestimation of FFR will occur because, due to the guiding catheter, coronary blood flow will not be as high as it could be without that guiding catheter. Consequently, the severity of the target lesion is underestimated. One can recognize this problem during PTCA by any sign of ventricularization of the arterial pressure signal, recorded by the guiding catheter during hyperemia. This problem cannot be solved by using guiding catheters with side holes because, in using those catheters, at hyperemia there is often an additional gradient between the side holes and the proximal coronary pressure at the tip of the guiding catheter[20]. Therefore, for physiologic measurements in coronary arteries, the use of 6F or 7F guidings without side holes is recommended. If 8F or 9F guidings have to be used, for reliable physiologic assessment of a stenosis and to prevent underestimation of its physiologic severity it is advisable to induce maximum hyperemia by intravenous adenosine and to pull back the guiding catheter slightly out of the coronary ostium during measurements.

At last, this study corroborates the fundamental physical principles underlying the concept of fractional flow reserve, stating that in case of maximum vasodilation the distribution of flow in the coronary circulation can be understood completely from pressure measurement, which constitutes a simple but practical tool to make the right decisions in the catheterization laboratory.

13.5 FFR and exercise-induced vasospasm.

In patients with normal coronary arteries, exercise and various forms of stress induce a vasodilation of the epicardial coronary arteries. In the presence of coronary atherosclerosis, a paradoxical vasoconstriction is sometimes present during exercise[21,22], during infusion of acetylcholine[23], during cold pressure test[24], but not during high dose dobutamine infusion[25,26] even though some heterogeneity in vasoactive response between coronary segments has been observed[27,28]. Exercise-induced paradoxical vasoconstriction is abolished by nitrates. Since it is good clinical practice to inject nitrates intracoronarily when entering the coronary tree with a guide wire, pressure-derived FFR is unlikely to take this vasospastic component into account. Therefore, the possibility exists that during pharmacologically induced hyperemia in the catheterization laboratory, the functional severity of the stenosis is less than during "real-life" exercise. This phenomenon might explain why in a few cases ischemia at exercise-testing may be present, whereas FFR measured at adenosine-induced hyperemia is above 0.75. In our practice, these patients are treated by calcium-antagonists and the exercise test is repeated thereafter, often reverting to negative in those cases.

13.6 FFR in long lesions and diffuse disease.

According to the fluid dynamic equation a progressive decline in pressure should be observed from the proximal to the distal part of a long narrowing. Nevertheless, in our clinical experience with intracoronary pressure measurements this phenomen is not always present. In long coronary stenoses a sudden pressure drop sometimes occurs at one particular point of the stenotic segment when the pressure sensor is slowly advanced or pulled back through the stenosis. In diffusely diseased vessels, even when no discrete 'significant' stenosis is visible at angiography, a marked pressure drop may exist between the proximal and the distal part of the artery, especially during hyperemia. The presence and the extent and the exact location of this decline in pressure is most often unpredictable from the angiogram. In these cases a pull-back maneuver of the pressure sensor under steady-state maximal hyperemia can be most useful: if this pressure drop is due to a focal stenosis an angioplasty can be considered; In contrast, when the pressure decline occurs gradually over the whole vessel length, it is unlikely that improving the conductance of a single segment may significantly improve myocardial perfusion. If in such a patient with angina pectoris and diffuse disease a considerable, gradual decline of coronary pressure is present along the coronary artery, resulting in a FFR < 0.75, a bypass graft on the distal part of the artery might be a better option. Such a dilemma what to do and how to solve this by coronary pressure measurements, is beautifully illustrated in chapter 17, case 16 and 17.

References.

1.   De Bruyne B, Baudhuin T, Melin JA, Pijls NHJ, SYS SU, Bol A, Paulus WJ, Heyndrickx GR, Wijns W. Coronary flow reserve calculated from pressure measurements in man. Validation with positron emission tomography. *Circulation* 1994;89:1013-1022.
2.   Pijls NHJ, Van Son JAM, Kirkeeide RL, De Bruyne B, Gould KL. Experimental basis of determining maximum coronary, myocardial, and collateral blood flow by pressure measurements for assessing function stenosis severity before and after percutaneous transluminal coronary angioplasty. *Circulation* 1993;87:1354-67.

3.   Hoffman JIE, Spaan JAE. Pressure-flow relations in coronary circulation. *Physiol Rev* 1990; 70:331-390.

4.   Di Mario C, Krams R, Gil R, Serruys PW. Slope of the instantaneous hyperemic diastolic coronary flow velocity-pressure relation. A new index for assessment of the physiological significance of coronary stenosis in humans. *Circulation* 1994;90:1215-1224.

5.   Lee KS, Marwick TH, Cook SA, Go RT, Fix JS, James KB, Sapp SK, MacIntyre WJ, Thomas JD. Prognosis of patients with left ventricular dysfunction, with and without viable myocardium after acute myocardial infarction. *Circulation* 1994;90:2687-2694.

6.   Califf RM, Topol EJ, Gersh BJ. From myocardial salvage to patient salvage in acute myocardial infarction: the role of reperfusion therapy. *J Am Coll Cardiol* 1989;14:1382-1388.

7.   Uren NG, Crake T, Lefroy DC, De Silva R, Davies GJ, Maseri A. Reduced coronary vasodilator function in infarcted and normal myocardium after myocardial infarction. *N Engl J Med* 1994; 331-222-227.

8.   Maseri A, Crea F, Kaski JC, Crake T. Mechanisms of angina pectoris in syndrome X. *J Am Coll Cardiol* 1991;17:499-506.

9.   Claeys MJ, Vrints CJ, Bosmans J, Krug B, Blockx PP, Snoeck JP. Coronary flow reserve during coronary angioplasty in patients with a recent myocardial infarction: relation to stenosis and myocardial viability. *J Am Coll Cardiol* 1996;28:1712-1719.

10. Pitt B. Evaluation of the postinfarct patient. *Circulation* 1995;91:1855-1860.

11. Kern MJ, Deligonul U, Tatineni S, Serota H, Aguirre FV, Hilton TC: Intravenous adenosine continous infusion and low dose bolus administration for determination of coronary vasodilatory reserve in patients with and without coronary artery disease. *J Am Coll Cardiol* 1991;18:718-729.

12. Uren NG, Camici PG, Melin JA, Bol A, De Bruyne B, Radvan J, Olivotto I, Rosen SD, Impallomeni M, Wijns W. Effect of aging on myocardial perfusion reserve. *J Nucl Med* 1995; 36:2032-2036.

13. Harris CN, Aronow WS, Parker DP, Kaplan MA. Treadmill stress in left ventricular hypertrophy. *Chest* 1973;63:353-359.

14. Marcus ML, Mueller TM, Gascho JA, Kerber RE. Effects of cardiac hypertrophy secondary to hypertension on the coronary circulation. *Am J Cardiol* 1979;44:1023-1031.

15. Hoffmann JIE: Maximal coronary flow and the concept of coronary vascular reserve. *Circulation* 1984;70:153-159.

16. De Bruyne B, Pijls NHJ, Heyndrickx GR, Hodeige D, Kirkeeide R, Gould KL. Pressure-derived fractional flow reserve to assess serial epicardial stenoses: theoretical basis and animal validation. *Circulation* 2000 (in press).

17. Vanoverschelde JL, Wijns W, Depre C, Essamri B, Heyndrickx GR, Borgers M, Bol A, Melin JA. Mechanisms of chronic regional post-ischemic dysfunction in humans. New insights from the study of non-infarcted collateral-dependent myocardium. *Circulation* 1993;87:1513-1523.

18. Gould KL. Coronary atherosclerosis and reversing atherosclerosis. 2nd Edition, Arnold Publishers, 1999; distributed by Oxford University Press.

19. Hanekamp C, Koolen JJ, Pijls NHJ, Bonnier JJRM, Michels HR. Comparison of quantitative coronary angiography, intravascular ultrasound, and pressure-derived fractional flow reserve to assess optimal stent deployment. *Circulation* 1999;99:1015-1021.

20. De Bruyne B, Stockbroeckx J, Demoor D, Heyndrickx GR, Kern MJ. Role of side holes in guide catheters: observations on coronary pressure and flow. *Cath Cardiov Diagn* 1994;33:145-152.

21. Gage JE, Hess OM, Murakami T, Ritter M, Grimm J, Krayenbuehl HP. Vasoconstriction of stenotic coronary arteries during dynamic exercise in patients with classic angina pectoris: reversibility by nitroglycerin. *Circulation* 1986;73:865-876.

22. Gordon JB, Ganz Peter, Nabel EG, Fish RD, Zebede J, Mudge GH, Alexander GW, Selwyn AP. Atherosclerosis influences the vasomotor response of epicardial coronary arteries to exercise. *J Clin Invest* 1989;83:1946-1952.

23. Ludmer PL, Selwyn AP, Shook THL, Wayne RR, Mudge GH, Alexander RW, Ganz P. Paradoxical vasoconstriction induced by acetylcholine in atherosclerotic coronary arteries. *N Engl J Med* 1986;315:1046-1051.

24. Nabel EG, Ganz P, Gordon JB, Alexander RW, Selwyn AP. Dilation of normal and constriction of atherosclerotic coronary arteries caused by the cold pressor test. *Circulation* 1988;77:43-52.

25. Bartunek J, Wijns W, Heyndrickx GR, De Bruyne B. Effects of dobutamine on coronary stenosis physiology and morphology. Comparison with intracoronary adenosine. *Circulation* 1999; 100: 243-249.

26. Wijffels E, Wijns W, Heyndrickx GR, De Bruyne B. Does high dose dobutamine induce a paradoxical coronary vasoconstriction of atherosclerotic arteries ? *Eur Heart J* 1998; 19: 334 (abstract).

27. Tamimi HE, Mansour M, Wargovich TJ, Hill JA, Kerensky RA, Conti R, Pepine CJ. Constrictor and dilator responses to intracoronary acetylcholine in adjacent segments of the same coronary artery in patients with coronary artery disease. *Circulation* 1994;89:45-51.

28. Penny WF, Rockman H, Long J, Bhargava V, Carrigan K, Ibriham A, Shabetal R, Ross J, Peterson KL. Heterogeneity of vasomotor response to acetylcholine along the human coronary artery. *J Am Coll Cardiol* 1995;25:1046-1055.

Chapter 14

FRACTIONAL FLOW RESERVE FOR EVALUATION OF CORONARY INTERVENTIONS

14.1 Fractional flow reserve after balloon angioplasty.

14.1.1 Introduction.

Are there any values of myocardial fractional flow reserve (FFR_{myo}) after a coronary intervention, indicating that the result of the procedure was excellent, moderate, or insufficient ?

In a diagnostic case, a value of FFR_{myo} of 0.75 accurately discriminates stenoses whether or not associated with inducible ischemia (chapter 11 and 12). This implies that after PTCA a value of FFR_{myo} < 0.75 definitely indicates an insufficient and unacceptable result, even if the angiogram looks satisfactory. The main question, therefore, remains how to discriminate patients with a moderate versus an excellent result after an intervention. In the first group, stent implantation or any other additional treatment may be desirable and in the second group, one could possibly refrain from stent implantation. The threshold value of FFR_{myo} indicating an *optimal PTCA-result,* will probably be higher than 0.75, which can be understood as follows: When a stable lesion in a diagnostic study has a value of FFR_{myo} of, for example 0.80, one can be reasonably sure that also next week or next month, this value will be approximately 0.80 and that no inducible ischemia will be present. However, after angioplasty, the well-recognized early loss of luminal gain[1-4] will most likely be paralleled by an early decrease of FFR_{myo}. Therefore, a value too close above that cut-off point of 0.75, may only be a too moderate physiologic result after PTCA.

Thus, it would be interesting to see if, in the presence of a satisfactory post-PTCA angiogram, there is a relation between FFR$_{myo}$ measured immediately after PTCA and the chance of early and late restenosis. Such a question is of direct clinical importance because a subgroup of patients could possibly be identified in whom stent implantation would be preferable and a subgroup which does not benefit from additional stent implantation. In this respect, those patients are especially interesting in whom both the angiographic and physiologic evaluation of the PTCA was excellent. In the recent DEBATE, DESTINY, and FROST trials, it was shown that in a particular subset of patients with a post-PTCA residual diameter stenosis of less than 35% by QCA and an absolute coronary flow velocity reserve (CFVR) of more than 2.5, the 6-month restenosis rate was only 10-15%, compared to 25-30% in the remaining population[5-8]. The predictive value of angiography alone or CFVR alone, was significantly weaker. Thus, these studies indicate that there is a complementary value of anatomic and physiologic evaluation methods of PTCA results.

In a similar way, we investigated the hypothesis if pressure-derived fractional flow reserve, being an even more lesion-specific index than CFR, has a complementary value to angiography in evaluating PTCA result. In other words, we investigated if a correlation was present between FFR measured directly after PTCA and long-term restenosis rate, and - if so - if a threshold value of FFR can be identified indicating particularly favorable long-term clinical outcome after plain balloon angioplasty.

14.1.2 Methods.

Study population. Because the threshold to place a stent after PTCA is currently very low, considerable bias would be introduced in studying an unstented patient cohort today. Such a group of patients would probably represent an extremely positive selection bias and would have a better prognosis anyway. Therefore, to investigate the relation between FFR after plain balloon angioplasty and clinical outcome, we studied a patient cohort that underwent PTCA in 1994, when stenting in our laboratory was performed only as bailout procedure and not as additional treatment after suboptimal PTCA. The study population consisted of 60 consecutive patients with single-vessel disease and normal left ventricular function who underwent plain balloon angioplasty of a single lesion. In all patients, a positive exercise test was available ≤ 24 hours before PTCA. In these patients, a pressure guide wire was used to record distal coronary pressure (P$_d$) and to calculate FFR before, during, and after the procedure. After successful PTCA, all medication was stopped except nifedipine 20 mg BID, which was stopped 48 hours later, and aspirin 80 mg/d, which was continued.

In those 58 patients with successful PTCA, the exercise test was repeated 5 to 7 days later. If the second exercise test was completely normal, from Bayesian considerations it was claimed that no inducible ischemia was present at that moment and that a positive exercise test later at follow-up would again indicate inducible ischemia.

Pressure measurement. During the PTCA, both aortic pressure (P_a) and distal (transstenotic) coronary pressure (P_d) were measured continuously by the guiding catheter and the pressure wire (Radi Medical Systems, Uppsala, Sweden), respectively. FFR was calculated 15 minutes after a satisfactory angiographic result had been obtained by FFR = P_d/P_a , where P_d and P_a were recorded simultaneously at maximum coronary vasodilation, induced by infusion of adenosine ($140\ \mu\ \cdot\ kg^{-1}\ \cdot\ min^{-1}$) into a femoral vein for 2 to 4 minutes[9,10] as described before.

Quantitative coronary angiography. QCA analysis was performed on the pre-PTCA angiograms and on the post-PTCA angiograms 15 minutes after the final balloon inflation, preferably in 2 orthogonal projections, with the Cardiovascular Angiography Analysis System[11]. With the guiding catheter as a scaling device, reference diameter, minimal lumen, diameter (MLD), and percentage diameter stenosis (DS) of the target lesion were calculated as the average value of both projections.

Follow-up and adverse cardiac events. Exercise testing was repeated after 5 to 7 days in all patients with successful PTCA. Follow-up visits were performed at 6,12, and 24 months. Adverse cardiac events were defined in a mutually exclusive hierarchic ranking order as death, myocardial infarction, unstable angina, coronary bypass surgery, repeated PTCA, and the recurrence of angina complaints accompanied by a positive exercise test, which was always performed in case of recurrent chest pain. No repeated angiography was performed, except in patients with recurrent chest pain to avoid bias and repeated PTCA based solely upon the oculo-stenotic reflex without presence of chest pain or documented ischemia.

Statistical analysis. Continuous data are reported as mean ± SD. Differences between subgroups were tested by use of paired or unpaired Student's *t* test when appropriate. Categorical differences between subgroups were tested by use of Fisher's exact test.

Univariate and multivariate logistic regression analyses were performed to determine independent predictors of an adverse cardiac event within 24 months of follow-up.

Table 14.1 *Baseline data of study patients.*

	Adverse Cardiac Event at follow-up		
	Yes (n = 16)	No (n = 42)	*P*
Male, n (%)	14 (88)	26 (62)	0.1101
Age, y	63 ± 10	60 ± 8	0.2213
Risk factors, n (%)			
Hypertension	5 (31)	14 (33)	1.0000
Diabetes	2 (13)	8 (19)	0.7105
Hypercholesterolemia	3 (19)	15 (36)	0.3417
Smoking	3 (19)	11 (26)	0.7360
Family history	5 (31)	19 (45)	0.1108
Previous PTCA, n (%)	0 (0)	1 (2)	1.0000
Previous aborted infarction, n (%)	2 (13)	8 (19)	0.7105
CCS class	2.7 ± 0.5	2.6 ± 0.6	0.7068
Duration of complaints, mo	14 ± 15	8 ± 8	0.1388
Drugs, n	2.8 ± 1.0	3.0 ± 0.8	0.3867
Angiographic data before PTCA			
LAD/LCX/RCA, No.patients	10/2/4	28/6/8	NS
Reference diameter, mm	2.93 ± 0.75	3.01 ± 0.48	0.6273
MLD, mm	1.38 ± 0.44	1.27 ± 0.41	0.3937
DS, %	53 ± 13	58 ± 11	0.0791
Pressure data before PTCA			
P_a , mmHg	93 ± 15	95 ± 16	0.6686
P_d , mmHg	47 ± 16	56 ± 16	0.0623
ΔP_{max} , mmHg	46 ± 16	39 ± 14	0.1092

CCS indicates Canadian Cardiology Society; LAD, left anterior descending; LCX, left circumflex; RCA, right coronary artery; and ΔP_{max} hyperemic transstenotic pressure gradient. N = 58.

By receiver-operating characteristic (ROC) analysis, the best threshold value of FFR to predict an adverse cardiac event was determined.

According to that value, patients were dichotomized into those with optimal and those with suboptimal functional results. Our study population was also subdivided into a subgroup with an optimal angiographic result, defined as a residual DS ≤ 35%, and into a subgroup with a suboptimal angiographic result, defined as a residual DS of 36% to 50%. Because detection of post-PTCA QCA variables with sufficient predictive diagnostic power would require a larger sample size, the choice for this DS cut-off value of 35% was based on the results of an earlier study that related residual DS after PTCA to restenosis chance[5].

Thus, our population was divided into 2 groups: group A, all patients in whom both the angiographic and functional results were optimal, and group B, the remaining patients in whom either the angiographic or functional result or both were suboptimal.

Event-free survival curves for both groups were constructed and compared by use of the log-rank test. A value of $P > 0.05$ was considered statistically significant.

14.1.3 Results.

Baseline data and procedural results. In 2 patients, no immediate satisfactory PTCA result could be achieved. Both patients underwent bypass surgery. Therefore, successful PTCA was performed in 58 patients, who were eligible for further follow-up.

The baseline clinical data and procedural results of these patients are summarized in table 14.1 and 14.2. In all 58 patients DS immediately after

Table 14.2 *Angiographic and pressure data before and after PTCA.*

Variable	Before	After	P
Pressure variables			
FFR	0.56 ± 0.14	0.88 ± 0.07	< 0.001
P_a, mmHg	94 ± 16	90 ± 16	< 0.006
P_d, mmHg	53 ± 17	79 ± 15	< 0.001
ΔP_{max}, mmHg	41 ± 15	11 ± 7	< 0.001
P_w, mmHg (during PTCA)	26 ± 11		
Angiographic variables			
Reference diameter, mm	2.99 ± 0.58	2.96 ± 0.52	0.729
MLD, mm	1.30 ± 0.42	2.19 ± 0.38	< 0.001
DS, %	57 ± 12	26 ± 9	< 0.001

P_w indicates coronary wedge pressure. N = 58.

PTCA was $< 50\%$; in 52 patients, DS was $\leq 35\%$. FFR increased from 0.56 ± 0.14 before PTCA to 0.88 ± 0.07 after the procedure ($P < 0.0001$). In all 58 patients, FFR immediately after PTCA was ≥ 0.75; in 29 patients, FFR was ≥ 0.90. In 56 of these 58 patients, the exercise test 5 to 7 days after PTCA reverted to negative.

Follow-up and predictive value of FFR and DS for adverse cardiac events.
A 24-month follow-up was obtained in all patients. During follow-up, 16 adverse cardiac events occurred, which are specified in table 14.3. FFR and mean hyperemic transstenotic pressure gradient (ΔP_{max}) in patients with or without an event at follow-up were significantly different. DS in this respect was not different between groups (table 14.4).

Multivariate logistic regression analysis of clinical, angiographic, and pressure variables demonstrated that post-PTCA FFR was the most significant independent predictor for adverse cardiac events (table 14.5). By ROC analysis, the best discriminating value of FFR with the highest sum of sensitivity and specificity was 0.89 (figure 14.1; ROC area, 68%; $P = 0.0103$). Therefore, FFR $\geq$ 0.90 was defined as indicating an optimal functional PTCA result, whereas $0.75 \leq$ FFR < 0.90 was defined as indicating an initially successful but suboptimal PTCA result.

Table 14.3 *Adverse cardiac events at 6, 12, and 24 months of follow-up.*

	6 months		12 months		24 months	
	A	B	A	B	A	B
Death	0	0	0	0	0	1
AMI	0	0	0	0	0	1
CABG	0	3	0	3	0	3
Repeated PTCA	1	5	1	6	2	6
Recurrent ischemia*	1	2	1	2	1	2
Total	2	10	2	11	3	13

AMI indicates acute myocardial infarction. A indicates the 26 patients in whom both optimal angiographic (residual DS $\leq$ 35%) and optimal functional (FFR $\geq$ 0.90) results were obtained. B indicates the remaining 32 patients in whom either the angiographic or functional result or both were suboptimal.
*Patients with a negative exercise test 5-7 days after the intervention and recurrent ischemia confirmed by a positive exercise test at follow-up.

Table 14.4 *Post-PTCA pressure and angiographic variables in patients with and without adverse cardiac event*

	Adverse Cardiac Event at follow-up		
	Yes (n = 16)	No (n = 42)	*P*
P_a , mmHg	92 ± 16	89 ± 15	0.5432
P_d , mmHg	78 ± 15	79 ± 15	0.6907
P_w , mmHg	23 ± 9	27 ± 12	0.1958
ΔP_{max} , mmHg	14 ± 7	10 ± 7	0.0273
FFR	0.84 ± 0.07	0.89 ± 0.07	0.0299
DS, %	28 ± 9	29 ± 8	0.6256

According to these cut-off values of 0.90 for FFR and 35% for DS, patients were then stratified into 4 subsets according to optimal versus suboptimal post-PTCA FFR and optimal versus suboptimal percentage DS. The result of this stratification in relation to the occurrence of cardiac adverse events is presented in figure 14.2. The restenosis rate for the patients with an excellent versus moderate functional result after PTCA are also presented as bar graphs in figure 14.3.

As shown in figure 14.4, event-free survival rates at 6, 12, and 24 months in patients with optimal functional and anatomic results were 92 ± 5%, 92 ± 5%, and 88 ± 6%, respectively, versus 72 ± 8%, 69 ± 8%, and 59 ± 9%, respectively, in the remaining patients (*P* = 0.047, *P* = 0.028, and *P* = 0.014, respectively). If the criterion of FFR ≥ 0.90 was used alone, an almost similar event-free survival was observed.

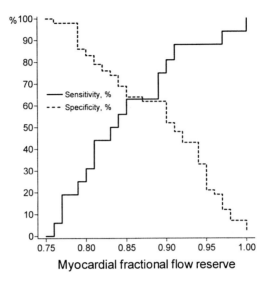

Figure 14.1 *ROC graph showing percentage correct prediction of event (sensitivity, %) and percentage correct prediction of no event (specificity, %) during follow-up of 24 months as function of post-PTCA FFR. Optimal cut-off value for FFR was chosen as point with highest sum of sensitivity and specificity.*

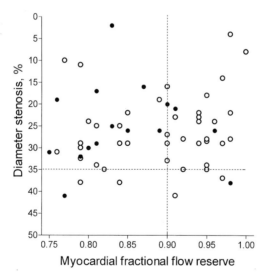

Figure 14.2. *FFR versus DS after PTCA. Separated by cut-off values for DS of 35% and FFR of 0.90, right upper quadrant represents 26 patients with both optimal angiographic and optimal functional results (group A); remaining 3 quadrants represent remaining patients in whom either angiographic or functional result or both were suboptimal (group B). Solid points indicate patients with adverse cardiac event during follow-up.*

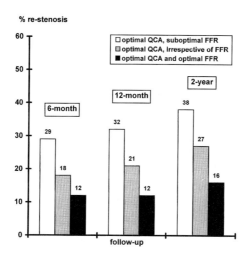

Figure 14.3. *Clinical restenosis rate after plain balloon angioplasty at 6-month, 1 year, and 2 year follow-up for patients with an optimal anatomic (residual DS < 35%) and functional result (FFR ≥ 0.90) versus patients with either suboptimal anatomic or functional result.*

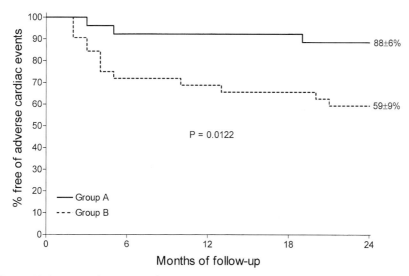

Figure 14.4 *Event-free survival curves. Group A indicates 26 patients in whom both optimal angiographic (residualDS ≤ 35%) and optimal functional (FFR ≥ 0.90) results were obtained. Group B indicates remaining 32 patients in whom either angiographic or functional result both were suboptimal.*

14.1.4 Discussion.

This retrospective study with 2 years of follow-up confirms the complementary value of anatomic and physiologic approaches in the evaluation of the PTCA result and indicates that a subgroup of patients (45% in this study) can be discriminated in whom an excellent long-term outcome with a low event rate can be obtained by regular balloon angioplasty. This study also confirms earlier results that the coronary angiogram alone is not able to predict clinical outcome[12,13]. The present data also show that $\approx 50\%$ of the patients with an angiographically optimal result (DS $\leq 35\%$) still have an FFR < 0.90 (figure 14.2).

The threshold value of 0.90, found in this study to correspond with favorable long-term outcome, needs further explanation. In diagnostic coronary catheterization, it has been established that an FFR of 0.75 reliably identifies lesions associated with reversible ischemia[9,10,14-16]. Therefore, immediately after PTCA, a value of FFR ≥ 0.75 will be sufficient to prevent inducible ischemia and can be called an initially successful functional result. However, when searching for a value of FFR indicating a sufficient long-term PTCA result, it can be expected that such a value must be > 0.75, because in the first days, weeks, and months after PTCA, considerable changes in stenosis morphology with some loss of the initial luminal gain may occur[17-19]. Dynamic processes like recoil, intimal hyperplasia, and smooth muscle cell proliferation may affect part of the initial gain and result in a decrease in FFR to values < 0.75 in a number of initially successfully dilated patients. Therefore, although reversible ischemia was absent shortly after PTCA in all patients with FFR ≥ 0.75 (as indicated by the reversal of the exercise test from positive to negative), in a number of patients, some decrease in FFR probably occurred during follow-up because of the dynamic processes described above. For this reason, it is conceivable that although FFR ≥ 0.75 is sufficient to prevent ischemia immediately after PTCA (as was the case in this study), an initially higher value is necessary in a dynamic situation to compensate for the anticipated changes in morphology and function and to minimize the chance of restenosis in the long run. In fact, such differences with respect to threshold values to be used either at diagnostic procedures or after coronary intervention have been established for most other anatomic and functional parameters, including QCA and Doppler flow velocity measurement[5,20,21].

The purpose of the present study was to investigate whether a particular predictive value of FFR somewhere between 0.75 and 1.00, can be identified above which clinical events become less likely. Our results suggest that such a value exists and equals 0.90. The observed differences were significant and maintained over a follow-up of 2 years. In those patients with optimal anatomic and functional results, event rate was low and comparable to event rates in stent studies like BENESTENT and STRESS[22-24].

14.1.5 Comparison with intravascular ultrasound.

The reasons why such a strong correlation is present between a high value of FFR and favorable outcome are not completely clear yet. However, from intracoronary ultrasound studies, it is known that even an almost normal angiographic luminogram after PTCA can be accompanied by considerable residual stenosis[25,26]. Tears and splits induced by balloon inflation may fill with contrast medium so that angiography is limited in the ability to assess short- and long-term benefits of angioplasty. This has been demonstrated recently in an elegant way by Akasaka[27] et al, who demonstrated by IVUS that in patients with a suboptimal FFR (0.71 ± 0.06) after plain balloon angioplasty, despite significant anatomic improvement, only cracks and tears were present and only little or no increase in IVUS luminal area was obtained (figure 14.5). After additional stent implantation, however, the lumen increased significantly and FFR increased accordingly to 0.86 ± 0.07. On the other hand, in those patients who already had a high value of FFR after PTCA (0.89 ± 0.04), IVUS showed a stent-like increase in luminal area from 2.0 ± 1.7 to 7.2 ± 2.3 mm^2 (table 14.5 and figure 14.6; courtesy of Dr.T.Akasaka, Kobe General Hospital). These data confirm that, in contrast to angiography, FFR reflects more accurately significant improvement of luminal area and the overall conductance of the dilated segment. Further studies comparing coronary pressure, and intravascular ultrasound are presently performed to support this position.

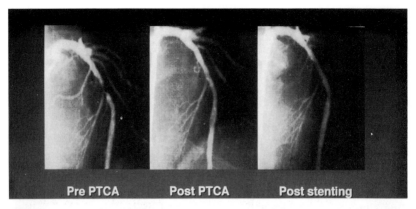

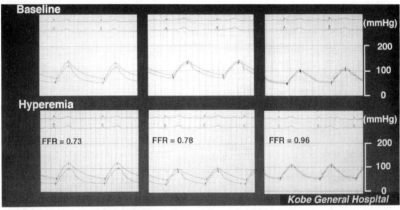

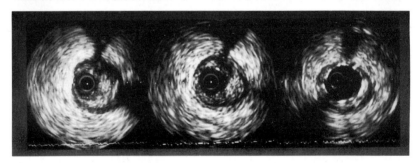

Figure 14.5 *Example of suboptimal FFR after PTCA and corresponding IVUS-findings, as well as the images after additional stenting. Although the angiography after regular balloon angioplasty shows an apparently successful result, FFR only increased minimally from 0.73 before to 0.78 after balloon angioplasty. By IVUS, it is confirmed that the angiographical improvement was only due to some cracks filling with contrast, without true improvement of the lumen (3.4 mm^2 before and 4.2 mm^2 after PTCA). After additional stenting, IVUS shows significant luminal increase from 4.2 to 7.9 mm^2, which is accompanied by complete normalization of FFR to 0.96 (Courtesy of T.Akasaka, MD, Kobe General Hospital).*

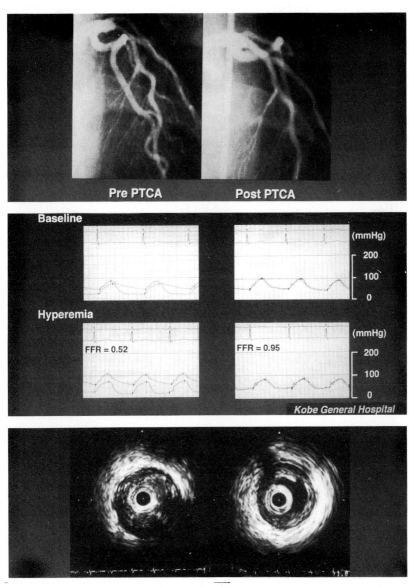

Figure 14.6 *Example of optimal FFR after PTCA and corresponding IVUS-findings. In this case, angiographically successful balloon angioplasty was accompanied by increase of FFR to 0.95, and no stent was placed. IVUS confirmed an excellent result with luminal increase from 1.9 to 7.2 mm². (Courtesy of T.Akasaka, MD, Kobe General Hospital).*

Table 14.5 *IVUS and FFR data after angiographically successful PTCA (N = 25).*

	Suboptimum FFR after PTCA (N=11) → addit.stenting	Optimum FFR after PTCA (N=14) → no stent
Coronary pressure (FFR)		
pre-PTCA	0.44 ± 0.21	0.45 ± 0.20
post-PTCA	0.71 ± 0.06	$0.89 \pm 0.04*$
post-stent	0.86 ± 0.07	-
IVUS lumen area (mm²)		
pre-PTCA	1.6 ± 0.4	2.0 ± 1.7
post-PTCA	4.4 ± 1.1	$7.2 \pm 2.3*$
post-stent	7.3 ± 2.0	-
IVUS symm index		
post-PTCA	0.6 ± 0.1	$0.8 \pm 0.1*$
post-stent	0.9 ± 0.1	
Cracks	9/11 (82%)	4/14 (29%)
Dissection > B	7/11 (64%)	1/14 (7%)

* P < 0.01 vs suboptimal FFR group   *From Akasaka et al, Kobe General Hospital*

14.1.6 Conclusions.

The studies described and referred to above, indicate that long-term clinical outcome after plain balloon angioplasty in patients with both FFR ≥ 0.90 and residual DS ≤ 35% is excellent and is comparable to the outcome observed after coronary stenting in patients with similar characteristics[22-24]. This suggests that in patients with an optimal functional and angiographic PTCA result, no further improvement in clinical outcome is expected from coronary stenting. Conversely, given the high event rate in patients with a suboptimal functional PTCA result reflected by FFR < 0.90, further action to improve the result seems most appropriate. The results from Akasaka's study with a close correlation between FFR and IVUS after PTCA, strongly support this position[27]. These conclusions are summarized and implemented in the guidelines in paragraph 14.5 at the end of this chapter.

14.2 Fractional flow reserve after stent implantation.

It is well known that coronary stent deployment may be incomplete in spite of normal angiographic images[9,10]. Therefore, methods to check complete deployment of a stent are important. So far, only intracoronary ultrasound has proven to be useful for that purpose and is considered as the gold standard in this respect. It enables visualization of complete apposition, symmetrical deployment of the stent, and confirmation of an internal stent diameter fitting the reference segments. However, IVUS is rather expensive and time-consuming and the interpretation of images is not trivial. Let's investigate, therefore, if coronary pressure is also a useful tool for evaluation of stent deployment and start with some background considerations with respect to this issue.

In the ideal case, coronary stenting should result in normalization of the conductance of the stented segment. Therefore, as myocardial fractional flow reserve (FFR_{myo}) is a specific index of that epicardial conductance, and as normal FFR_{myo} equals 1.0, it seems to be logical to propose FFR_{myo} as an index of optimal stent deployment. Any decreased value of FFR_{myo} would indicate subnormal epicardial conductance and therefore sub-optimal deployment of the stent. In contrast to other functional methods, such as Doppler and videodensitometry, there is no variation of normal values or confounding by distal small vessel disease and even if the microvasculature does not function normally immediately after PTCA, FFR_{myo} associated with a well-deployed stent is expected to be 1.0. In the present paragraph it will be validated that epicardial segmental conductance completely normalizes indeed after optimum stent deployment and vice versa, that incomplete stent deployment is associated with a residual hyperemic gradient across the stent. At first, a recent study will be described comparing QCA, IVUS and coronary pressure measurement side-to-side in 30 patients undergoing a coil stent implantation. Next, the results of a large database will be presented of patients who underwent coronary pressure-guided stent implantation.

14.3 Comparison of QCA, intravascular ultrasound, and coronary pressure measurement to assess optimum stent deployment.

14.3.1 FFR as a specific index of epicardial conductance.

Notwithstanding the benefits of coronary stenting during coronary intervention in terms of a better initial result and lower restenosis rate, the use of coronary stents has also been associated with some major concerns, i.e. the risk of (sub) acute stent closure despite optimum anticoagulation and in-stent restenosis which can be difficult to treat[22,23,28,29]. Studies with intracoronary ultrasound (IVUS) have shown that despite an apparently satisfying angiographic result, stents are often insufficiently deployed and high pressure balloon inflation may be necessary to achieve complete stent expansion[30]. However, unnecessary high pressure inflation bears the risk of damaging the adjacent wall, disturbing the configuration of the stent, protruding the plaque remnants through the stent struts, and inducing inappropriate intimal hyperplasia[31]. Therefore, the importance of methods to guide optimum stent deployment is indisputable and the usefulness of IVUS in this respect is unsurpassed so far. However, IVUS is expensive, requires exchange of the balloon for the IVUS catheter, and can be time consuming[31,32]. Therefore, it would be useful to have available a cheaper and more simple alternative method of evaluating optimum stent deployment.
Pressure-derived myocardial fractional flow reserve (FFR_{myo}) has emerged as an easily obtainable, accurate, and lesion-specific index of the functional severity of a coronary stenosis, not affected by hemodynamic variability such as changes of heart rate and blood pressure[9,10,14,15]. FFR_{myo} has an unequivocal normal value of 1.0 for every patient and every coronary artery, and is a specific index of the conductance of the epicardial coronary artery. As discussed in chapter 14.1 during percutaneous transluminal coronary angioplasty, FFR_{myo} quantifies subsequent changes in maximum achievable blood flow[13,15]. Because the purpose of coronary stenting is normalization of the conductance of the stented epicardial segment, it has been hypothesized that FFR_{myo} after coronary stenting should return to normal, or at least that if disease is present elsewhere in the same coronary artery, no hyperemic gradient should persist across a well-stented segment[33]. The opposite (i.e. the question of whether the absence of a hyperemic gradient is always associated with complete stent deployment) has not been investigated so far and is less trivial. Therefore, the purpose of this study was to compare in a

side-by-side manner the value of QCA, IVUS, and coronary pressure measurement for assessment of optimum stent deployment.

14.3.2 Methods.

Study population. Thirty patients who were scheduled for elective coronary angioplasty and primary stenting of a de novo lesion in the proximal part of a native coronary artery with a reference diameter of ≥ 3.0 mm were selected for inclusion in the study. After written informed consent had been obtained, these patients were treated and underwent implantation of a Wiktor-i stent (Medtronic) according to the procedure described below. The study protocol was approved by the institutional ethical review board .

Angioplasty and stent implantation. After the introduction of a 6-8F guiding catheter into the left femoral artery and the introduction of a 5F sheath into the femoral vein, 10.000 IU heparin iv was administered, repeated by an additional 5000 IU every hour. The guiding catheter was advanced into the coronary artery, and after intracoronary administration of 300 µg of nitroglycerin, angiograms were made from two orthogonal projections at an acquisition rate of 25 frames/s. Determination of the appropriate stent size was performed with the use of on-line quantitative coronary angiography (QCA) measurement. After appropriate predilatation, a Wiktor-i stent was implanted using an inflation pressure of 6 Atm, after which deployment was assessed consecutively by QCA, IVUS, and pressure measurement. For all these three investigational modalities, criteria for optimum stent deployment were defined in advance. If optimum stent deployment was not achieved with any of these 3 methods, inflation pressure was increased with steps of 2 Atm and stent deployment was reassessed by the use of all three investigational modalities after every step, until all criteria for optimum stent deployment were met by all methods (figure 14.7), or until the treating cardiologist decided to accept the result. If no optimum result could be achieved, a larger balloon size could be chosen to repeat the sequence above. After stent implantation, all patients were treated by ticlopidine 250 mg daily for 28 days and aspirin 80 mg indefinitely.

Quantitative coronary angiography. Coronary angiograms were made from preferably two orthogonal views before the procedure, after predilatation, and after every step of stent deployment. For all angiograms, 10 mL (right coronary artery) or 12 mL (left coronary artery) of the contrast agent iomeprol (Iomeran) with an iodine content of 350 mg/mL was injected with the use of a power injector at an injection rate of 4 mL/s. QCA was both performed on-line and repeated off-line, using the QCA-CMS 3.0 system

(CMS-MEDIS)[34]. For automated edge detection, the gradient field transform algorithm of this system for complex lesion analysis was used[35]. It has been shown that with radiopaque stents, like the Wiktor stent, accurate edge detection can be performed in this way, provided that a high iodine contrast agent is used with rapid and complete filling of the epicardial segment, as was the case in this study[36]. Reference diameter, minimal luminal diameter, and percentage diameter stenosis were calculated as the average value of the two views analyzed off-line. Optimum stent deployment according to QCA was defined as a residual diameter stenosis of < 10 %.

Intravascular ultrasound imaging (IVUS). Intravascular ultrasound imaging was performed using a 2.9F single element 30 MHz beveled transducer imaging catheter (Cardiovascular Imaging Systems Inc., Sunnyvale. CA, U.S.A.) or a 3.0F phased-array transducer (Endosonics, Rancho Cordova, CA). At every step of evaluation the catheter was withdrawn with a speed of 0.5 mm/s , by using a motorized automatic pull-back device. Stent deployment was assessed on-line and defined as optimum if, and only if, all of the following criteria were fulfilled[37]:

1. *complete apposition of all stent struts against the vessel wall;*
2. *symmetry index ≥ 0.7 (the ratio of the minimal in-stent lumen diameter to the maximal in-stent lumen diameter);*
3. *in-stent minimal cross-sectional area (CSA) ≥ 90 % of the average reference CSA, or ≥ 100% of the smallest reference segment CSA.*

All studies were recorded on videotape, and re-analyzed off-line.

Coronary pressure measurement and calculation of FFR$_{myo}$.
During the procedure, aortic pressure (P_a) and distal (transstenotic) coronary pressure (P_d) were measured continuously by the guiding catheter and a 0.014-in pressure guide wire (PressureWire, RADI Medical Systems, Uppsala, Sweden), respectively. Before angioplasty and after every step of in-stent balloon inflation, steady-state maximum hyperemia was induced by intravenous infusion of adenosine 140 µg.kg^{-1}.min^{-1}, through the femoral venous sheath and myocardial fractional flow reserve (FFR$_{myo}$) was calculated by:

$$FFR_{myo} = P_d / P_a$$

where P_a and P_d are recorded simultaneously at maximum hyperemia. After the predilatation, a pull-back pressure curve was made to detect disease elsewhere in the artery. *In case of unexpected coronary artery disease elsewhere in the vessel,* which was the case in 3 patients, *FFR$_{myo}$ was replaced by the ratio of the hyperemic pressure just distal to the stent to the hyperemic pressure just proximal to the stent.* Because FFR$_{myo}$ in true normal coronary arteries equals 0.94 -1.00 (chapter 10), and because normalization of epicardial conductance is expected by optimum stent implantation, optimum stent deployment according to coronary pressure measurement was defined as a value of FFR_{myo} (or a distal-to-proximal hyperemic pressure ratio) of ≥ 0.94.

Statistical analysis. The values of angiographic and pressure indexes are given as mean $\pm$ SD. All data for QCA and IVUS refer to the off-line analysis. The relations between IVUS and FFR, QCA and IVUS, and QCA and FFR were analyzed with use of the χ^2 (Chi-square) test. The inflation pressures necessary to obtain optimum results were compared by use of the unpaired *t*-test. Receiving Operator Characteristics (ROC) analysis was performed to establish the value of FFR most predictive for optimum stent deployment according to the combined IVUS criteria. Statistical significance was considered to be present at $P < 0.05$.

14.3.3 Results .

Baseline characteristics and procedural results. In our study population (mean age, 60 ± 8 years, 24 males and 6 females), 30 Wiktor-i stents with a diameter of 3.5 ± 0.3 mm were successfully implanted; 10 in the left anterior descending artery, 11 in the left circumflex artery, and 9 in the right coronary artery.

A total of 93 balloon inflations for stent deployment at different inflation pressures of 6 to 14 Atm were performed, according to the study protocol. Ultimately, optimum stent deployment was obtained in 24 patients according to QCA criteria, in 17 patients according to IVUS criteria, in 17 patients according to FFR_{myo} criteria, and in 13 patients according to all 3 investigation modalities. In other words, optimization of stent deployment according to all 3 investigational modalities was not obtained in 17 patients, as specified in table 14.6.

Twenty-nine patients could be discharged uneventful within 24 hours after the procedure. One patient experienced an enzymatic non Q-wave myocardial infarction, and was discharged 7 days later in good condition.

Quantitative coronary angiography. Reliable QCA measurements were performed after 92 of the 93 balloon inflations used for stent deployment. Optimum stent deployment according to QCA was achieved in 24 of the 30 patients at a mean inflation pressure of 8.4 ± 2.0 Atm. The distribution of inflation pressures and QCA results are presented in table 14.6.

Intravascular ultrasound imaging (IVUS). Reliable IVUS imaging could be performed after 87 of the 93 inflations. Reasons for not having performed

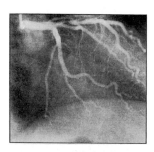
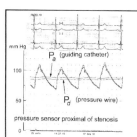
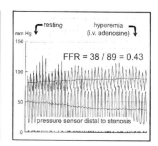

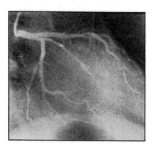
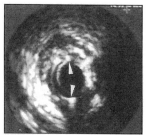
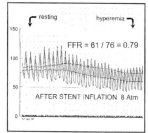

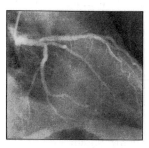
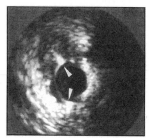
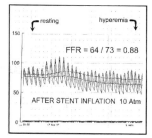

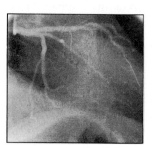
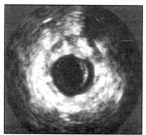
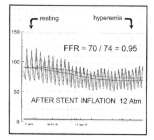

Figure 14.7 (opposite page) *Coronary angiograms, simultaneously obtained aortic (P$_a$) and distal coronary (Pd) pressures, and IVUS images during successive steps of protocol in a 49-year-old man. Top row, Angiogram and pressure tracings before intervention. Identical pressures are recorded by guiding catheter and pressure sensor, located just proximal of stenosis. After the sensor has been advanced across the lesion, considerable decrease of transstenotic pressure occurs, which further decreases during administration of intravenous adenosine at infusion rate of 140 mg · kg^{-1} · min^{-1} to induce steady-state maximum coronary hyperemia. FFR is calculated as the ratio of hyperemic distal to proximal pressure and equals 0.43. Three bottom rows, coronary angiogram, IVUS images, and pressure recordings after stent inflation with, 8, 10, and 12 Atm, respectively. At 8 Atm, although residual stenosis by QCA is < 10%, IVUS image shows incomplete apposition of several stent struts, and there still is a considerable pressure drop provocable across the stented segment, resulting in a FFR value of 0.79. At 10 Atm, both IVUS image and pressure recordings have improved, but they are still suboptimum. At 12 Atm, IVUS and pressure measurement show optimum results according to study criteria.*

IVUS imaging after 6 inflations were stent deformation (n = 2), length of the procedure (n = 3), and technical failure of the equipment (n = 1). All three IVUS criteria for optimum stent deployment were met after 19 inflations in 17 patients, at an average inflation pressure of 11.8 ± 0.7 Atm. After the last inflation, complete apposition of all stent struts against the vessel wall, symmetric stent expansion, and sufficient cross sectional area (CSA) surface were obtained in 18, 30, and 22 of the 30 patients, respectively. IVUS data are summarized in table 14.6.

Myocardial fractional flow reserve. Reliable hyperemic pressure measurements and calculation of FFR$_{myo}$ were performed after 87 of the 93 inflations. Reasons for not having obtained pressure measurements after the remaining 6 inflations were technical problems with the signal in 3 cases and doubt about the presence of sufficient hyperemia in 3 other cases. FFR$_{myo}$ increased from 0.49 ± 0.17 before intervention to 0.93 ± 0.07 at the final measurement. Finally, complete normalization of FFR$_{myo}$ (i.e., a value ≥ 0.94) was obtained in 17 patients at an average inflation pressure of 11.5 ± 0.9 Atm. *In those patients, in whom an hyperemic pressure gradient was still present after the last balloon inflation, a slow pull-back curve across the stent at steady-state hyperemia was always performed to confirm the presence of a pressure drop within the stented segment.* In a few patients, it was even possible to correlate a discrete pressure drop to the site of incomplete apposition of 1 of the struts. An interesting observation was deterioration of FFR$_{myo}$ in 2 patients, after initial improvement, when

Table 14.6 *QCA measurements, IVUS results, and Coronary Pressure-Derived*
FFR_{myo} *after successive stent inflations.*

| | No. of Dilations | QCA | | IVUS | | | | FFR_{myo} | | QCA, IVUS, FFR_{myo} Optimal Stent Deployment* |
		% DS	DS <10%*	Apposition	S >0.7*	CSA*	All*	Mean±SD	FFR_{myo} ≥0.94*	
Preintervention	30	78.93±8.60	...	...	...	...	...	0.49±0.17	...	...
6 atm	30	10.83±8.93	13	3	24	8	3	0.84±0.12	4	2
8 atm	25	9.73±10.11	19	6	28	13	6	0.87±0.10	7	4
10 atm	21	5.84±8.93	2	12	29	20	10	0.88±0.09	11	6
12 atm	14	4.26±10.93	24	18	30	21	17	0.91±0.10	17	13
14 atm	3	8.42±1.81	24	18	30	22	17	0.80±0.05	17	13

% DS indicates percentage diameter stenosis; SI, symmetry index; CSA, cross-sectional area; and asterisk, cumulative number of patients fulfilling the respective criteria.

inflation pressure was increased further. FFR_{myo} data are summarized in table 14.6.

Relation between QCA, IVUS, and FFR_{myo}. In table 14.7, QCA, IVUS, and FFR_{myo} are compared side-by-side with respect to optimum stent deployment. Concordance between IVUS and FFR_{myo} was found in 91% of the paired observations. Only after 7 out of 81 inflations discordance was present between IVUS and FFR_{myo}. In 5 of these 7 outliers , FFR_{myo} had already normalized, whereas IVUS was still suboptimum: in 3 cases, there was incomplete apposition of the struts, and in 2 cases, there was both incomplete strut apposition and insufficient in-stent CSA. In 4 of these 5 cases, concordance was still achieved at the next step, after inflation at a 2 Atm higher pressure. In the 2 cases with optimum IVUS and suboptimum FFR_{myo}, the latter value was 0.89 and 0.91, respectively. In these cases, a hyperemic pressure drop of 7 and 9 mmHg, respectively, was still detectable on the pressure pull-back curve across the stent at maximum hyperemia, at a discrete location within the stent, without any visible abnormality at IVUS. By ROC analysis, the most accurate value of FFR to predict optimum stent deployment by IVUS, was 0.94, corresponding exactly to the lower limit of the normal range as found in earlier studies (figure 14.8)

The correlations between IVUS and QCA, and between FFR_{myo} and QCA were significantly worse: 48% and 46% concordance rates, respectively.

Table 14.7 *Relations among QCA, IVUS, and pressure-derived FFR.*

	FFR+	FFR-		QCA+	QCA-		QCA+	QCA-
IVUS+	14	2	IVUS+	15	3	FFR+	14	3
IVUS-	5	60	IVUS-	42	27	FFR-	42	25
Concordance	91%			48%			46%	

+ indicates optimum stent deployment according to the respective criteria; -, suboptimum stent deployment. Note the large number of observations in which the QCA result of stent deployment was already optimum, whereas IVUS and FFR still yielded suboptimum stent deployment.

The majority of the discordant observations were caused by an already optimum QCA result but still suboptimum IVUS or still depressed FFR_{myo}, respectively.

Optimum inflation pressure and specificity of the different IVUS criteria.
In figure 14.9, the cumulative distribution of observations with optimum stent deployment according to the different evaluation modalities is presented in relation to the inflation pressure. It can be observed how FFR provides similar information as provided by the most stringent IVUS criteria, being complete apposition of all struts. In those patients in whom optimum stent expansion of the Wiktor-i stent was not obtained at 12 Atm, it was also not obtained at 14 Atm, and in 2 cases either stent deformation or decrease of FFR occurred at that last step. It is interesting to observe in figure 14.9 that a satisfactorily symmetry index by IVUS is achieved rather easy, that achieving a sufficient cross-sectional area is more difficult, and that achievement of complete strut apposition by IVUS is the most difficult and only obtainable in approximately 50% of the patients in this study.

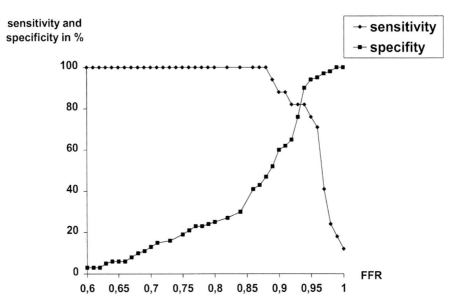

Figure 14.8 *ROC analysis to establish the FFR value most predictive for optimum stent deployment according to all IVUS criteria.*

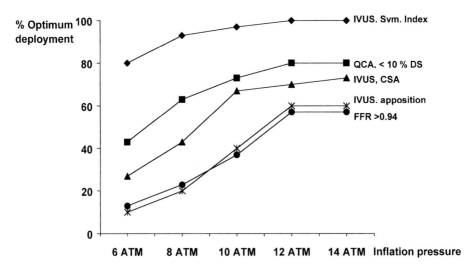

Figure 14.9 *Cumulative distribution of observations with optimum stent deployment according to different evaluation modalities in relation to inflation pressure. It is important to note that optimum FFR corresponds with the most stringent IVUS criterion, being complete apposition of all struts.*

14.3.4 Discussion.

This study demonstrates a high concordance rate of 91% between IVUS and FFR_{myo} for the purpose of evaluating optimum stent deployment. As shown in this study, QCA alone is obviously insufficient for that purpose.

Several investigators have shown that in case of IVUS-guided stent placement, instead of QCA alone, better acute results are obtained and that warfarin anticoagulation can be replaced by antiplatelet therapy without increasing the incidence of stent thrombosis. It has also been shown that the inflation pressures necessary to obtain optimum stent deployment as assessed by IVUS are higher than the pressures needed for optimum deployment as assessed by QCA only, which was confirmed for the Wiktor-i stent in the present study (figure 14.9). However, due to financial constraints, time limitation, and the increasing number of stents used, IVUS guided stent implantation is not routinely performed in the majority of catheterization laboratories. Therefore, angiography-guided stent implantation with high-pressure balloon inflation without IVUS guidance has been proposed as an alternative[39]. Although this has significantly reduced acute stent thrombosis, some negative effects of blind, unnecessarily high pressure inflation have been suggested, such as adjacent vessel wall damage and augmentation of neointimal proliferation[40,41].

Coronary pressure derived FFR_{myo} is a specific index of the conductance of the epicardial coronary artery. In contrast to other functional methods, such as Doppler velocimetry and videodensitometry, FFR_{myo} shows no variation of normal values, is not confounded by distal small vessel disease, and not influenced by hemodynamic variations. Therefore it is a specific measure of the functional state of the stented segment. As demonstrated in the present study, pressure measurements indeed correlate very well with IVUS imaging with respect to suboptimum or optimum stent deployment.

The disconnectable pressure wire can be used as a primary guidewire throughout a coronary intervention, facilitating easy, rapid, and safe assessment of the hyperemic pressure gradient across the stented segment. Because the sensor is located 3 cm from the floppy tip, it can be pulled back and advanced across the stented segment time and again, without the necessity of crossing the stent with the tip of the wire. Multiple passages with potential damage or dislocation of the stent can be avoided in that way[42]. An interesting observation in this study was the fact that optimum stent deployment according to IVUS or FFR_{myo} could only be achieved in approximately 60% of the patients. Although in early reports it was claimed that optimum deployment could be achieved in the majority of stented patients, recent literature is more doubtful on that point and our present study supports that position[43]. It is unclear yet, if there are differences in that respect between coiled wire stents as used in this study, and slotted tube stents. In a former study by Vrints et al [44], it was shown that Doppler flow velocity measurements after stenting yielded higher values of coronary flow reserve for slotted tube stents than for coiled wire stents. From our own database, presented in chapter 14.4, we found that FFR after stent implantation in unselected patients between January 1998 and May 1999 was 0.93 ± 0.05 for slotted tube stents (n = 65) and 0.93 ± 0.06 for coiled wire stents (n = 50; NS).

In some patients in our present study, stent deployment even deteriorated at higher pressure, suggesting that unlimited high pressure might be deleterious, especially when applied without adequate control. It is unknown whether this problem is specifically related to the Wiktor-i stent used in this study, or should be extrapolated to other types of stents. Another interesting observation was that the maximum inflation pressure for optimum inflation of the Wiktor-i stent, never exceeded 12 Atm in this study, although upsizing of the balloon was necessary in some patients.

It is interesting to observe in the present study that even small abnormalities in stent deployment, such as poor apposition of a few struts, resulted in the majority of cases in hemodynamic consequences reflected by an abnormal FFR (figure 14.7).

Study limitations. Due to the extensive study protocol, the number of patients in this study was rather small, which was partly compensated by the stepwise inflation protocol, providing a sufficient number of paired observations of IVUS and pressure, QCA and pressure, and IVUS and QCA, respectively. Only a selective group of patients was investigated with a single stenosis in the proximal part of a large vessel and only one type of stent was investigated. Data on smaller vessels and different types of stents, are presented in chapter 14.4. Furthermore, there are no data relating optimum initial deployment as investigated in this study to long-term outcome. To address this issue, studies with large numbers of patients are required.

Finally, although coronary pressure measurement seems to be equally effective for assessment of stent deployment as IVUS, in case of insufficient deployment it does not elucidate the cause of the problem. In contrast to IVUS, no data are obtained about vessel wall and plaque morphology, malformation of the stent, malapposition of the struts, hidden disease in the adjacent vessel parts, or other morphologic parameters.

Clinical implications and conclusion. In this study the usefulness of coronary pressure measurement to guide optimum stent deployment was comparable to intravascular ultrasound imaging. Concordance between both techniques was present in 91% of all observations. Because a single pressure guide wire can be used to perform the interventional procedure and to perform the pressure recordings, coronary pressure measurement can be suggested as a rapid and cheap alternative for IVUS to assess stent deployment without the necessity to use additional equipment, to perform exchange procedures, or to cross the stented lesion.

One important note has to be made: in case of diffuse disease or more than one stenosis within the coronary artery, FFR_{myo} for evaluation of the stented segment should be calculated by the ratio of hyperemic pressure just distal to the stent to hyperemic pressure just proximal to the stent, in order to eliminate error due to disease elsewhere in the vessel. This is further discussed at the end of paragraph 14.5.

14.4 Stent database.

Between January 1998 and May 1999, coronary pressure guided stent implantation was performed in 125 patients. All possible efforts were made in those patients to achieve a hyperemic distal to proximal pressure ratio across the stent as close to 1.0 as possible. The baseline data of these patients as well as the angiographic and hemodynamic results are presented in table 14.8.

It is interesting to note that a value ≥ 0.94 (indicating completely normalized epicardial conductance and corresponding with optimum IVUS according to the stringent MUSIC criteria) could be achieved in approximately 70% of the patients only. This is in correspondence with our earlier data in the QIF study and data of other groups[45,46]. As a consequence, it should be realized that completely optimum stent deployment cannot be achieved in 30% of the patients, despite high pressure balloon inflations and other efforts.

Table 14.8 *Coronary pressure guided stent implantation. Patient characteristics and result.*

	Coil stent	Slotted tube
patients (#)	50	65
male (#)	30	51
age	61 ± 9	59 ± 9
LAD/CX/RCA	20/16/14	36/9/20
ref $\varnothing$ before PTCA (mm)	3.1 ± 0.5	3.2 ± 0.7
% DS before PTCA	72 ± 14	59 ± 13
mld before PTCA (mm)	0.9 ± 0.4	1.3 ± 0.4
ref $\varnothing$ post-stent (mm)	3.2 ± 0.4	3.3 ± 0.5
% DS post-stent	9 ± 11	10 ± 9
mld post-stent (mm)	3.0 ± 0.5	2.9 ± 0.5
FFR before procedure	0.54 ± 0.19	0.53 ± 0.15
FFR post-stent	0.93 ± 0.06	0.93 ± 0.05
stent $\varnothing$	3.4 ± 0.3	3.3 ± 0.4
max infl.press	9.8 ± 2.2	11.1 ± 2.6
final FFR ≥ 0.94	66%	68%
final FFR ≥ 0.90	82%	86%

There is no significant difference for any of the variables.

Because after a classical PTCA, a FFR value of ≥ 0.90 indicates a favourable long-term outcome, as discussed in paragraph 14.1, we also investigated in how many patients it was possible to achieve a post-stent hyperemic distal to proximal pressure ratio across the stent of ≥ 0.90. That was the case in 82% of the coil wire stents and in 86% of the slotted tube stents (NS). The cumulative distribution of FFR values after stenting, are presented in figure 14.10. There are no long-term follow-up data of these patients yet and, although it seems to be plausible, the relation between post-stent FFR ≥ 0.90 and favorable long-term outcome remains to be established.

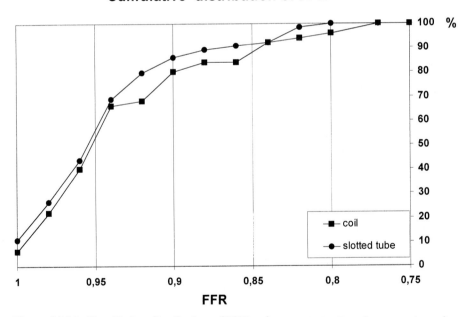

Cumulative distribution of FFR

Figure 14.10 *Cumulative distribution of FFR values post-stenting. In approximately 85% of the patients, a FFR value ≥ 0.90 was achievable and in 70% a value ≥ 0.94. No differences were observed between coil wire and slotted tube stents.*

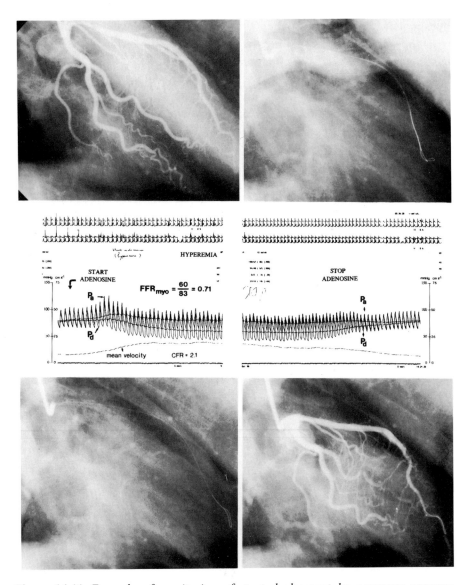

Figure 14.11 *Example of monitoring of stent deployment by coronary pressure measurements in a 53-year-old male with a 70% proximal LAD-stenosis (panel A). Both a pressure guide wire and a Doppler wire are advanced into the distal*

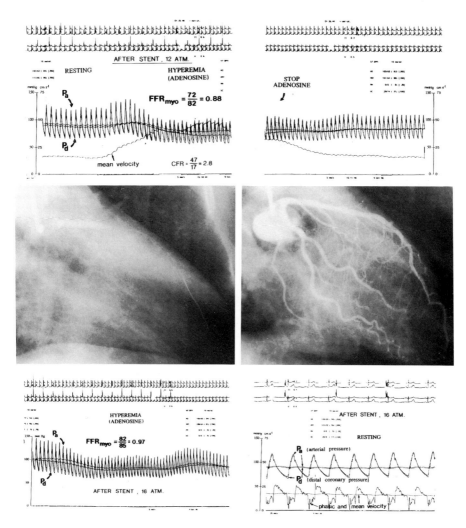

coronary artery (panel B) and simultaneous pressure and velocity recordings are
made. Before PTCA, FFR$_{myo}$ equals 0.71 and CFVR 2.1 (panel C and D). After
stent implantation with 12 atm, an excellent angiogram is observed (panel F) and
CFVR has increased to 2.8. Nevertheless, stent deployment must be suboptimal
because FFR$_{myo}$ is still outside the normal range (panel G and H). After high
pressure inflation by 16 atm (panel I), the angiogram looks unchanged (panel J) but
FFR$_{myo}$ completely returns to normal, indicating a complete restoration of normal
epicardial conductance and optimal stent deployment (panel K).

14.5 Guidelines and recommendations for using coronary pressure in monitoring coronary interventions.

From the studies described in this chapter, the following conclusions can be drawn with respect to on-line evaluation of a coronary intervention by coronary pressure measurements in the catheterization laboratory:

Regular Balloon Angioplasty:

   ♦ *post-PTCA FFR < 0.75:*
      → unsuccessful PTCA; further action is required irrespective
         of the angiographic result.

   ♦ *post-PTCA FFR 0.75 - 0.89:*
      → moderate functional result. Restenosis rate at 6 months
         is approximately 30%, even if the angiogram is satisfactory.
      → consider stent or other additional action.

   ♦ *post-PTCA FFR$_{myo}$ ≥ 0.90:*
      → excellent functional result. If this is accompanied by a
         residual diameter stenosis ≤ 35% and the absence of
         a dissection type C to F, clinical restenosis rate is only
         12% at 6-month follow-up and 16% at 2-year follow-up.
      → no additional benefit by stenting.

Stent Implantation.

   ♦ *post-stent FFR < 0.90:*
      → suboptimal result; insufficient stent deployment.

   ♦ *post-stent FFR ≥ 0.90:*
      → acceptable result, achievable in 85% of the patients.

   ♦ *post-stent FFR ≥ 0.94:*
      → optimum stent implantation, corresponding to all IVUS
         criteria for optimum stent deployment. Such a result,
         however, is achievable in 70% of the patients only.

Important note: After stent implantation, FFR should be calculated as the ratio of hyperemic pressure just distal and just proximal to the stented segment. In case of a residual gradient within a coronary artery, it should be realized that such a gradient can be created by disease elsewhere in the vessel. Plaques or diffuse disease in the proximal part of the vessel, may not result in a gradient before dilatation of a severe stenosis further on, but after increase of blood flow by dilating or stenting the most severe stenosis, disease more proximal in the vessel may be unmasked and a hyperemic gradient can be present now. Examples to illustrate this phenomenon are presented in figure 10.5 and in chapter 17, case 17.

To avoid confounding and misinterpretation of stent deployment, it is preferable to induce sustained hyperemia by i.v. adenosine or ATP infusion and to analyze the pressure pull-back recording across the stented segment, and more proximal if applicable. If intracoronary adenosine is used, which is too short-acting to make a pressure pull-back recording, coronary pressure after i.c. adenosine administration should be measured once with the pressure sensor just distal to the stent and once with the sensor just proximal to the stent.

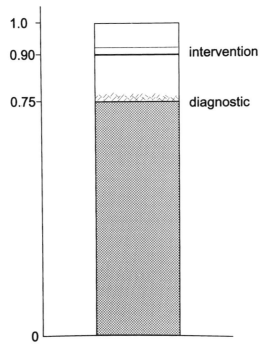

Figure 14.12 *Threshold values of FFR to be used in the catheterization laboratory (courtesy of P.Yock, MD, Stanford, CA).*

References.

1. Libby P, Warner SJC, Salomon RN, Birinyi LK. Production of platelet-derived growth factor-like mitogen by smooth muscle cells from human atheroma. *N Engl J Med* 1988; 318: 1493-1498.
2. Rensing BJ, Hermans WRM, Beatt KJ, Serruys PW. Quantitative angiographic assessment of elastic recoil after PTCA. *Am J Cardiol* 1990; 66: 1039-1044
3. Essed CE, Van den Brand M, Becker AE. Transluminal coronary angioplasty and early restenosis: fibrocellular occlusion after wall laceration. *Br Heart J* 1983; 49: 393-396.
4. Serruys PW, Straus BH, Van Beusekom H, Van der Giessen WJ. Stenting of coronary arteries: has a modern Pandora's box been opened ? *J Am Coll Cardiol* 1991; 17: 143B-154B.
5. Serruys PW, Di Mario C. Prognostic value of coronary flow velocity and diameter stenosis in assessing the short and long-term outcome of balloon angioplasty: The Debate study (Doppler Endpoint Balloon Angioplasty Trial Europe). *Circulation* 1997; 96: 3369-3377.
6. Di Mario C and the DESTINI-CFR study group. Doppler and QCA guided aggressive PTCA has the same target lesion revascularization as stent deployment: 6-month-results of the DESTINI-study. *J Am Coll Cardiol* 1999; 33: 47A.
7. De Bruyne B and Debate II investigators. A randomized study to evaluate provisional stenting after guided balloon angioplasty. *Circulation* 1998; 98: I-498.
8. Lafont A and the FROSST study group. The French optimal stenting trial: a multicenter, prospective, randomized study comparing systematic stenting to angiography/coronary flow reserve guided stenting: 6-month clinical and angiographic follow-up. *J Am Coll Cardiol* 1999; 33: 89A.
9. Pijls NHJ, Van Gelder B, Van der Voort P, Peels K, Bracke FALE, Bonnier HJRM, El Gamal MIH. Fractional flow reserve: a useful index to evaluate the influence of an epicardial coronary stenosis on myocardial blood flow. *Circulation*, 1995: 92: 3183-3193.
10. Pijls NHJ, De Bruyne B, Peels K, Van der Voort PH, Bonnier HJRM. Bartunel J, Koolen JJ. Measurement of fractional flow reserve to assess the functional severity of coronary stenoses. *N Engl J Med.* 1996; 334: 1703-1708.
11. Reiber JHC, Serruys PW, Kooijman CJ, Wijns W, Slager CJ, Gerbrands JJ, Schuurbiers JCH, Den Boer A, Hugenholtz PG. Assessment of short-, medium-, and long-term variations in arterial dimensions from computer-assisted quantification of coronary cineangiograms. *Circulation*, 1985; 71: 280-288.
12. Rensing Bj, Hermans WR, Vos J, Tijssen JG, Rutsch W, Danschin N, Heyndrickx GR, Mast EG, Wijns W, Serruys PW, for the Coronary Artery Restenosis Prevention on Repeated Thromboxane Antagonism (CARPORT) Study Group. Luminal narrowing after percutaneous transluminal coronary angioplasty: a study of clinical, procedural, and lesional factors related to long-term angiographic outcome. *Circulation* 1993; 88: 975-985.
13. Strauss BH, Escaned J, Foley DP, Di Mario C, Haase J, Keane D, Hermans WRM, De Feyter PJ, Serruys PW. Technologic considerations and practical limitations in the use of quantitative angiography during percutaneous coronary recanalization. *Prog Cardiovasc Dis.* 1994; 36: 343-362.
14. De Bruyne B, Bartunel J, Sys SU, Pijls NHJ, Heyndrickx GR, Wijns W. Simultaneous coronary pressure and flow velocity measurements in humans, feasibility, reproducibility, and hemodynamic dependence of coronary flow velocity reserve, hyperemic flow versus pressure slope index, and fractional flow reserve. *Circulation* 1996; 94: 1843-1849.

15. De Bruyne B, Bartunek J, Sys SU, Heyndrickx GR. Relation between myocardial fractional flow reserve calculated from coronary pressure measurements and exercise-induced myocardial ischemia. *Circulation* 1995; 92: 39-46.

16. Bech GJW, De Bruyne B Bonnier HJRM, Bartunek J, Wijns W, Peels K, Heyndrickx GR, Koolen JJ, Pijls NHJ. Long-term follow-up after deferral op percutaneous transluminal coronary angioplasty of intermediate stenosis on the basis of coronary pressure measurement. *J Am Coll Cardiol* 1998; 31: 841-847.

17. Serruys PW, Luijten HE, Beatt KJ, Geuskens R, De Feyter PJ, Van den Brand M, Reiber JHC, Ten Katen HJ, Van Es GA, Hugenholtz PG. Incidence of restenosis after successful coronary angioplasty: a time-related phenomenon: a quantitative angiographic study in 342 consecutive patients at 1, 2, 3, and 4 months. *Circulation* 1988; 77: 361-371.

18. Mintz GS, Popma JJ, Pichard AD, Kent KM, Lowell SF, Chuang YC, Griffin J, Leon M. Intravascular ultrasound preictors of restenosis after percutaneous transcatheter coronary revascularization. *J Am Coll Cardiol* 1996; 27: 1678-1687.

19. Kimura T, Kaburagi S, Tamura T, Yoki H, Nakagawa Y, Yokoi H, Hamasaki N, Nosaka H, Nobuyoshi M, Mintz GS, Popma JJ, Leon MB. Remodeling of human coronary arteries undergoing angioplasty or atherectomy. *Circulation* 1997; 96: 475-483.

20. Kern MJ, De Bruyne B, Pijls NHJ. From research to clinical practice: current role of intracoronary physiologically based decision making in the cardiac catheterization laboratory. *J Am Coll Cardiol* 1997; 30: 613-620.

21. Gould KL, Kelly KO, Bolson EL. Experimental validation of quantitative coronary angiography for determining pressure flow characteristics of coronary stenosis. *Circulation* 1982; 66: 930-937.

22. Serruys PW, de Jaegere P, Kiemeney F, et al, for the Benestent study group. A comparison of balloon-expandable-stent implantation with balloon angioplasty in patients with coronary artery disease. *N Engl J Med* 1994; 331: 489-495.

23. Fischman DL, Leon MB, Baim DS et al. A randomized comparison of coronary stent placement and balloon angioplasty in the treatment of coronary artery disease. *N Engl J Med* 1994; 331: 496-501.

24. Serruys PW, Van Hout B, Bonnier H, Legrand V, Garcia E, Macaya C, Sousa E, Van der Giessen W, Colombo A, Seabra-Gomes R, Kiemeneij F, Ruygrok P, Ormiston J, Emanuelsson H, Fajadet J, Haude M, Klugmann S, Morel MA. Randomized comparison of implantation of heparin-coated stents with balloon angioplasty in selected patients with coronary artery disease (BENESTENT II). *Lancet* 1998; 352: 673-681.

25. Honye J, Mahon DJ, Jain A, White CJ, Ramee SR, Wallis JB, Al-Zarka A, Tobis JM. Morphological effects of coronary balloon angioplasty in vivo assessed by intravascular ultrasound imaging. *Circulation* 1992; 85: 1012-1025.

26. Hodgson JM, Reddy KG, Suneja R, Nair RN, Lesnefsky EJ, Sheehan HM. Intracoronary ultrasound imaging: correlation of plaque morpholopy with angiography, clinical syndrome and procedural results in patients undergoing coronary angioplasty. *J Am Coll Cardiol* 1993; 21: 35-44.

27. Akasaka. (*personal communication*).

28. Kimura T, Yokoi H, Nakagawa Y, Tamura T, Kaburagi S, Sawade Y, Sato Y, Hamasaki N, Nosaka H, Nobuyoshi M. Three-year follow-up after implantation of metallic coronary artery stents. *N Engl J Med* 1996; 334: 561-566.

29. Reimers B, Moussa I, Akiyama T, Tucci G, Ferraro M, Martini G, Blengino C, Di Mario C, Colombo A. Long-term clinical follow-up after successful repeat percutaneous intervention for stent restenosis. *J Am Coll Cardiol* 1997; 30: 186-192.

30. Colombo A, Hall P, Nakamura S, Almagor Y, Maiello L, Martini G, Gaglione A, Goldberg SL, Tobis JM. Intravascular stenting without anticoagulation, accomplished with intravascular ultrasound guidance. *Circulation* 1995; 91: 1676-1688.

31. Serruys PW, Di Mario C. Who was thrombogenetic: the stent or the docter ? *Circulation* 1995; 91: 1891-1893.

32. Gorge G, Haude M, Ge J, Voegele E, Gerber T, Rupprecht HJ, Meyer J, Erbel R. Intravascular ultrasound after low and high inflation pressure coronary stent implantation. *J Am Coll Cardiol* 1995; 26: 725-730.

33. Kern MJ, De Bruyne B, Pijls NHJ. From research to clinical practice: current role of physiologically based decision making in the catheterization laboratory. *J Am Coll Cardiol* 1997 (in press).

34. Hausleiter J, Nolte CWT, Jost W, Wiese B, Sturm M, Lichtlen PR. Comparison of different quantitative coronary analysis systems: ARTEK, CAAS and CMS. *Cathet Cardiovasc Diagn* 1996; 36: 14-22.

35. Van der Zwet PMJ, Reiber JHC. A new approach for the quantification of complex lesion morphology: the gradient field transform-basic principles and validation results. *J Am Coll Cardiol* 1994; 24: 216-224.

36. Serruys PW, de Jaegere P, Bertrand M, Kober G, Marquis JF, Piessens J, Uebis R, Valeix B, Wiegand V. Morphologic change in coronary artery stenosis with the Medtronic Wiktor stent: initial results from the core laboratory for quantitative angiography. *Cathet cardiovasc Diagn* 1991; 24: 237-245.

37. Di Mario C. gorge G, Peters R, Kearney P, Pinto F, Hausmann D, van Birgelen C, Colombo A, Mudra H, Roelandt J, Erbel R. Clinical applications and image interpretation in intracoronary ultrasound. *Eur Heart J* 1998; 19: 207-229.

38. Schomig A, Neumann FJ, Kastrati A, Schuhlen H, Blasini R, Hadamitzky ????, Walter H, Zitmann-Roth EM, Richardt G, Alt E, Schmitt C, Ulm K. A randomized comparison of antiplatelt and anticoagulant therapy after the placement of coronary-artery stents. *N Engl J Med* 1996; 334: 1084-1089.

39. Nakamura S, Hall P, Gaglione A, Tiecco F, Di Maggio M, Maiello L, Martini G, Colombo A. High pressure assisted coronary stent implantation accomplished without intravascular guidance and subsequent anticoagulation. *J Am coll Cardiol* 1997; 29: 21-27.

40. Fernandez-Avilles F, Alonso JJ, Duran JM, Gimeno F, Garcia-Moran R, Paniagua J, Garcimartin I. High pressure increase late loss after coronary stenting. *J Am Coll Cardiol* 1997; 29: 369A. abstract.

41. Savage MP, Fischman DL, Douglas JS, Pepine CJ, Werner JA, Bailey SR, Rake R Goldberg S. The dark side of high pressure stent deployment. *J Am Coll Cardiol* 1997; 29: 368A. abstract.

42. Nicosia A, van der Giessen WJ, Airiian SG, von Birgelen C, de Feyter PJ, Serruys PW. Is intravascular ultrasound after coronary stenting a safe procedure ? Three cases of stent damage atributable to ICUS in a tantalum coil stent. *Cathet Cardiovasc Diagn* 1997; 40: 265-70.

43. Werner GS, Gastmann O, Ferrari M, Schuenemann S, Knies A, Diedrich J, Kreuzer H. Risk factors for acute and subacute stent thrombosis after high pressure stent implantation: a study by intravascular ultrasound. *Am Heart J* 1998; 135: 300-309.

44. Vrints CJ, Claeys MJ, Bosmans J, Conraads V, Snoeck JP. Effect of stenting on coronary flow velocity reserve: comparison of coil and tubular stents. *Heart* 1999; 82: 465-470.

45. Hanekamp CEE, Koolen JJ, Pijls NHJ, Michels HR, Bonnier JJRM. Comparison of QCA, intravascular ultrasound, and coronary pressure measurement to assess optimum stent deployment. *Circulation* 1999; 99: 1015-1021.

Chapter 15

FRACTIONAL FLOW RESERVE AND CLINICAL OUTCOME

15.1 Introduction

There is ample inferential evidence that patients with physiologically significant stenoses are at increased risk[1]. Patients with proven coronary artery disease and in whom signs of myocardial ischemia are observed at low workload have an adverse event rate which is four times higher than in those with similar stenoses but in whom ischemia can only be provoked during exercise[2,3]. This relationship between inducible ischemia and poor prognosis has led to the wide acceptance of treating functionally important stenoses even though their angiographic appearance is mild or moderate. The converse, not treating angiographically significant but functionally mild lesions, remains more controversial. The prevalence of angiographically significant lesions in an arbitrary population of 60-year-old asymptomatic males, is 20% and many of these lesions have probably no functional significance[4]. However, cardiologists are reluctant to leave untreated an angiographically significant stenosis, even when no objective signs of ischemia can be induced. This explains, at least in part, why a considerable number of angioplasties are performed without proof of reversible myocardial ischemia[5]. It is likely that a number of these angioplasties are based on an "oculo-stenotic" reflex and are possibly unnecessary.

Should an angiographically significant but physiologically mild stenosis be treated or not? Does treatment improve the prognosis or just worsen it by triggering a detrimental restenosis process in a previously stable lesion ?

The present chapter reports on three studies performed to answer these questions.

15.2   Retrospective analysis of patients outcome after deferred angioplasty based on FFR$_{myo}$.

15.2.1 Study design.

Between May 1993 and May 1997 guide-wire based coronary pressure measurements for the determination of FFR$_{myo}$ were performed in our labs in over 600 patients, either at diagnostic or at interventional catheterization. From this group of patients all records were reviewed for selecting the first 100 patients who fullfilled the following inclusion criteria: (1) Patients were referred for an intervention of one stenosis in the mid or proximal part of a native coronary artery; (2) The myocardial territory depending on the stenosed target vessel was normokinetic as assessed by visual estimation of the ventriculogram; (3) The planned intervention was deferred based upon a pressure derived FFR$_{myo}$ of more than or equal to 0.75, determined during the control-angiogram just prior to the planned PTCA.

Distal coronary pressure measurements were performed with a pressure monitoring guide wire. Maximum arteriolar vasodilation was obtained with either intracoronary or intravenous adenosine or intracoronary papaverine. Myocardial fractional flow reserve was calculated as the average of two consecutive measurements not differing from each other by more than 5%. The practical details of coronary pressure measurement, of maximum coronary vasodilation, and of the calculation of myocardial fractional flow reserve have been described in chapters 4 and 5.

Before coronary pressure measurement, intracoronary or sublingual nitrates were administered and a coronary angiogram was obtained in at least two projections. Using the guiding catheter as a scaling device, the reference diameter of the target vessel, minimal luminal diameter, percent diameter stenosis and percent area stenosis of the stenotic segment were determined in all patients by quantitative coronary angiography [6,7].

Baseline data included the risk factors, anginal status (CCS class), number of anti-anginal medications, results of non-invasive stress tests (if available), left ventricular ejection fraction and quantitative angiographic indexes.

Follow-up clinical data were obtained in all patients by patient interview and by written correspondence with the cardiologist who was presently treating or had last treated the patient. Clinical events were mutually exclusive and were defined in the following ranking order as death, myocardial infarction, unstable angina, coronary bypass surgery and coronary angioplasty. Death was considered cardiac, unless proven otherwise. Coronary events were subclassified into target vessel related or target vessel unrelated.

The decision not to perform the planned angioplasty required extensive explanation to the patient and to the referring cardiologist. In particular, it was explained that the decision to defer the intervention was based on coronary pressure measurements indicating adequate myocardial perfusion and that the operator had concluded that the lesion could not be held responsible for the patient's chest pain. Decisions regarding the medical treatment of the patients after the deferral of PTCA were left to the referring physician.

15.2.2 Results.

Baseline characteristics. The clinical characteristics of the study patients are shown in Table 15.1. At least one noninvasive stress test had been performed in 64 patients of whom 28 had a positive result for ischemia. Therefore, in a total of 72 patients, noninvasive stress tests for ischemia were negative (n=30), inconclusive (n=6), or not available (n=36). In those patients, the decision to schedule PTCA had been based solely on persistent chest pain and the presence of an angiographically suspect lesion. Ten patients were in CCS class 1 but were referred for an intervention on the basis of coincident positive stress test results and the presence of an intermediate stenosis.

Angiographic characteristics and FFR$_{myo}$. The lesion characteristics as well as the results of the pressure measurements are shown in Table 15.2. The target lesion was located in the proximal or midsection of the left anterior descending coronary artery in 64 patients, the left circumflex coronary artery in 10 patients and in the right coronary artery in 26. Quantitative coronary angiographic analysis of the reference diameter of the adjacent normal segment, minimal stenosis lumen diameter, percent diameter stenosis and percent area stenosis resulted in average values of 3.17 ± 0.67 mm, 1.68 ± 0.45 mm, 46.9 ± 9.4 % and 68.5 ± 10.5 %, respectively. In 40 patients percent diameter stenosis was >50 %. In 35 patients minimal lumen diameter was <1.5 mm. The average FFR$_{myo}$ was 0.87 ± 0.07 (range 0.75 to 1.00). The average peak hyperemic transstenotic pressure gradient was 12 ± 6 mmHg (range 0 to 24).

Procedural safety and follow-up. There were no procedural complications related to the catheterization or coronary pressure measurements. Complete clinical follow-up was obtained in all patients. The average follow-up period was 18 ± 13 months (range 3 to 42) and was >6 months in 79 patients.

Table 15.1 *Baseline clinical characteristics of the patients in whom the planned PTCA was deferred based upon coronary pressure measurements (n=100)*

Age (yr)	61 ± 11
Range	33 - 83
Man	69
Baseline CCS class	1.9 ± 1.2
Estimated LVEF (%)	66 ± 12
Patients with:	
Diabetes Mellitus	17
Hypertension	37
Smoking, ever and current	39
Hypercholesterolemia	37
Family hx of CAD	43
Previous coronary events	41
Previous angioplasty of target vessel	22
Previous angioplasty of other vessel	9
Previous CABG other vessel(s)	5
Previous infarction related to other vessel	6
Previous aborted infarction related to target vessel	8
Atypical complaints	41
Typical complaints	59
One vessel disease	64
Two vessel disease	30
Three vessel disease	6
Pre PTCA stress test result available	64
Pre PTCA stress test result	
Positive	28
Negative	30
Inconclusive	6
Patients using:	
Aspirin	83
Beta blockers	58
Calcium Antagonists	49
Nitrates	45
Antianginal drugs at baseline	2.4 ± 1.2

Data presented are mean value ± SD, range or number of patients. Ca: calcium; CABG: coronary artery bypass grafting; CAD: coronary artery disease; CCS: Canadian Cardiovascular Society; Hx : history; LVEF: left ventricular ejection fraction; MI: myocardial infarction.

Table 15.2 *Angiographic characteristics and myocardial fractional flow reserve (n=100).*

Involved coronary artery:	
LAD/LCX/RCA	64/10/26
QCA:	
Ref diam (mm)	3.17 ± 0.67
MLD (mm)	1.68 ± 0.45
% DS	46.9 ± 9.4
% area stenosis	68.5 ± 10.5
Patients with:	
% DS > 50%	40
MLD < 1.5 mm	35
FFR_{myo}	0.87± 0.07
Range of FFR_{myo}	0.75-1.00
Peak hyperemic transstenotic pressure gradient	12 ± 6
Range of hyperemic gradient	0 - 24

Data presented are mean value ± SD, range or number of patients. DS: diameter stenosis; FFR_{myo} : myocardial fractional flow reserve; LAD: left anterior descending coronary artery; LCx: left circumflex coronary artery; MLD: minimal lumen diameter; QCA: quantitative coronary arteriography; RCA: right coronary artery; Ref diam: reference diameter.

During follow-up period, two patients died from noncardiac causes after 3 and 10 months, respectively. The first death was a 49-year old man with atypical complaints and a mild aortic stenosis (mean gradient 12 mm Hg), who committed suicide 3 months after the catheterization. The second was a 77-year old man who died from a gastric cancer. In this patient, with chest complaints and known coronary disease, a gastrectomy was considered. Intracoronary pressure measurements were performed to evaluate the need for a preoperative PTCA of the stenosis. PTCA was deferred based on an FFR_{myo} of 0.89. No cardiac-related deaths occurred.

In eight patients coronary events occurred, four of which were target vessel related. The average interval to a target vessel-related incident was 27 months, whereas the average interval to incidents not related to the target vessel was 11 months. Only two coronary events occurred within 6 months after deferral, and both were unrelated to the target vessel. There was no difference in QCA variables (p=0.909) or in FFR_{myo} (p=0.374) at the initial

Anginal Status

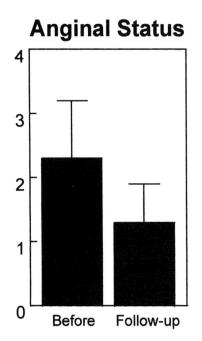

Medication

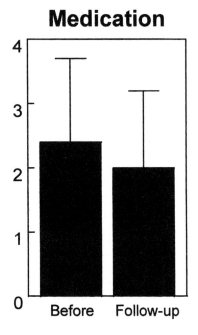

Figure 15.1 *CCS class of angina (left) and average number of anti-anginal medications taken by the patients (right) before the deferred angioplasty and at follow-up.*

assessment between patients with an event at follow-up and the remaining group.

The average CCS class in the event-free group (90 patients) decreased from 2.0 ± 1.2 at baseline to 0.7 ± 0.9 at follow-up (p<0.0001). The average number of used antianginal drugs in these 90 patients decreased from 2.4 ± 1.2 at baseline to 1.9 ± 1.2 at follow-up (p=0.0022). At follow up, 81 patients were in CCS class I or had no chest pain (figure 15.1).

Survival and event-free survival. As analyzed by the Kaplan-Meier method, at 42 months the percentage estimated survival (± SEM) after deferral of PTCA was 97 ± 2%, survival free from death or target vessel-related events was 84 ± 7%, and survival free from death or any coronary event was 78 ± 7% (figure 15.2).

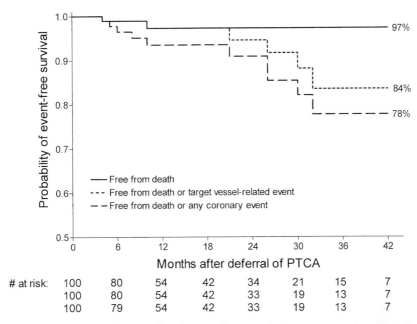

Figure 15.2 *Estimated survival and event-free survival curves (Kaplan-Meier) of all patients in whom the planned PTCA of an intermediate coronary stenosis was deferred on the basis of a pressure-derived FFR$_{myo}$ ≥0.75. Numbers below the x-axis represent patients at risk at 0, 6, 12, 18, 24, 30, 36 and 42 months after deferral of angioplasty for survival, survival free of target vessel-related event, and survival free of any coronary event, respectively.*

15.2.3 Comments.

Favourable outcome without intervention. The present study suggests that it is safe to defer angioplasty of an intermediate stenosis, if that stenosis has no physiologic importance, as assessed by pressure-derived FFR$_{myo}$ ≥0.75.
No cardiac-related deaths occurred in our deferred group, and during an average follow-up of 18 months, a target vessel-related event occurred only in 4 of 100 patients. Only one patient experienced a myocardial infarction after 26 months because of disease progression in the target vessel. The average reference diameter of the coronary arteries in the present study was >3 mm, indicating that these were all large vessels and that the favourable outcome was not due to inclusion of smaller vessels that would have had a good outcome in any case.
Evidence of reversible ischemia as a prerequisite for performing PTCA. In the present study, 72 patients had been scheduled for angioplasty only on the

basis of clinical and visual angiographic criteria. Stress testing in these patients was either negative, inconclusive or not performed. Although our study cohort was restricted to patients with intermediate stenoses, their data are comparable to those of a general PTCA population, as reported by Topol et al[5], indicating that in the United States, more than 60% of coronary interventions are performed without objective proof of reversible ischemia.

By QCA, 40 of 100 stenoses in the present study group appeared to be > 50% in diameter stenosis, the anatomic cutoff value generally accepted for discriminating between "significant" and "nonsignificant" lesions. Such lesions would have been routinely dilated if only angiographic criteria had been applied.

Although the rate of clinical events in the present study is markedly lower than that usually reported after angioplasty, it may be argued that in recent angioplasty trials, lesions undergoing a coronary intervention were on average more symptomatic, had a larger degree of obstruction as assessed by quantitative coronary angiography, and were all associated with positive exercise tests. Nevertheless, it is noteworthy that in those studies a coronary event rate of approximately 30% was reported within 12 months after balloon angioplasty alone and approximately 15% after stenting[8]. In the present study, no target vessel-related events occurred within the first 6 months of follow-up and only in 10% of this study group events occurred after an average follow-up of 18 months. This event rate is only slightly higher than in an asymptomatic 60-year-old population of approximately 2 to 3% a year and in accordance with previous studies[9,11] in similar patient groups where intervention was deferred on the basis of physiologic measurements of either coronary blood flow velocity or coronary pressure.

In 28 patients the pre-PTCA exercise test was positive despite a FFR_{myo} >0.75. Exercise-induced spasm may have played a role in some patients, and the exercise test could have been false positive in others. It is well known that the accuracy of exercise testing in patients with moderate stenosis is low and that false positive results may occur in up to 20% of these patients[12]. Moreover, as described earlier, in 10 of these 28 patients no complaints were present and the indication for angiography, which revealed the intermediate stenosis, had been the positive exercise test itself. In those patients the rate of false positive exercise tests must have been higher than usual[11]. Two of these 28 patients experienced a coronary event, respectively, at 20 and 24 months, both target vessel related. This long event-free interval suggests that these events may have been related to the natural progression of atherosclerotic disease rather than incorrect initial diagnosis.

In the 90 event-free patients, anginal class improved significantly at follow-up despite a decrease in the average number of antianginal medications taken by these patients. This improvement is possibly related to patient

reassurance by explaining that the lesion was not clinically important and that the chest pain could very well be of other than cardiac origin. This decrease of symptoms after reassurance supports the idea that in many of these patients the chest complaints were not caused by the coronary lesion, underlining that deferral of the planned PTCA had been the correct decision.
Conclusions. Because this study is retrospective, non-randomized, and does not provide comparative data from a control group of patients in whom angioplasty was actually performed, it is impossible to establish the clinical event rate that would have occurred had angioplasty actually been performed. Nevertheless, it can be concluded that in patients with chest pain who are scheduled for PTCA of an intermediate coronary stenosis, deferral of PTCA on the basis of an $FFR_{myo} > 0.75$ is safe, irrespective of the noninvasive stress test result, and is associated with a very low coronary event rate of approximately 5% a year, much lower than expected had PTCA been performed in all these patients.

To confirm these observations, a large randomized prospective study was mandatory. Such a study has been performed in the meantime and the preliminary results are presented below.

15.3 Prospective analysis of FFR-based decision-making to perform or defer a coronary intervention: The DEFER study.

The results of the retrospective study presented above suggest that it is safe to defer a planned angioplasty of a physiologically non-significant stenosis. As the latter study is retrospective, the clinical outcome of these patients in the hypothetical case angioplasty would have been performed remains unknown. Therefore, a randomized prospective study was warranted to evaluate the clinical outcome of performing versus deferring coronary angioplasty (and stenting) of physiologically non-significant coronary stenoses. This was the purpose of the DEFER study, a randomized multicenter study which has been completed recently. Some preliminary results of this study are reported here.

The primary objective of the trial was to test the hypothesis that in patients, admitted for a coronary intervention without clear evidence of reversible ischemia, deferring the PTCA based upon a FFR larger than 0.75 is safe and at least as good as performing it both in terms of prognosis and quality of life. The secondary objective was to compare the cost-effectiveness of these two strategies (perform versus defer angioplasty).

Study design. Patients were included in this study if they fulfilled the following two criteria: (1) referral for elective angioplasty of one coronary stenosis with a diameter stenosis by visual assessment of at least 50% in a native coronary artery with a reference diameter of more than 2.5 mm; (2) no objective signs of reversible myocardial ischemia within the last two months. Non-invasive tests was either negative, non-conclusive, equivocal, or simply not available for whatever reason. Patients with multivessel disease were not excluded but should be referred for angioplasty of only one single stenosis. A total of 325 patients were included.

Figure 15.3 shows the flow chart of the DEFER study. The randomization was performed in the catheterization laboratory, *just prior to angiography*, to avoid any bias. Diameter stenosis (%) was calculated off-line by quantitative coronary angiography. Coronary pressure measurements for the calculation of myocardial fractional flow reserve were performed on-line as described in chapter 5. When FFR was smaller than 0.75, the planned angioplasty was performed irrespective of the randomization. In contrast, when FFR was larger than 0.75, the randomization was applied and the patients either underwent the planned angioplasty or were treated medically. In case of angioplasty, any type of coronary intervention was allowed. The operator was urged to achieve the best possible result based on the subjective analysis of the angiogram. At the end of the angioplasty, the result was *not* evaluated by pressure measurements to avoid any bias. All patients included in the study were followed-up clinically for 1 year. A coronary angiogram was performed only when clinically indicated. The clinical end-points included death, myocardial infarction, CABG and target lesion revascularization.

Preliminary results. Out of the 325 patients, 185 (57%) had a FFR of the target lesion larger or equal to 0.75. The patients with a FFR larger than 0.75 had similar baseline characteristics, risk factors and lesion distribution as patients with a FFR smaller than 0.75.

On the average, the percent diameter stenosis was smaller in patients with a FFR larger than 0.75 than in patients with a FFR smaller than 0.75 (48 ± 9% versus 57 ± 12%, respectively). However, there was a major overlap between the data from these two patients groups and by angiography alone it was impossible to predict if an individual patient belonged to one or the other group. Thirty-one percent of patients with a FFR larger than 0.75 had an angiographic diameter stenosis of more than 50%, while 26% of patients with a FFR smaller than 0.75 had an angiographic diameter stenosis of less than 50%.

The stenting rate was 53% in patients with a FFR larger than 0.75 who were randomized to angioplasty and 66% in patients with a FFR smaller than

0.75. The post-angioplasty diameter stenosis was similar in these two groups (17 ± 12% and 18 ± 13%, respectively).

Among patients with a FFR larger than 0.75, there was no significant difference in improvement in anginal class (CCS) between patients randomized to angioplasty (average decrease 0.5 ± 0.3 CCS class) and patients in whom the angioplasty was deferred (average decrease 0.8 ± 0.4 CCS class). In contrast, patients with a FFR smaller than 0.75 (and in whom angioplasty was performed anyway) improved significantly more (decrease 1.1 ± 0.5 CCS class) than patients with a FFR larger than 0.75.

After a mean clinical follow-up of 8 months up to now, the event rate was 16% in patients with a FFR smaller than 0.75, 9% in patients with a FFR larger than 0.75 who were randomized to angioplasty and 3% in patients with FFR larger than 0.75 in whom angioplasty was deferred. In other words, in patients with FFR < 0.75, PTCA could be performed with an event rate as usual in PTCA of single vessel disease and a significant functional

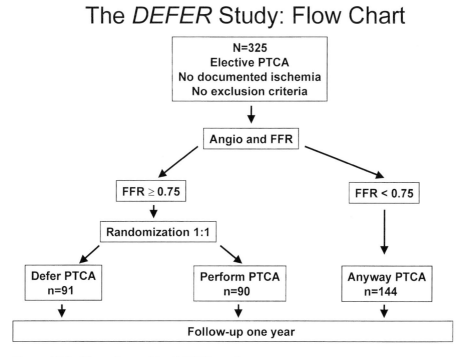

Figure 15.3 *Flow chart of the DEFER study.*

improvement as indicated by a decrease of CCS class by 1.1 ± 0.5 class. On the contrary, in patients with FFR > 0.75, no benefit at all was achieved by the intervention neither in terms of prognosis, nor in terms of CCS class, and a slightly higher event rate was observed in the first year as compared to patients in whom the PTCA was deferred.

These *preliminary results* indicate the following: (1) in roughly 50% of patients with stable thoracic complaints scheduled for coronary angioplasty without objective proof of reversible myocardial ischemia, the stenosis is found hemodynamically non-significant; (2) the distinction between significant and non-significant lesion cannot be done on the basis of coronary angiography alone; (3) in patients with a FFR smaller than 0.75 (i.e. hemodynamically significant stenoses) coronary angioplasty seems to be warranted as the functional class of these patients significantly improves at follow-up; (4) patients with a FFR larger than 0.75 (i.e. lesions which are hemodynamically non-significant) do not benefit from angioplasty as both their complaints and the occurrence of cardiac events are similar whether or not angioplasty has been performed.

Therefore, in patients scheduled for angioplasty without documented reversible myocardial ischemia, FFR appears to be an ideal tool to identify those patients who will benefit from angioplasty and, conversely, to avoid unnecessary angioplasty in the other patients.

The final results of the DEFER study will be available and probably be close to publication at the time of publication of this book.

15.4 FFR and clinical outcome in patients with intermediate left main stenosis.

The presence of left main coronary artery (LM) stenosis has major prognostic and therapeutical consequences and is often decisive in the choice for surgical versus non-surgical therapy[14]. It is generally accepted to perform a bypass operation in patients with LM stenosis > 50% clearly visible by angiography and associated with reversible ischemia by non-invasive tests[14-17]. However, in clinical practice angiographically intermediate stenosis of the LM is not uncommon. It is unclear whether the prognosis of these patients will be improved by bypass surgery. Plaque rupture at the site of a hemodynamically non-significant stenoses may have dramatic consequences. Yet, CABG of mild stenoses leads to inappropriate use of availabe grafts and premature occlusion of either the native vessel or the graft(s), leaving the risk of acute occlusion unaffected[18]. This problem is further complicated because reliable angiographic quantification of a LM stenosis is often difficult[19,20], because classical non-invasive tests to document reversible ischemia are often unable to differentiate between ischemia caused by the LM itself or by accompanying other stenoses elsewhere in the coronary arteries[21,22], and because bypass surgery in LM disease is not without risk[23]. In case of doubt, surgical revascularization is often chosen.

Accordingly, a prospective study was designed to investigate the usefulness of pressure-derived FFR for clinical decision making in patients with equivocal left main disease.

Methods. All patients were eligible for this study who underwent diagnostic catheterization in our hospital between 1994 and 1998 and in whom a LM stenosis was present of 40 to 60 % by visual estimation. Furthermore patients were only eligible if no other angiographic abnormalities were present which indicated bypass surgery anyway. In other words, when e.g. in addition to the presence of an equivocal LM stenosis, three vessel disease was present implicating bypass surgery anyway, the patient was not eligible for this study. If, in addition to the presence of an equivocal LM stenosis, a stenosis suitable for PTCA was present elsewhere in the coronary tree, the patient was eligible for this study. After informed consent had been obtained, coronary pressure measurement and calculation of FFR associated with the LM stenosis was performed and the decision either to perform or to defer surgery was based upon FFR below or above 0.75, respectively. Quantitative coronary arteriography analysis was performed on the control cine angiograms, obtained just prior to the intra-coronary pressure measurements.

Table 15.3 *Baseline clinical, angiographic, and pressure data of 52 patients with an equivocal left main coronary artery stenosis in whom bypass surgery was either deferred (Group A, n=22) or performed (Group B, n=30) on the basis of coronary pressure measurement and the myocardial fractional flow reserve threshold value of 0.75.*

	Group A	Group B
	≥ 0.75 (n=22)	< 0.75 (n=30)
Male, n (%)	16 (73)	26 (87)
Age, y	61 ± 9	63 ± 9
Risk factors, n (%)		
Hypertension	4 (18)	9 (30)
Diabetes	8 (36)	6 (20)
Cholesterol	8 (36)	14 (47)
Smoking	7 (32)	19 (63)*
Family Hx of CAD	4 (18)	16 (53)*
Previous PTCA, n (%)	2 (9)	4 (13)
Previous infarction, n (%)		
LCA area	6 (27)	1 (3)*
RCA area	2 (9)	4 (13)
CCS class	2.8 ± 1.0	3.4 ± 0.9
Stress test performed, n(%)	13 (59)	10 (33)
pos/neg/inconcl	8/1/4	7/1/2
LVEF (%)	55 ± 8	57 ± 6
Additional disease, n (%)		
1/ 2 vessel disease	9/6	10/13
angiographic data		
Ref diam, mm	4.05 ± 0.74	3.45 ± 0.59*
MLD, mm	2.40 ± 0.49	1.95 ± 0.39*
DS, %	40 ± 9	43 ± 10
Pressure data		
P_a, mmHg	90 ± 13	95 ± 18
P_d, mmHg	80 ± 9	63 ± 14 *
ΔP_{max}, mmHg	9 ± 6	32 ± 11*
FFR	0.90 ± 0.06	0.67 ± 0.09*

Data presented are number and percentage of patients and mean value ± SD. CCS: Canadian Cardiology Society; DS: diameter stenosis; Hx: history; LCA: left coronary artery; LVEF: left ventricular ejection fraction; MLD: minimal lumen diameter; P_a : mean aortic pressure; P_d : mean distal coronary pressure; ΔP_{max}: hyperemic transstenotic pressure gradient; PTCA: percutaneous transluminal coronary angioplasty; RCA : right coronary artery; Ref diam: reference diameter; FFR: myocardial fractional flow reserve. *= p < 0.05 versus group A.

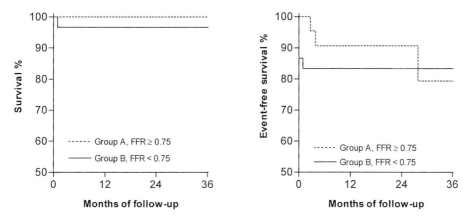

Figure 15.4 *Event-free survival after 3 years of follow-up in intermediate left main stenosis. Group A indicates 22 patients with an equivocal left main stenosis in whom bypass surgery was deferred based upon FFR ≥ 0.75. Group B indicates 30 patients with an equivocal left main stenosis in whom bypass surgery was performed based on a FFR ≤ 0.75.*

All patients were followed up at least once a year and data on anginal status and medication usage were obtained at all follow-up visits. Major adverse events were mutually exclusive and defined in the following ranking order as death, myocardial infarction, unstable angina, coronary bypass surgery or redo-surgery and coronary angioplasty. Angiographic follow-up was only performed in case of recurrent complaints or coronary events.

Baseline characteristics and procedural results. A total of 52 patients were included in the study. Baseline characteristics of the study population are listed in table 15.3. Except for smoking, a family history of coronary heart disease, and the presence of a Q wave myocardial infarction in the area of the left coronary artery no significant differences in base-line demographic and clinical data were present between those patients with a functionally insignificant (FFR ≥ 0.75: Group A, n=22) versus functionally significant LM stenosis (FFR < 0.75: Group B, n=30) as assessed by FFR. Although the LM percent diameter stenosis was similar in both groups A and B (40% versus 43%, NS), the average reference diameter (4.1 ± 0.7 versus 3.5 ± 0.6, $p < 0.01$) and minimal lumen diameter (2.4 ± 0.5 versus 2.0 ± 0.4, $p < 0.001$) were significantly larger in group A, albeit with a large overlap of angiographic parameters. The average number of risk factors was significantly higher in group B (1.8 ± 1.4) versus group A (1.1 ± 1.1, p = 0.03). There were no complications related to the catheterization nor to the coronary pressure measurement. Bypass surgery was performed in all 30 patients in group B and deferred in all 22 patients of group A. In this latter group, 5 patients underwent PTCA of an other lesion (LAD 3 times, LCX 2 times), 16 patients were treated medically, and 1 patient underwent aortic valve replacement without bypass surgery. Some examples from patients in this study are shown in chapter 17, case 10, 11, and 12.

Follow-up. Follow-up was obtained in all patients. Average follow-up was 24±14 months ranging from 2 to 56 months with 38 patients having a follow-up of more than 1 year. In group A, the conservative group, CABG was performed in 1 patient after more than 2 years of follow-up because of disease progression and in 2 patients in this group re-PTCA of the LAD was performed. In group B, the surgical group, 1 patient died 29 days after surgery because of respiratory failure due to acute respiratory distress syndrome and pneumonia, in 1 patient a large anterior wall myocardial infarction occurred perioperatively, and in 3 patients early re-thoracotomy was necessary in the first hours after surgery, twice because of recurrent ischemia (treated by additional placement of a saphenous vein graft on the LAD), and once because of intractable mitral valve regurgitation treated by mitral valve replacement. In none of the patients of the surgical group, any event occurred during the remaining follow-up. Average CCS class decreased from 2.8 ± 1.0 at baseline to 1.6 ± 0.7 at the last follow-up visit in group A (P < 0.001) and from 3.4 ± 0.9 to 1.5 ± 0.8 in group B (P < 0.001). At follow up, 43 out of 52 patients were in CCS class 2 or less. In group A, the average number of used anti-anginal drugs decreased from 2.1 ± 1.2 to 1.5 ± 1.1 (P < 0.01) and in group B from 2.1 ± 1.5 to 1.1 ± 0.9 (P < 0.001). This decrease in medication use was not significantly different between both groups.

Survival and cardiac event-free survival. As analyzed by the Kaplan-Meier method, at 3 years of follow-up after deferral (group A) versus performance of CABG (group B) the estimated percent survival (±SEM) was respectively 100 ± 0% and 90 ± 4% (NS); survival free from death or any major adverse cardiac event was respectively 81 ± 8% and 79 ± 12% (NS) (figure 15.4).

Discussion. This study shows that among patients with an intermediate LM stenosis (40 – 60% diameter stenosis), about half of these narrowings (59%) can be considered as physiologically significant (FFR < 0.75) and half (41%) cannot. In the first group CABG was performed based upon earlier studies, in the second group no surgery was performed. This strategy was accompanied by an excellent survival and freedom of events up to 4 years after the diagnostic procedure.

At follow-up average CCS class decreased significantly in both groups. However, this improvement was largest in the group of patients with a FFR below 0.75, suggesting that their complaints were related to the LM stenosis and that CABG was justified indeed.

Although percentage stenosis severity was equal in both groups the patients with FFR < 0.75 had a smaller reference diameter by QCA and accordingly a smaller MLD. It is likely that in those patients diffuse LM disease was present which was not detected by angiography. This phenomenon of diffuse LM disease is well known from intravascular ultrasound studies which have shown that hidden left main disease is more frequent than generally appreciated[24].

Despite the lower mean reference diameter and minimal luminal diameter in patients in whom the stenosis was functionally significant, angiography was not able in individual patients to predict which stenosis was functionally significant and which was not.

Clinical implications. This study indicates that in patients with intermediate left main coronary artery disease intracoronary pressure measurement and calculation of FFR is feasible and useful for deciding whether or not CABG should be performed. The present data extend the usefulness of the cut-off FFR value of 0.75 to patients with a left main stenosis. In patients with a left main coronary artery FFR ≥ 0.75, CABG may be deferred and inappropriate usage of graft material is avoided. A medical approach, as well as watchful waiting and regular follow-up of these patients seems most appropriate. In patients with a left main coronary artery FFR < 0.75, the equivocal LM stenosis bears functional significance and therefore CABG is justified. Finally this study confirms the inability of angiography and QCA to discriminate between physiologically significant and insignificant equivocal LM lesions.

15.5   Practical consequences for the routine use in the catheterization laboratory.

Both from the retrospective and prospective studies in almost 500 patients presented in this chapter, it will be clear that, before performing a coronary intervention, it is generally mandatory to have objective evidence that the lesion to be dilated can be held responsible for reversible ischemia. If such evidence is not available by non-invasive tests, it can be obtained in the catheterization laboratory - right on the spot - by invasive functional testing. Because of its simplicity and accuracy, coronary pressure measurement is the best method to obtain such evidence in the catheterization laboratory presently. If the lesion can be shown to be associated with reversible ischemia, indicated by FFR < 0.75, PTCA can be performed within the same session, using the pressure wire as angioplasty guide wire. PTCA in such patients results in a similar functional improvement as usual in PTCA-patients and can be performed at a similar risk and clinical restenosis rate. In case of multiple lesions or left main disease, aortocoronary bypass surgery can be considered. On the contrary, if by invasive testing it is unlikely that the respective stenosis can be held responsible for reversible ischemia, indicated by FFR ≥ 0.75, it is safe to defer the planned intervention. In those patients with FFR ≥ 0.75, the event rate in the next year is lower without PTCA and there is no advantage of PTCA in terms of functional improvement as CCS class improves to a similar degree in those patients whether or not PTCA is performed.

Finally, these studies make clear that in patients with multivessel disease, determination of the culprit lesion(s) by pressure measurement is extremely useful and helps in the decision to perform PTCA of 1 or 2 stenoses versus CABG of 2 or more vessels.

References.

1.   Wilson RF. Assessing the severity of coronary artery stenoses. *N Engl J Med* 1996;334:1735-1737.
2.   McNeer JF, Margolis JR, Lee KL, et al. The role of the exercise test in the evaluation of patients for ischemic heart disease. *Circulation* 1978;57:64-70.
3.   Brown KA. Prognostic value of thallium-201 myocardial perfusion imaging: a diagnostic tool comes of age. *Circulation* 1991;83:363-381.

4. Chaitman BR, Bourassa MG, Davis K, Rogers WJ, Tyras GH, Berger R, Kennedy JW, Fisher L, Judkins MP, Mock MB, Killip T: Angiographic prevalence of high-risk coronary artery disease in patients subsets. *Circulation* 1981; 64: 360-367.

5. Topol EJ, Ellis SE, Cosgrove DM, Bates ER, Muller DWM, Schork NJ, Schork MA, Loop FD. Analysis of coronary angioplasty practice in the United States with an insurance-claims data base. *Circulation* 1993;87:1489-1497.

6. Reiber JHC, Serruys PW, Kooijman CJ, Wijns W, Slager CJ, Gerbrands JJ, Schuurbiers Jch, den boer A, Hugenholtz PG. Assessment of short-, medium- and longterm variations in arterial dimensions from computer-assisted quantification of coronary cineangiograms. *Circulation* 1985;71:280-288.

7. Haase J, Di Mario C, Slager CJ, van der Giessen WJ, den Boer A, de Feyter PJ, Reiber JH, Verdon PD, Serruys PW. In vivo validation of on-line and off-line geometric coronary measurements using insertion of stenosis phantom in porcine coronary arteries. *Cath Cardiovasc Diagn* 1992;27:16-27.

8. Macaya C, Serruys PW, Ruygrok p, et al. Continued benefit of coronary stenting versus balloon angioplasty: one-year clinical follow-up of Benestent trial. *J Am Coll Cardiol* 1996;27:255-61.

9. Lesser JR, Wilson RF, White CW. Physiologic assessment of coronary stenoses of intermediate severity can facilitate patients selection for coronary angioplasty. Coronary Artery Disease. *J Am Coll Cardiol* 1990;1:697-705.

10. Kern MJ, Donohue TJ, Aguirre FV, et al. Clinical outcome of deferring angioplasty in patients with normal translesional pressure-flow velocity measurements. *J Am Coll Cardiol* 25:178-86.

11. Fleg JL, Gerstenblith G, Zonderman AB, et al. Prevalence and prognostic significance of exercise-induced silent myocardial ischemia detected by thallium scintigraphy and electrocardiography in asymptomatic volunteers. *Circulation* 1990;81:428-36.

12. Pijls NHJ, De Bruyne B, Peels K, et al. Measurement of fractional flow reserve to assess the functional severity of coronary-artery stenoses. *N Eng J Med* 1996; 334:1703-8.

13. Bech GJW, De Bruyne B, Pijls NHJ. Comparison of deferral verus performance of based upon fractional flow reserve: the DEFER study. *J Am Coll Cardiol* 1999; 33: 89A.

14. Caracciolo EA, Davis KB, Sopko G, et al, for the CASS investigators. Comparison of surgical and medical group survival in patients with left main coronary artery disease. *Circulation* 1995;91:2325-34.

15. Takaro T, Peduzzi P, Detre KM, et al. Survival in subgroups of patients with left main coronary artery disease: Veterans Administration cooperative study of surgery for coronary arterial occlusive disease. *Circulation* 1982;66:14-21.

16. European Coronary Surgery Study Group: Long-term results of prospective randomized study of coronary artery bypass surgery in stable angina pectoris. *Lancet* 1982;2:1173-80.

17. Mock MB, Killip T. Effect of coronary bypass surgery on survival patterns in subsets of patients with left main coronary artery disease: report of the collaborative study in coronary artery surgery (CASS). *Am J Cardiol* 1981;48:765-77.

18. Lust RM, Zeri RS, Spence PA, et al. Effect of chronic native flow competition on internal thoracic artery grafts. *Ann Thorac Surg* 1994;57:45-50.

19. Isner JM, Kishel J, Kent KM, Ronan JA, Ross AM, Roberts WC. Accuracy of angiographic determination of left main coronary arterial narrowing. *Circulation* 1981;63:1056-64.

20. Cameron A, Kemp HG, Fisher LD, et al. Left main coronary artery stenosis: angiographic determination. *Circulation* 1983;3:484-9.

21.   Janosi A, Vertes A. Exercise testing and left main coronary artery stenosis: can patients with left main disease be identified? *Chest* 1991;100:227-9.

22.   Gibbons RJ, Fyke FE 3d, Brown ML, Lapeyre AC 3d, Zinsmeister AR, Clements IP. Comparison of exercise performance in left main and three vessel coronary artery disease. *Cathet Cardiovasc Diagn* 1991;22:14-20.

23.   Chaitman BR, Rogers WJ, Davis K, Tyras DH, Berger R, Bourassa MG. Operative risk factors in patients with left main coronary artery disease. *N Engl J Med* 1980;303:953-7.

24.   Nishimura RA, Higano ST, Holmes DR. Use of intracoronary ultrasound imaging for assessing left main coronary artery disease. *Mayo Clin Proc* 1993;68(2):134-40.

Chapter 16

ASSESSMENT OF COLLATERAL BLOOD FLOW BY CORONARY PRESSURE MEASUREMENT

16.1 Assessment of collateral circulation.

Although the importance and protective role of the collateral circulation of the heart have been recognized for decades, no methods have been available so far for quantitative assessment of collateral blood flow in conscious humans[1-4].

The value of distal coronary occlusion pressure as an index of collateral flow at coronary occlusion, has been investigated by Schaper in experimental models and was recognized by Gruentzig, King, Meier, and other investigators in the early days of angioplasty[5-8]. Its clinical usefulness, however, remained limited because no consistent scientific model was available for the interpretation of data.

In the present chapter, the background theory and experimental and clinical validation will be presented as to how quantifying collateral blood flow by guide wire based coronary pressure measurements, not only at coronary artery occlusion, but also before and after angioplasty. A number of examples will be discussed in detail to clarify the method, which looks complex at first but is really simple to apply in clinical practice.

16.2 Fractional collateral blood flow.

The concept of fractional flow reserve provides a theoretical and experimental basis for the assessment of coronary collateral blood flow by coronary pressure measurement. As explained in chapter 4 and 7, by combining coronary wedge pressure (P_w) with simultaneously recorded aortic pressure (P_a) and central venous pressure (P_v) at maximum coronary

vasodilation, a quantitative index of collateral flow can be calculated both
before and after PTCA, and also maximum recruitable collateral blood flow
at coronary artery occlusion can be assessed. That index, called fractional
collateral blood flow, expresses actual collateral flow (Q_c) as a ratio to
normal maximum myocardial perfusion (Q^N) as follows:

$$Q_c/Q^N = FFR_{myo} - FFR_{cor} \qquad \textit{(general form)}$$

$$= \frac{(P_d - P_v)}{(P_a - P_v)} - \frac{(P_d - P_w)}{(P_a - P_w)}$$

$$= \frac{(P_w - P_v)(P_a - P_d)}{(P_a - P_v)(P_a - P_w)}$$

It should be emphasized that for calculation of fractional collateral blood
flow - also if there is no coronary occlusion - it is mandatory to know the
virtual value of P_w as it should be at the current P_a and P_v. For that purpose,
the constancy of the ratio $(P_w - P_v)/(P_a - P_v)$ has to be used. Because that ratio
is constant irrespective of the current hemodynamic conditions (figure 7.4),
it is possible to calculate the virtual value of P_w at every given value of P_a
and P_v, from the values of P_a, P_v, and P_w recorded during any coronary artery
occlusion.
The mathematical derivation of the equations above as well as the proof of
the constancy of the ratio $(P_w - P_v)/(P_a - P_v)$, is derived in chapter 4.7 and
experimental evidence of its correctness has been presented in chapter 7.3.2.
At coronary occlusion, P_d equals P_w by definition and therefore the formula
for fractional collateral flow is further simplified to:

$$Q_c/Q^N = \frac{P_w - P_v}{P_a - P_v} \qquad \textit{(coronary occlusion)}$$

The last equation, representing recruitable collateral flow at coronary
occlusion, can also be intuitively understood by figure 16.1: At maximum
vasodilation of the coronary circulation, maximum flow is determined by

myocardial perfusion pressure, which equals $(P_a - P_v)$ if no stenosis is present at all. At total occlusion of the supplying coronary artery, myocardial perfusion pressure equals $(P_w - P_v)$. Because at maximum vasodilation, myocardial flow is proportional to driving pressure, it is clear that maximum recruitable collateral flow as a ratio to normal maximum myocardial blood flow, can be expressed by the equation above.

In this context, it is important to note that fractional collateral flow is a more relevant clinical parameter than absolute collateral flow. Absolute flow, expressed in ml/min is meaningless because the myocardial distribution to be perfused, is unknown and varies widely between different arteries and different subjects. Moreover, absolute collateral flow is dependent on current blood pressure whereas fractional collateral flow is not, as shown in chapter 7.

In summary:

♦ fractional collateral flow expresses collateral blood flow as a fraction of normal maximum myocardial blood flow.

♦ fractional collateral blood flow can be calculated not only at balloon occlusion but also before and after an intervention.

♦ In all cases, however, it is necessary to have recorded P_w at balloon occlusion at least once. Therefore, this method for collateral flow assessment will remain limited to interventional procedures.

♦ Recruitable fractional collateral blood flow at coronary occlusion, is obviously the most relevant clinical parameter and is easily obtained by the ratio $(P_w - P_v)/(P_a - P_v)$.

♦ Fractional collateral flow outside coronary occlusion, is calculated by $FFR_{myo} - FFR_{cor}$. If current P_a and P_v are different from P_a and P_v at occlusion (which is generally the case), the constancy of $(P_w - P_v)/(P_a - P_v)$ is used to calculate the virtual value of P_w needed.

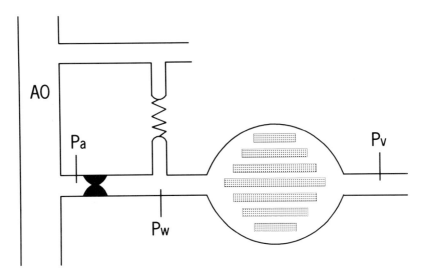

Figure 16.1 *Model of the coronary circulation at total occlusion of the coronary artery. Perfusion pressure over the myocardium, provided by the collaterals, equals $(P_w - P_v)$; whereas normal perfusion pressure at maximum vasodilation would be $(P_a - P_v)$. Abbreviations: AO: aorta; P_a: mean aortic pressure; P_w: mean distal coronary pressure in the occluded coronary artery (coronary wedge pressure) at maximum vasodilation of the myocardial vascular bed; P_v: central venous pressure.*

16.3 Calculation of fractional collateral blood flow in clinical practice.

Example 1.

This theory can be best further clarified by discussing some examples. At first, it is recommended to study example 1 in paragraph 4.5. That example treats the theoretical simple case where aortic and venous pressures do not change during a PTCA procedure.

The next example, presented below, demonstrates the calculations when systemic pressures do change during PTCA, as is usually the case:

Example 2.

Suppose that a PTCA is performed in one of the coronary arteries. At maximum coronary hyperemia (induced by i.c. papaverine or i.c. or i.v. adenosine), mean arterial pressure is 96 mmHg before PTCA and 80 mmHg at the measurement after PTCA; distal coronary pressure P_d equals 51 mmHg before PTCA and 65 mmHg thereafter, corresponding with an hyperemic gradient of 45 mmHg and 15 mmHg, respectively; venous pressure is 6 mmHg before and 5 mmHg after PTCA. Pw during balloon inflation equals 23 mmHg. Mean arterial pressure during balloon inflation is 92 mmHg and mean venous pressure during balloon inflation is 6 mmHg. In this case, with changing P_a and P_v, the value of P_w should first be calculated as it would be at the particular P_a and P_v as present before and after PTCA. That can be done by using the constancy of $(P_w - P_v)/(P_a - P_v)$ and results in a virtual value of P_w of 24 mmHg before PTCA and 20 mmHg after PTCA (see also paragraph 16.4.1). The recorded pressures can then be tabulated as follows:

	Before PTCA	At occlusion	After PTCA
P_w	96	92	80
P_d	51	-	65
P_v	6	6	5
P_w	24	23	20

Next, FFR_{myo} and FFR_{cor} are calculated by their respective equations:

Before PTCA : $FFR_{myo} = (51 - 6) /(96 - 6)$ $= 0.50$
  $FFR_{cor} = (51 - 24)/(96 - 24)$ $= 0.375$

and therefore : fractional collateral flow (Q_c/Q^N):
  $= FFR_{myo} - FFR_{cor}$
  $= 0.50 - 0.375 = 0.125$

After PTCA   : $FFR_{myo} = (65 - 5) \ /(80 - 5) = 0.80$
                    $FFR_{cor} = (65 - 20)/(80 - 20) = 0.75$

and therefore : fractional collateral flow (Q_c/Q^N):
                     $= FFR_{myo} - FFR_{cor}$
                     $= 0.80 - 0.75 = 0.05$

This means that the functional significance of that particular coronary stenosis before PTCA, was such that maximum myocardial blood flow was reduced to 50% of the value it would be if the artery were completely normal. Moreover, of every 50 ml blood flowing to the supplied myocardium, 37.5 ml came from the stenotic coronary artery itself and 12.5 ml was provided by the collateral circulation.

After PTCA, maximum myocardial flow has increased to 80% of its normal value and this time, out of every 80 ml of blood streaming to that myocardial distribution, 75 ml of blood arrives there by the dilated coronary artery and 5 ml by the collaterals.

At last, maximum recruitable collateral blood flow at coronary occlusion, is calculated by $(23 - 6)/(92 - 6) = 0.20$, and equals therefore 20% of normal maximum myocardial perfusion.

These data are summarized in a matrix as shown below:

	Before PTCA	At occlusion	After PTCA
FFR_{myo}	0.50	0.20	0.80
FFR_{cor}	0.375	0.00	0.75
Q_c/Q^N	0.125	0.20	0.05

Such a matrix completely describes the distribution of flow in the coronary circulation and is not dependent on changes in blood pressure, heart rate, or contractility.

Example 3.

After having studied this theoretical example, it is recommended to look at example 2 in paragraph 4.5, which is taken from real practice. The pressure recordings of that patient are presented in figure 4.9. The pressures before PTCA, at occlusion, and after PTCA, recorded after administration of an adequate hyperemic stimulus, are:

	Before PTCA	At occlusion	After PTCA
P_a	101	108	97
P_d	53	-	94
P_v	5	6	5
P_w	(22)	24	(21)

and the respective values of FFR_{myo}, FFR_{cor}, and fractional collateral flow Q_c/Q^N can be summarized in the matrix:

	Before PTCA	At occlusion	After PTCA
FFR_{myo}	0.50	0.18	0.97
FFR_{cor}	0.39	0.00	0.96
Q_c/Q^N	0.11	0.18	0.01

Example 4 and 5.

Some further examples illustrating the calculations to assess myocardial, coronary, and collateral fractional flow reserve before and after PTCA, are presented in chapter 17, case 22 and 23.

16.4 Some further aspects of fractional collateral flow.

In this paragraph, some in depth notes are made and some further aspects of fractional collateral flow are discussed, which are interesting but not particularly important for clinical application of the method. Reading of this paragraph can be omitted without influencing the general understanding of this chapter.

16.4.1 The constant relation between P_a, P_v, and P_w.

It has already been noted several times that the ratio $(P_w - P_v)/(P_a - P_v)$ is constant. The mathematical proof of that constancy is given in paragraph 4.7. This means in fact that in one particular patient and one particular coronary artery and myocardial distribution, the relation between P_a, P_v and P_w at hyperemia is fixed. Any change in 2 of these parameters, will result in a predictable change in the third parameter. At a first glance, this may seem somewhat surprising, but thinking about this issue, one will realize that this fact reflects the development of the collateral circulation in that vascular bed at that very moment. As shown in paragraph 4.7, the ratio $(P_w - P_v)/(P_a - P_v)$ describes the relation between minimal myocardial resistance and minimal resistance of the collateral system and, as those numbers are constant, it is not surprising that only two degrees of freedom are present in the set of the three variables, P_a, P_v, and P_w. This has also been proved experimentally in dogs, as illustrated in figure 7.3 and 7.4. In those figures, irrespective of changes in P_a (and subsequent changes in P_v), the relation between $(P_a - P_v)$ and $(P_w - P_v)$ remains constant. The slope of the regression line is given by $(R + R_c)/R$ and is inversely proportional to the extent of collateral development.

All theory mentioned above refers to a stable situation with respect to collateral development. If the collateral circulation improves further over time, R_c changes and a new situation occurs. If one could investigate a patient twice with a sufficient time interval between, and could do a balloon occlusion at both opportunities, a unique model is present to quantify the development of the collateral circulation over time. Such a model could become important in the near future in evaluating the effects of growth factors and gen-therapy and to follow angiogenesis.

16.4.2 Maximum hyperemia at coronary occlusion.

By definition, it is mandatory to induce maximum coronary and myocardial hyperemia to calculate FFR_{myo} and FFR_{cor}. When coronary occlusion occurs, one can argue that, in case of ischemia of the myocardium supplied by the occluded artery, the distal bed will already be maximally dilated and no additional stimulus is necessary. This is indeed the case as long as the maximum recruitable collateral flow is insufficient to protect the myocardium at rest. However, if the collateral circulation is developed so well that collateral flow can exceed resting myocardial blood flow, the value of Q_c/Q^N calculated at occlusion may underestimate maximum recruitable collateral flow when no additional hyperemic stimulus is given. In the case of assessment of FFR_{myo} and FFR_{cor}, the hyperemic stimulus can be administered either intravenously or intracoronary. If one decides to administer the stimulus at coronary occlusion, however, the only available route will be the intravenous, and adenosine or ATP infusion is mandatory.

For answering the clinical question if a patient is sufficiently protected by collaterals in the case of coronary artery occlusion, an extra hyperemic stimulus at balloon occlusion is not germane in our opinion: if the collateral flow is insufficient to protect the myocardium at rest, maximum hyperemia will be present, induced by ischemia. In that case, collateral flow is correctly calculated by measuring $(P_w - P_v)/(P_a - P_v)$. If, on the other hand, collateral flow is sufficient to protect the myocardium at rest, fractional collateral flow will be underestimated but the calculated value is still above the critical threshold and informs the investigator about sufficient protection. For clinical research on collateral blood flow, administration of i.v. adenosine during balloon occlusion is advisable. Also, reading of paragraph 4.6.3 is advised with respect to this issue.

16.4.3 Is it necessary to measure venous pressure for collateral flow assessment ?

In the equation for FFR_{myo}, the central venous pressure can generally be neglected without affecting the calculation. Because P_v is low compared to P_a and P_d, only very small mistakes are made as long as P_v is not elevated.

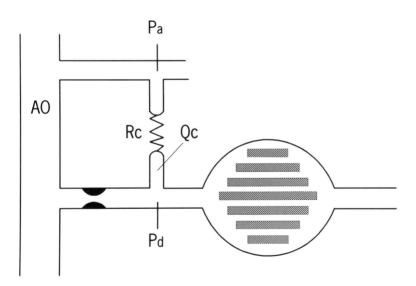

Figure 16.2 *Equivalent of figure 4.7, clarifying the proportionality between pressure gradient and collateral blood flow. Abbreviations: AO: aorta; P_a: mean aortic pressure, which is equal to mean distal coronary pressure in a normal coronary artery; P_d: mean pressure distal to the coronary stenosis, measured at maximum coronary hyperemia; R_c: minimal resistance of the collaterals; Q_c: maximum achievable collateral blood flow.*

(As an illustration, in example 3 in paragraph 16.3, FFR_{myo} equals 0.50 before PTCA and 0.97 after PTCA. If P_v is neglected, these values are 0.52 and 0.97 respectively).

In calculating fractional collateral flow, however, the mistakes by neglecting P_v may be larger. Because in that equation, P_v is compared to P_w (which may be low itself) considerable mistakes may be made, especially in the case of recruitable collateral flow at occlusion. In example 3 of paragraph 16.3, Q_c/Q^N equaled 0.11 before PTCA and 0.18 at balloon occlusion. If P_v were neglected, these values would have been 0.13 and 0.23 respectively. Therefore, when calculating recruitable collateral blood flow during balloon inflation, we recommend measuring P_v also. The rationale behind using P_v and not zero flow pressure, has been discussed already in paragraph 4.3.

16.4.4 Collateral flow at different degrees of stenosis.

The relation between collateral blood flow at different degrees of stenosis, can be obtained immediately by looking at figure 16.2, which is the equivalent of figure 4.7. From that figure it is clear that $Q_c = (P_a - P_d)/R_c$. Therefore, when the superfix$^{(1)}$ relates to one degree of stenosis (eg. before PTCA) and the superfix$^{(2)}$ to another degree of stenosis (eg. after PTCA), the relation between the collateral flow at the different degree of stenosis, is given by:

$$\frac{Q_c^{(2)}}{Q_c^{(1)}} = \frac{(P_a^{(2)} - P_d^{(2)})/R_c}{(P_a^{(1)} - P_d^{(1)})/R_c} = \frac{\Delta^{(2)}P}{\Delta^{(1)}P}$$

In other words, decrease of hyperemic ΔP after PTCA is directly proportional to decrease of collateral blood flow, provided that the artery giving the collaterals, is normal. It should be noted that when changes in P_a have occurred between situation (2) and (1), the ratio $\Delta^{(2)}P/\Delta^{(1)}P$ represents the absolute ratio of $Q_c^{(2)}/Q_c^{(1)}$.

For a "fair" comparison, that index should be made independent of the change in driving pressure by taking:

$$\frac{Q_c^{(2)}}{Q_c^{(1)}} = \frac{\Delta^{(2)}P}{P_a^{(2)} - P_v^{(2)}} : \frac{\Delta^{(1)}P}{P_a^{(1)} - P_v^{(1)}}$$

Example 1: In example 1 in chapter 4.5), hyperemic ΔP was 50 mmHg before PTCA and 10 mmHg thereafter. Therefore, $Q_c^{(2)}/Q_c^{(1)}$ is expected to be 1 : 5. It was already directly calculated in that example that fractional collateral flow was 0.03 after PTCA and 0.15 before, which is indeed 1 : 5.

Example 2: In example 2 in paragraph 12.3, hyperemic ΔP was 45 mmHg before PTCA and 15 mmHg thereafter. Because P_a and P_v changed during the procedure, the expected ratio is given by:

$$\frac{Q_c^{(1)}}{Q_c^{(1)}} = \frac{15}{80-5} \; ; \; \frac{45}{96-6} = 0.2 : 0.5 = 0.4$$

It was already calculated in that example that fractional collateral flow was 0.05 after PTCA and 0.125 before, which is indeed a ratio of 0.4.

16.5 Potential of recruitable collateral blood flow to predict future ischemic events.

16.5.1 Introduction.

In this paragraph an important clinical application of collateral blood flow assessment by coronary pressure measurements is described.

It is well known that a coronary artery may become gradually or even suddenly occluded without causing myocardial infarction or even left ventricular dysfunction. Therefore, in a number of patients collateral flow must be at least sufficient to meet the metabolic demands of the myocardium at rest. As shown by Schaper and Weihrauch in a number of species and by Vanoverschelde and Wijns in selected patients, collateral perfusion in the distribution of a totally occluded artery can vary widely, from almost no collateral flow up to 60% of normal maximum perfusion[5,9].

It would be of great clinical importance if, at the time of a PTCA, prognostic information could be obtained about the risk in case that the dilated artery would occlude in the future. Patients with a low recruitable collateral blood flow, who are at particular risk for extensive infarction in case of re-occlusion, could be better identified then and treated without any delay in case of recurrent symptoms. Especially in some European countries, with waiting lists for PTCA, this would be a relevant issue.

For those reasons, a prospective study was performed to determine whether the assessment of fractional collateral blood flow at the time of angioplasty, is useful to predict a future ischemic event in case of restenosis or occlusion of the dilated artery. As will be shown, this study also provided the opportunity to collect further evidence regarding the validity of the equations for collateral flow calculations in man, and to compare fractional collateral blood flow to other indexes of collateral perfusion.

16.5.2 Study design.

One hundred and twenty consecutive patients (age 59 ± 9 y, range 31-79; 91 males, 29 females) accepted for elective PTCA of single vessel disease (LAD: n=48; LCX: n=35; RCA: n=37), were included in this study who fullfilled two criteria:

First, stable angina pectoris class III had to be present for at least 3 months. Second, the regular exercise test prior to PTCA had to be clearly positive. As will be discussed later, the first inclusion criterion is necessary to be reasonably sure that the collateral circulation had been well-developed and that collateral development had reached a steady state level[1,10-12]. The second inclusion criterion is necessary to ensure a completely reliable means of discriminating between the presence or absence of ischemia in the distribution of the coronary artery at balloon inflation.

Patients with previous infarction or other conditions interfering with unequivocal interpretation of exercise testing, were excluded. All patients received aspirin 80 mg daily from at least 24 hours before PTCA. No restrictions were made with respect to other concommittant medication.

Before PTCA, collaterals to the involved artery on the diagnostic angiogram were classified as grade 0 (no visible collaterals), grade 1 (faintly visible collaterals without filling of the stenotic epicardial vessel), grade 2 (partial filling) or grade 3 (complete filling of the stenotic vessel up to the stenosis) according to Rentrop[13].

At the time of the PTCA, a 6F multipurpose catheter was introduced into one of the femoral veins and advanced into the right atrium for central venous pressure recording (P_v). The PTCA guiding catheter was introduced into one of the femoral arteries and advanced into the ostium of the coronary artery. A regular guide wire and balloon catheter were advanced and the balloon was positioned into the stenosis as usual. Just before inflation, the guide wire was removed, enabling reliable pressure recording through the central lumen of the balloon catheter during the subsequent balloon infla-tions. Because the only distal pressure measured in this study, was occlusion pressure P_w, no mistakes are made by measuring that pressure through the balloon lumen. All inflations lasted 2 minutes and P_a, P_w, and P_v were simultaneously recorded during all inflations. Both frontal and precordial leads were used to monitor the ECG during balloon inflations, enabling recognition of ischemia by comparison to the available exercise ECG.

If the operator wished to evaluate the result, the guide wire was introduced again, the balloon was pulled back, and contrast injections were performed. If more balloon inflations were deemed necessary, the whole sequence was repeated. After a satisfactory result had been obtained, the procedure was finished. Patients were discharged 36-48 hours after the procedure. Recruitable collateral blood flow was calculated by the equation:

$Q_c/Q^N = (P_w - P_v)/(P_a - P_v)$ and correlated to the absence or presence of ischemia on the ECG during balloon occlusion. Also the visibility of collaterals on the angiogram, chest pain, and a P_w-value of less or more than

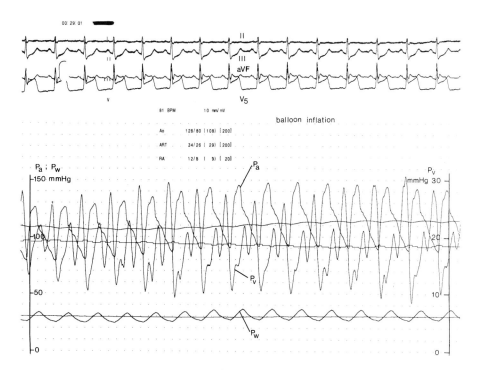

Figure 16.3 *Example of the simultaneous recording of arterial (P_a), central venous (P_v), and coronary wedge pressure (P_w) during balloon inflation. Although mean P_w equals approximately 30 mmHg, fractional collateral blood flow, represented by (P_w - P_v)/(P_a - P_v) equals only 21% and ischemia is present, as revealed by the ECG.*

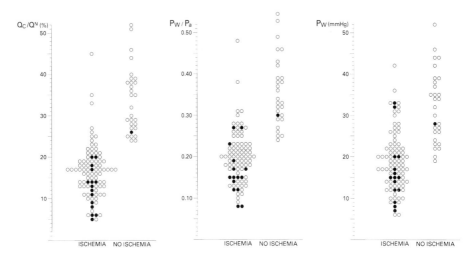

Figure 16.4 *Left panel: Individual values of collateral blood flow (Q_c) during coronary artery occlusion, expressed as a percentage of normal maximum myocardial blood flow (Q^N), and its relation to the presence or absence of ischemia on the ECG. The solid points indicate those patients who experienced an acute ischemic event during the follow-up of 6-22 months. Middle panel: Corresponding values of P_w/P_a ratio. Right panel: Corresponding values of coronary wedge pressure, showing considerably more overlap than Q_c/Q^N and P_w/P_a.*

28 mmHg, were correlated to the presence or absence of ischemia at balloon occlusion. These correlations were evaluated by X^2-tests. A P-value of $<$ 0.05 was considered significant.

Moreover, receiver operating characteristic curves (ROC-curves) were constructed for Q_c/Q^N, P_w, and the degree of collaterals seen on the angiogram and the areas under these curves were calculated. In those patients in whom more balloon inflations were performed, intra-class correlation (ICC) was performed to investigate differences between the subsequent inflations.

During a mean follow-up of 16 months (range 6-22 months), death, myocardial infarction, and unstable angina with acute ischemia on the resting ECG and followed by angiography, were monitored as ischemic events and correlated to Q_c/Q^N as calculated at the time of PTCA.

16.5.3 Results.

Pressure derived recruitable collateral flow data were successfully obtained in 119 patients. An example of such pressure recordings at balloon inflation is shown in figure 16.3.

P_a during balloon occlusion showed a wide inter-individual variation with a range of 61-141 mmHg; for P_w this range was 6-59 mmHg and for P_v 2 - 11 mmHg. The values of recruitable collateral flow, calculated from those pressures and expressed as a percentage of normal maximum myocardial perfusion, are displayed in figure 12.4. In 90 patients, ischemia was present at balloon inflation and in 87 of these patients, Q_c/Q^N was less than or equal to 28%. On the other hand, in all 29 patients without ischemia, Q_c/Q^N exceeded 24%. Stated another way, $Q_c/Q^N > 0.28$ excluded ischemia in 88% of the patients and $Q_c/Q^N < 0.24$ was always accompanied by ischemia at balloon occlusion. The small range between 0.24 and 0.28 is the grey zone of overlap.

The individual values of P_w at balloon occlusion are also displayed in figure 16.4. The best separation is achieved at a P_w-value of 29 mmHg. The overlap between ischemic and non-ischemic values, however, is considerably larger than is the case for Q_c/Q^N.

Because in clinical practice, P_v is not routinely measured during PTCA, we also evaluated the ratio P_w/P_a to indicate presence or absence of ischemia during balloon occlusion. For that index, the best seperating value was 0.30 with only little overlap (figure 16.4, middle column and table 16.1).

In our population, 2 balloon inflations with simultaneous pressure recordings were performed in 50 patients and 3 or more inflations in 19 patients. Fractional collateral flow at the first, second and third inflation was 20.7 ± 10.2% (n=119), 20.5 ± 11.7% (n=50), and 20.6 ± 13.7% (n=19), respectively (figure 16.5). The difference between Q_c/Q^N at the first and second inflation, and second and third inflation was 2.0 ± 2.3% and 1.4 ± 1.4% respectively (N.S.), indicating that at least during the procedure no further recruitment of collaterals occurred.

In table 16.1, the relation is given between presence or absence of ischemia on the ECG and Q_c/Q^N, the P_w/P_a ratio, visibility of collaterals at the angiogram, P_w alone (without taking into account P_a and P_v), and chest pain, respectively. The area under the ROC-curve was, 0.97, 0.93, 0.88, and 0.64 respectively for Q_c/Q^N, P_w/P_a, P_w, and visibility of collaterals. A perfect test would have an area of 1.0. Therefore Q_c/Q^N is the best of these indexes to correctly predict sufficient or insufficient collateral blood flow. But, if P_v is not measured individually and not elevated, also the P_w/P_a index suffices well.

During a mean follow-up of 16 months (range 6-22), ischemic events occurred in 16 patients (table 16.2). None one of them belonged to the group with $Q_c/Q^N > 0.28$ and all except one of them had a value of $Q_c/Q^N < 0.24$, definitely indicating insufficient collateral blood flow at balloon inflation at the time of the previous PTCA. (Relative risk 7.9; $X^2 = 5.38$; $P < .05$).

Similarly, all of the patients with an adverse event at follow-up except one, had a P_w/P_a value < 0.30, indicating the usefulness of that somewhat simpler index (relative risk 5.4 in patients with $P_w/P_a \leq 30$ vs those with $P_w/P_a > 30$).

Finally, the relation between the degree of collaterals on the angiogram and the calculated value of Q_c/Q^N was investigated and is presented in figure 16.6. As shown, the absence of visible collaterals on the angiogram (degree 0) is often associated with low fractional collateral flow. On the contrary, however, visible collaterals degree 1 or 2 do not guarantee sufficient fractional collateral flow as indicated by the Q_c/Q^N index. Remarkably, 3 of the 16 patients with an ischemic event during follow-up had visible collaterals degree ≥ 2 on the angiogram.

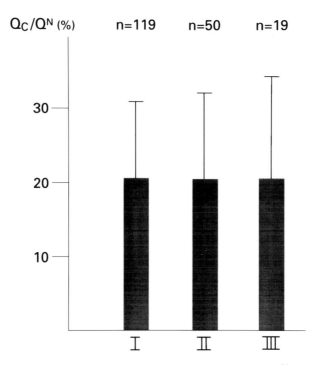

Figure 16.5 *Recruitable fractional collateral blood flow (Q_c/Q^N), at the consecutive balloon inflations (mean $\pm$ SE).*

16.5.4 Discussion.

Methodology to assess coronary collateral blood flow in the human catheterization laboratory, is far behind compared to the experimental environment. There is an immense gap between detailed and advanced basic scientific data about growth, development, recruitment, derecruitment, and neurohumoral regulation of collateral flow in isolated preparations and animal models, and its practical use in conscious man[14-16].

The method used in this study to derive an index of collateral flow from simultaneous pressure recordings, is rapid and relatively simple to apply with standard equipment. It is well-known that in healthy persons, hyperemic blood flow equals approximately 3-5 times resting blood flow with quite a variability depending on inter-individual variation, age, and hemodynamic loading conditions[17-19]. Therefore, one would roughly expect that if recruitable collaterals at coronary occlusion are able to provide approximately 25-30% of normal maximum myocardial perfusion, the myocardium is protected at rest. The value of 28%, found in this study, is very close to that theoretically expected value and gives further evidence for the correctness of this method in conscious man.

Because fractional collateral flow is independent on age, absolute values, and loading conditions, it can be understood why we found such a well demarcated range of sufficient and insufficient collateral blood flow values with little overlap.

If the P_w/P_a index is used to assess the extent of recruitable collateral circulation, a value of 0.30 was found to discriminate patients protected by collaterals or not. This number is remarkably close to earlier studies by Meier et al and later studies by Piek et al, showing that a P_w/P_a value of 0.31 and 0.30, respectively, had a predictive value of approximately 90% and 84%, respectively, to indicate protection against ischemia[6,7,20]

In our study population, with angina class III for at least 3 months, it was assumed that recruitable collateral blood flow to the jeopardized myocardium had been well developed to a steady state. This assumption was based upon experimental data[10-12,20,21] and seemed to be confirmed in our population by the observation that in those patients with multiple balloon inflations, no further increase in collateral contribution was observed (figure 16.5).

Strictly speaking, all pressure measurements in this study should have been performed at maximum vasodilation of the arteriolar bed distal to the site of balloon occlusion as outlined in paragraph 16.4.2. Because we assumed that coronary artery occlusion in itself is a potent vasodilatory stimulus, no extra vasodilatory drugs were administered. In about 25% of our patients,

Table 16.1 *Relation between presence or absence of ischemia on the ECG and recruitable fractional collateral flow (Q_c/Q^N), The P_w/P_a ratio, visibility of any collaterals on the angiogram, chest pain at balloon inflation, and coronary wedge pressure (P_w) alone, respectively.*

	Q_c/Q^N $\leq 28\%$	Q_c/Q^N $> 28\%$
ISCHEMIA +	87	3
ISCHEMIA -	8	21

$$X^2 = 62.9$$

	$P_w/P_a \leq 0.30$	$P_w/P_a > 0.30$
ISCHEMIA +	83	7
ISCHEMIA -	9	20

$$X^2 = 44.5$$

	NO VISIBLE COLLATERALS	VISIBLE COLLATERALS
ISCHEMIA +	72	18
ISCHEMIA -	9	20

$$X^2 = 25.8$$

	PAIN +	PAIN -
ISCHEMIA +	76	14
ISCHEMIA -	14	25

$$X^2 = 16.8$$

	$P_w \leq 29$	$P_w > 29$
ISCHEMIA +	80	10
ISCHEMIA -	13	16

$$X^2 = 27.4$$

Table 16.2

Pat #	Gender (M/F)	Age (Y)	Collat. angio	Q_c/Q^N (%)	P_w/P_a	P_w (mmHg)	Type of event	T (days)
12	M	58	0	13	0,14	15	UAP	477
14	M	54	0	6	0.08	8	AMI	2
23	M	60	0	9	0,12	12	AMI	574
26	M	62	1	12	0,15	9	UAP	1
31	M	60	3	17	0,19	33	AMI	4
47	F	61	2	14	0,15	15	AMI	189
48	M	78	2	26	0,30	28	UAP	468
72	M	53	1	5	0,14	12	UAP	3
76	M	57	0	8	0,12	15	UAP	108
79	M	63	0	20	0,27	20	UAP	220
80	F	45	1	14	0,15	16	AMI	1
85	F	53	0	20	0,27	32	UAP	151
90	M	48	0	11	0,17	14	UAP	29
91	M	46	0	6	0,08	7	UAP	78
99	F	46	0	18	0,23	20	UAP	176
103	F	48	0	14	0,17	17	UAP	165

Characteristics of the patients, having an ischemic event at follow-up.

AMI: acute myocardial infarction; Collat.angio: degree of collaterals on the angiogram; P_w: coronary wedge pressure at balloon occlusion; P_a : mean aortic pressure; Q_c/Q^N: recruitable collateral blood flow, expressed as a percentage of normal maximum myocardial blood flow; T: time between PTCA and ischemic event at follow-up; UAP: unstable angina pectoris.

however, no ischemia at balloon inflation was observed, which could mean that the occlusion in itself was a suboptimal hyperemic stimulus. If an additional vasodilatory stimulus would have been administered, an even higher value of Q_c/Q^N could have been observed in those patients. Therefore, the values in the right column of the left panel of figure 12.4 could be underestimated. Because the separation between sufficient and insufficient collateral flow would have been even better in that case, we believe that the conclusions of our study are still valid despite not using additional pharmacologic agents to achieve vasodilation.

To perform this study, it was necessary to have at our disposal a completely reliable method to confirm or exclude ischemia at balloon occlusion. This was achieved by selecting the patients on a basis of well-recognizable reversible ECG abnormalities at ischemia. Because in all of our patients, a recent positive exercise ECG was available, and because we used those ECG leads during PTCA which showed the ischemic abnormalities in an optimum way, by comparison to that exercise ECG, the ECG at coronary artery occlusion could be used as a standard for presence or absence of ischemia at balloon inflation. Not only fractional collateral flow was compared to that standard, but also previously used indexes of collateral flow such as visibility of collaterals on the angiogram, chest pain, and coronary wedge pressure alone. All of these parameters were inferior to Q_c/Q^N in correctly predicting ischemia.

16.5.5 Comparison of Q_c/Q^N to visibility of collaterals and long-term follow-up.

As shown in figure 16.6, the relation between degree of visibility of collaterals on the angiogram and calculated value of fractional collateral flow, is rather variable and warns against relying upon the angiogram alone to assess the risk in case of occlusion of the dilated artery. A more reliable relation is found when contrast injection in the contralateral artery is performed during balloon inflation, as shown by Piek et al[12,22]. However, their methodology requires 2-sided femoral artery canulation and is not feasible on a routine basis.

From our equation for recruitable collateral blood flow at coronary artery occlusion, it can also be understood why P_w alone was found in the past to have only a limited value for estimating recruitable collateral blood flow: According to the equation, $P_w = 20$ mmHg in an individual with a mean arterial pressure of 90 mmHg and central venous pressure of 10 mmHg, indicates a recruitable collateral flow of only 12.5% of normal maximum myocardial perfusion whereas the same P_w in another individual with a

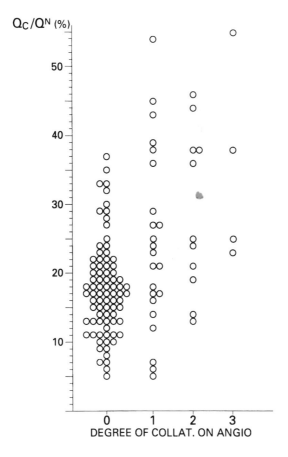

Figure 16.6 *Relation between degree of visible collaterals on the coronary angiogram, according to Rentrop , and the calculated value of fractional collateral blood flow Q_c/Q^N.*

simultaneously measured arterial pressure of 70 mmHg and central venous pressure of 0 mmHg, results in a collateral contribution of 29% of normal maximum myocardial perfusion. This example demonstrates that P_w alone does not reliably reflect the extent of collateral circulation, as assumed in some previous studies. In fact, the dependence of classical indexes of collateral flow on actual hemodynamic status, is illustrated by this example. By using the P_w/P_a ratio, better correlations were obtained because variations in blood pressure are compensated for by this index. For clinical purposes, therefore, use of the P_w/P_a index seems to be sufficient and has considerable prognostic value with respect to long-term follow-up. For scientific purposes, true fractional collateral flow (Q_c/Q^N) has the preference.

During the follow-up of 6-22 months, 16 ischemic events occurred: All of these patients had a recruitable fractional collateral blood flow less than 28%. (relative risk 7.9) and 15 of them had P_w/P_a value ≤ 30 (relative risk 5.4). Therefore, although in the long term natural progression or changes in coronary artery disease may occur, $Q_c/Q^N > 28\%$ or $P_w/P_a > 30$ can be considered as significant predictors of protection against myocardial infarction in case of future occlusion of the coronary artery. This follow-up has been extended recently up to 5 years without affecting the conclusions of this study.

16.5.6 Clinical implications and limitations.

The method described in this study required removal and re-introduction of the guide wire through the balloon catheter. We had to do this because at the time of this study, pressure monitoring guide wires were still in a developmental phase. With the present availability of first line sensor tipped guide wires, the procedure becomes much simpler and except introduction of a central venous catheter no further manipulations are necessary anymore at all. Collateral flow assessment by pressure measurements can be routinely applied now in interventional procedures with minimal cost within minutes by just using a pressure guide wire instead of a regular guide wire.

This study has several clinical implications. First, it provides insight into the distribution of recruitable collateral flow in a patient population with stable angina pectoris. As shown, fractional collateral flow in this study ranged from 5% to 56% of normal maximum myocardial perfusion (figure 16.4). This means that collateral flow is not negligible, as is sometimes assumed for the purpose of simplicity[23,24]. Present methods for coronary flow assessment in the clinical catheterization laboratory, such as videodensitometry and Doppler flow velocimetry, are limited by considerable overlap between normal and pathologic values[23-25]. As may be clear now, this overlap may be due in part to not taking into account the contribution of collateral flow by those methods.

Second, during PTCA, those patients at particular risk for extensive myocardial infarction in case of future occlusion of the dilated coronary artery, can be better identified. Just simply measuring P_w at balloon occlusion and calculating fractional collateral flow or P_w/P_a discriminates patients with a > 5x higher risk for a coronary event in the next years ! This is important clinical information which becomes available within minutes !

Third, this method may be useful in quantitation and follow-up of collateral blood flow for a number of investigational purposes such as stimulation of

Table 16.3 *Pressure-derived indexes for assessing collateral blood flow.*

ADVANTAGES

♦   *quantitative assessment of collateral blood flow*
♦   *easily applicable in routine interventional procedures*
♦   *independent of blood pressure and other hemodynamic variations*
♦   *excellent reproducibility*
♦   *relevant clinical information: $P_w/P_a \geq 0.30$ means 5x lower clinical event rate at 5-year follow-up than $P_w/P_a \leq 0.30$*

LIMITATIONS

♦   *coronary wedge pressure (P_w) is always necessary → only applicable at PTCA*
♦   *measurement of central venous pressure (P_v) is mandatory in case this pressure is expected to be elevated*

collateral development by growth factors and the effect of drugs on recruitment. The major limitation of this method is, that it can only be applied during PTCA and not as a diagnostic procedure because P_w has to be recorded at coronary artery occlusion. Moreover, for exact calculation of fractional collateral flow, measurement of P_v and use of central venous catheter, is necessary. The advantages and limitations of coronary pressure measurements to assess collateral blood flow, are summarized in table 16.3.

References.

1. Sasayama S, Fujita M. Recent insights into coronary collateral circulation. *Circulation* 1992; 85: 1197-1204.
2. Mizuno K, Horiuchi K, Matui H. Role of coronary collateral vessels during transient coronary occlusion during angioplasty assessed by hemodynamic, electrocardiographic, and metabolic changes. *J Am Coll Cardiol* 1988; 12: 624 - 628.

3. Pijls NHJ, Bech GJW, El Gamal MIH, Bonnier JJRM, De Bruyne B, Van Gelder B, Michels HR, Koolen JJ. Quantification of recruitable coronary collateral blood flow in conscious humans and its potential to predict future ischemic events. *J Am Coll Cardiol* 1995; 25: 1522 - 1528.
4. Pijls NHJ, Bracke FALE. Damage to the collateral circulation by PTCA of an occluded coronary artery. *Cath Cardiov Diagn* 1995; 34: 61 - 64.
5. Schaper J, Weihrauch D. Collateral vessel development in the porcine and canine heart. In: Schaper W and Schaper J, eds. *Collateral Circulation*. Boston MA: Kluwer Academic Publishers, 1993: 65-102.
6. Meier B, Luethy P, Finci L, Steffenino GD, Rutishauser W. Coronary wedge pressure in relation to spontaneously visible and recruitable collaterals. *Circulation* 1987; 75: 906-13.
7. De Bruyne B, Meier B, Finci L, Urban P, Rutishauser W. Potential protective effect of high coronary wedge pressure on left ventricular function after coronary occlusion. *Circulation* 1988; 78: 566-72.
8. King SB, Douglas JS, Gruentzig AR. Percutaneous transluminal coronary angioplasty, in: King SB and Douglas JS (eds), Coronary arteriography and angioplasty. *Mc Graw Hill*, New York 1985; pp 433-460.
9. Vanoverschelde JLJ, Wijns W, Deprez JC. Mechanisms of chronic regional post-ischemic dysfunction in humans. New insights from the study of noninfarcted collateral-dependent myocardium. *Circulation* 1993; 87: 1513-23.
10. Fujita M, Sasayama S, Ohno A, Nakajima H, Asanoi H. Importance of angina for development of collateral circulation. *Br Heart J* 1987; 57: 139-43.
11. Longhurst JC, Symons JD. Function and development of coronary collateral vessels. In: Schaper W and Schaper J,eds. Collateral Circulation. Boston MA: *Kluwer Academic Publishers* 1993: 195-214.
12. Piek JJ, Koolen JJ, Hoedemaker G, David GK, Visser CA. Severity of single-vessel coronary arterial stenosis and duration of angina as determinants of recruitable collateral vessels during balloon angioplasty occlusion. *Am J Cardiol* 1991; 67:13-17.
13. Rentrop KP, Thornton JC, Feit F, Van Buskirk M. Determinants and protective potential of coronary arterial collaterals as assessed by an angioplasty model. *Am J Cardiol* 1988; 61: 677-684.
14. Schaper W, Görge G, Winkler B, Schaper J. The collateral circulation of the heart. *Prog cardiov Dis* 1988; 31:57-77.
15. Pupita G, Maseri A, Kaski JC. Myocardial ischemia caused by distal coronary artery constriction in stable angina pectoris. *N Engl J Medic* 1990; 323: 514-20.
16. Harrison DG, Simonetti I. Neurohumoral regulation of collateral perfusion. *Circulation* 1991; 83: (suppl III): 62-7.
17. Gould KL, Lipscomb K, Hamilton GW. Physiologic basis for assessing critical stenosis: instantaneous flow response and regional distribution during coronary hyperemia as measures of coronary flow reserve. *Am J Cardiol* 1974; 33: 87-94.
18. Hoffman JIE. Maximal coronary flow and the concept of coronary vascular reserve. *Circulation* 1984; 70: 153-59.
19. Gould KL, Kirkeeide RL, Buchi M. Coronary flow reserve as a physiologic measure of stenosis severity. *J Am Coll Cardiol* 1990; 15: 459-74.
20. Piek JJ, van Liebergen RAM, Koch KT, Peters RJG, David GK. Clinical, angiographic, and hemodynamic predictors of recruitable collateral flow assessed during balloon angioplasty coronary occlusion. *J Am Coll Cardiol* 1997; 29: 275-282.

21. Yamamoto H, Tomoike H, Shimokawa H, Nabeyama S, Nakamma M. Development of collateral function with repetitive coronary occlusion in a canine model reduces myocardial reactive hyperemia in the absence of significant coronary stenosis. *Circ Res* 1984; 55: 623-32.

22. Piek JJ, Koolen JJ, Metting van Rijn AC. Spectral analysis of flow velocity in the contralateral artery during coronary angioplasty: a new method for assessing collateral flow. *J Am Coll Cardiol* 1993; 21: 1574-82.

23. Pijls NHJ, Aengevaeren WRM, Uyen GJH, et al. Concept of maximal flow ratio for immediate evaluation of percutaneous transluminal coronary angioplasty result by video-densitometry. *Circulation* 1991; 83: 854-65.

24. Hess OM, McGillen MJ, De Boe SF, Pinto IMF, Gallagher KP, Mancini GBJ. Determination of coronary flow reserve by parametric imaging. *Circulation* 1990; 82: 1438-48.

25. Ofili EO, Labovitz AJ, Kern MJ. Coronary flow velocity dynamics in normal and diseased arteries. *Am J Cardiol* 1993; 71: 3D - 9D.

Chapter 17

CLINICAL CASES

In this chapter, a selection of instructive clinical cases is presented. In each case, a short overview is given of the patient's history, the clinical question which had to be solved, the solution provided by pressure measurement, and the subsequent treatment. Going through these cases will familiarize the reader with the applications and features of coronary pressure measurement and fractional flow reserve.

A number of instructive cases have already been presented in the previous chapters of this book, such as *intermediate stenosis* (figure 4.4 and 4.5; figure 12.1), *monitoring of PTCA* (figure 4.8 and 4.9), and *evaluation of adequate stent deployment* (figure 14.7 and 14.11). Also, a number of instructive pressure curves and *pitfalls* have been discussed in detail in chapter 5 and 6.

The abbreviations used in this chapter, are explained in the list of abbreviations at the beginning of this book.

17.1 Intermediate stenosis.

Case 1:

Case history: A 51-year-old man presented with typical exercise-induced angina. The regular exercise test was positive, as was thallium scintigraphy. At coronary angiography, however, only a long, apparently insignificant lesion was seen with an estimated diameter stenosis of approximately 30% (panel A and B).

Problem: Is this lesion functionally significant and should it be treated ?

Solution: The answer is given in panel C. At rest, only a small gradient is present, but at hyperemia a rather large gradient is unmasked and FFR_{myo} equals 0.67, confirming that this anatomically mild but long stenosis is responsible for the patient's complaints and the positive non-invasive tests. The patient underwent bypass surgery, whereafter the exercise-thallium test normalized, and is free of complaints 2 years later.

Comments: Although not expected by angiography, such a long but anatomically insignificant lesion may significantly decrease maximum blood flow.

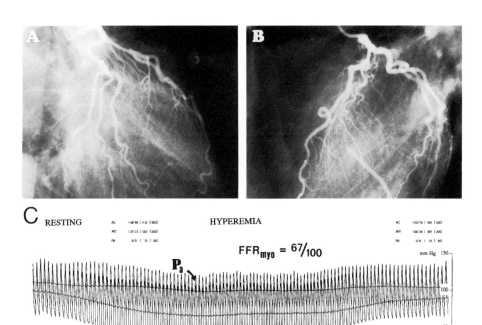

Case 2:

Case history: 46-year-old long distance runner admitted because of aborted sudden death. Cardiopulmonary resuscitation was initiated by the patient's son and when the medical emergency team arrived, ventricular fibrillation was present. The ECG performed after defibrillation did not show clear signs of myocardial infarction. Left heart catheterization was performed 48 hours later. The left ventricular angiogram showed a normal global left ventricular function (ejection fraction: 58%) with an asynchronous relaxation of the antero-lateral segments. An angiographically mild stenosis in the proximal LAD (diameter stenosis 42% and mld 2.3 mm was observed (panel A).

Problem: Is the stenosis in the proximal LAD hemodynamically significant and responsible for the circulatory arrest ?

Solution: The intracoronary pressure tracings obtained at rest and during maximum hyperemia are shown in panel B. When the pressure sensor crosses the proximal segment of the LAD (arrows), a brisk pressure gradient of 35 mmHg appears. The FFR calculated during hyperemia was 0.52.

Comments: Accordingly, a 3.5 mm stent was deployed in the proximal LAD with an excellent angiographic and functional result. Six months later, the patient was asymptomatic without anti-anginal medication and had resumed intense sport activities. A maximal exercise ECG was normal. However, a control angiogram (panel C) showed an angiographically similar stenosis (diameter stenosis 47% and minimal luminal diameter 2.3 mm by quantitative coronary angiography). In contrast, pressure measurement in the LAD (panel D) showed no gradient at rest and a FFR of 0.86 at maximum hyperemia. Therefore, despite an angiographically similar stenosis, no functional significance of the lesion could be demonstrated this time which is in accordance with the clinical status and exercise test. Accordingly, no further treatment was undertaken.

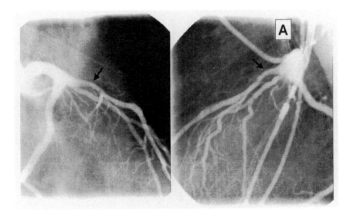

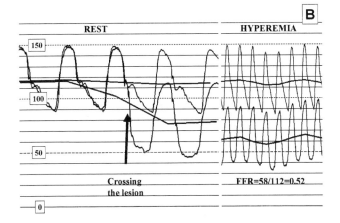

B

REST HYPEREMIA

150

100

50

Crossing
the lesion FFR=58/112=0.52

0

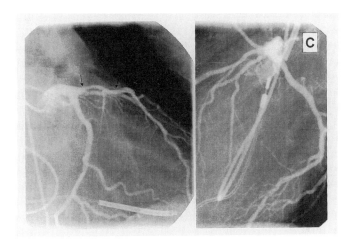

C

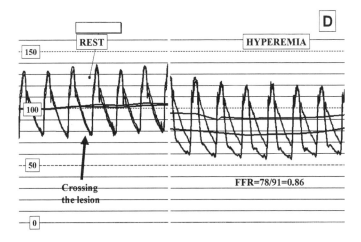

D

REST HYPEREMIA

150

100

50

Crossing
the lesion FFR=78/91=0.86

0

Case 3:

Case history: A 76-year-old lady who underwent bypass operation 8 years earlier presented at the out-patient clinic with atypical chest pain and arterial hypertension. No non-invasive stress testing had been performed. At coronary angiography, the venous bypass to the RCA and the LIMA to the LAD were both nicely patent. In a large marginal branch of the LCX which had not been bypassed, an angiographically 'intermediate' stenosis was present (panel A).

Problem: Is this stenosis responsible for the complaints of the patients ? Is PTCA indicated ?

Solution: Pressure measurements (panel B) showed that this lesion was hemodynamically not significant and no angioplasty was performed.

Comments: This case illustrates the poor relationship between angiographic assessment (even when quantitative coronary angiography is applied) of stenosis severity and FFR which is a more specific index of epicardial conductance.

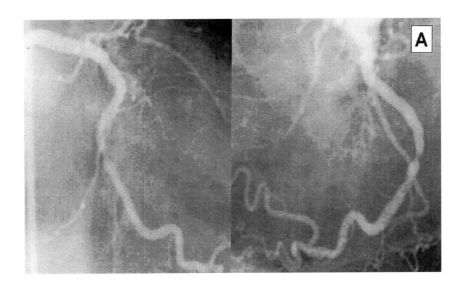

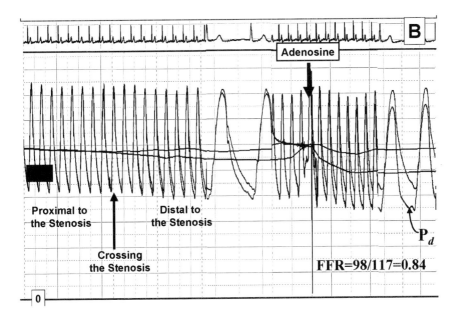

Case 4:

Case history: A 52-year-old woman presented with atypical chest pain, a positive exercise test at 80% of the expected exercise tolerance, and negative thallium scintigraphy. At angiography, an intermediate proximal RCA stenosis was observed with a diameter stenosis of 39% at QCA (left upper panel).

Problem: Is this intermediate lesion in the RCA functionally significant and should it be treated ? And is the thallium scintigram false negative ? Or is that lesion not functionally significant, the thallium scintigram true negative, and the regular exercise test false positive ?

Solution: The middle panel shows indisputably that maximum achievable blood flow to the myocardium supplied by the RCA is significantly decreased, as reflected by a value of FFR_{myo} of 0.65. PTCA was performed subsequently, with a good angiographic result (right upper panel) but a moderate functional result (lower panel). Nevertheless, the exercise test reverted to negative.

Five weeks later, recurrent chest pain occurred, the exercise test was positive again, and a successful re-PTCA of a significant restenosis was performed, followed again by normalization of the exercise test.

Comments: Obviously, the regular exercise test was true positive and thallium scintigraphy was false negative in this patient. It should be realized that in a number of patients, perfusion *differences* of at least 25-35% are required to be visible at perfusion scintigraphy. Because inducible ischemia is mostly present below a value of FFR_{myo} of 0.75, it is clear that there is a grey zone with respect to perfusion scintigraphy in a number of patients, especially those with intermediate stenoses and a FFR_{myo} somewhere between 0.65 and 0.75. In those patients, inducible ischemia is generally present but may be missed by perfusion scintigraphy.

This shortcoming of perfusion scintigraphy is even more pronounced, when not only a significant lesion is present in one vessel, but also less severe abnormalities in other vessels, as is often the case. If, for example, FFR_{myo} equals 0.85, 0.80, and 0.70 for the RCA, LCX, and LAD, respectively, the LAD-lesion is functionally significant and capable to cause reversible ischemia, but will generally be missed by the present imaging techniques.

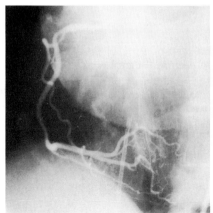
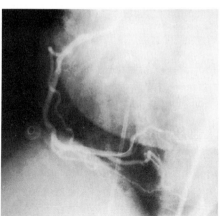

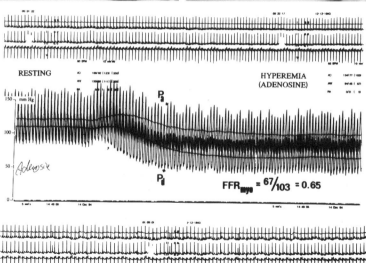

RESTING   HYPEREMIA
                           (ADENOSINE)

P$_a$

150 mm Hg

100

50

Adenosine

P$_d$

$$FFR_{myo} = \frac{67}{103} = 0.65$$

RESTING   HYPEREMIA

P$_a$

150 mm Hg

100

50

P$_d$

$$FFR_{myo} = \frac{72}{93} = 0.78$$

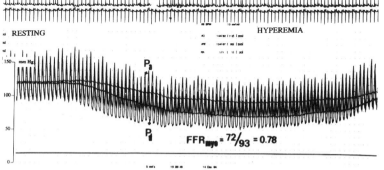

17.2 Long lesion.

Case 5:

Case history: A 46-year-old man presented with typical chest pain. Exercise thallium scintigraphy, however, was negative. Because of persistent, typical, exercise-related symptoms, coronary angiography was performed, revealing a long but apparently only mildly narrowed segment in the proximal LAD (panel A and B). The patient was reassured and sent home. One week later, he was re-admitted after an out-of-hospital cardiac arrest during cycling.

Problem: Is the LAD lesion responsible for the exercise-induced ischemia and the out-of-hospital cardiac arrest ?

Solution: Coronary pressure measurements show a large pressure drop when the sensor crosses the stenosis (panel C). After administration of adenosine, a further decline of distal LAD pressure occurs (panel D), resulting in a FFR_{myo} of 0.65. Dipyridamole thallium scintigraphy was performed but negative again. Dobutamine stress-echocardiography, on the contrary, showed severe hypokinesis of the anterior wall at 40 µg/kg/min of dobutamine and a heart rate of 167 bpm. Coronary bypass surgery was performed, whereafter no symptoms were present anymore. The stress-echocardiogram, performed 9 weeks later, was normal.

Comments: Both exercise thallium scintigraphy and dipyridamole thallium scintigraphy failed to show reversible ischemia. As shown by a FFR_{myo} of 0.65 and by the reversal of the stress-echocardiogram after revascularization, the lesion was significant and almost resulted in the death of this young patient. If pressure measurements in this intermediate lesion had been performed straight at the initial coronary angiography, much trouble and risk would have been avoided. Obviously, in this patient thallium scintigraphy was false negative and stress-echocardiography was true positive. We have also observed cases in whom the opposite was true. A series of 45 similar difficult cases in whom both exercise thallium scintigraphy, stress-echocardiography, and invasive assessment of FFR_{myo} was performed within an interval of 48 hours, is described in chapter 12.

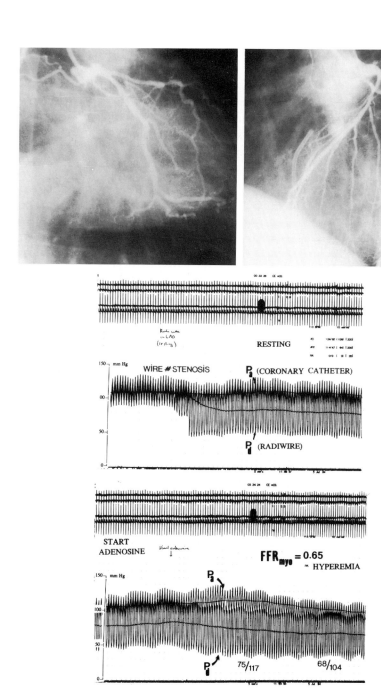

17.3 Difficult coronary anatomy.

Case 6:

Case history: A 51-year-old man was admitted because of typical chest pain at rest and transient T-wave abnormalities on the ECG in the anterior leads. At catheterization, an abnormality was only seen in the LAO 45/20 view with respect to the LAD artery and both diagonal branches. All other views seemed to be normal.

Problem: Are any of these three branches (D1, D2, or LAD) abnormal and responsible for the chest pain and ECG-changes ?

Solution: At first, the pressure wire is advanced to the tip of the guiding catheter and it is confirmed that equal pressures are measured at that location and that no gradient is present proximal to the trifurcation (panel A). After the wire has been advanced into the first diagonal branch, hyperemia is induced and it can be easily observed that fractional flow reserve of the myocardium supplied by that branch, equals 0.88 (panel B). Therefore, although some plaque must be present with some influence on maximum achievable blood flow, this diagonal branch cannot be responsible for the reversible ischemia in this patient, because FFR_{myo} well exceeds the cut-off value of 0.75. FFR_{myo} of the second diagonal branch is 1.0 (panel C) and therefore, that branch is completely normal with respect to flow. After introduction of the pressure wire into the LAD, however, it is demonstrated that FFR_{myo} of the LAD-dependent myocardium is severely depressed to

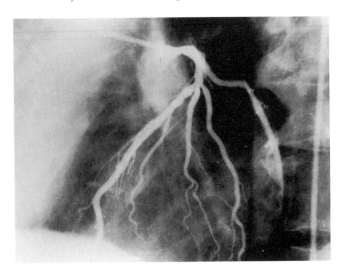

0.42 (panel D) and therefore it is the LAD itself which is responsible for the inducible ischemia in this patient and needs to be revascularized.

Comments: This patient illustrates how in cases of difficult interpretation of angiography (overprojection, bi- or trifurcations, foreshortening, etc.) pressure recordings clearly reveal the presence or absence of significant disease. When, in such cases, a pull-back curve is made at continuous maximum hyperemia (see figure 12.1 or case 7 of this chapter), the exact location of the stenosis can be identified, even when it is not visible by angiography.

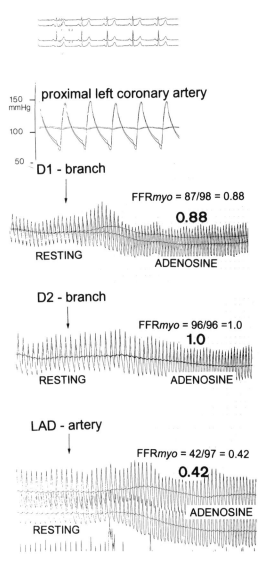

Case 7:

Case history: A 53-year old male presented with typical chest pain at moderate exercise. Thallium-exercise testing was clearly positive with a reversible perfusion defect in the anterior wall. At coronary angiography, a severe stenosis was seen in the mid-LAD segment and a mild lesion was present in the very proximal LAD. The patient was referred for PTCA of the mid-LAD stenosis.

Problem: How can we be sure that only the mid-LAD stenosis is the culprit lesion and that PTCA of that stenosis will be a sufficient treatment indeed ?

Solution: A 0.014" pressure wire was placed in the distal LAD, continuous hyperemia was induced by i.v. adenosine infusion, and a slow pull-back pressure recording was made. Indeed, there is a pressure drop at the location of the mid-LAD lesion, but an even larger drop is present at the very proximal LAD. FFR of both lesions together equals $58/110 = 0.53$. It is clear that also the proximal stenosis has functional significance and that PTCA of the mid-LAD stenosis alone cannot completely relieve the inducible ischemia in this patient. Therefore, this patient underwent minimal invasive bypass surgery and the left internal mammarian artery was placed on the distal LAD. Thallium scintigraphy, performed 6 weeks later, was negative.

Comments: This case illustrates the value of coronary pressure measurements to investigate the coronary artery along its complete length and to indicate both the exact location and the severity of different stenoses. Also lesions located at bifurcations and often difficult to assess by angiography, can be reliably interrogated in that way. In this patient, PTCA of the mid-LAD stenosis could not have relieved the inducible ischemia of this patient and was avoided, and the most appropriate treatment - minimal invasive bypass surgery - was chosen on the basis of the pressure measurement.

Note: In case a like this, there is also a mutual influence of one stenosis on the hemodynamic manifestation of the other. This issue is further clarified in chapter 13.4 and in cases 18 and 19 in this chapter.

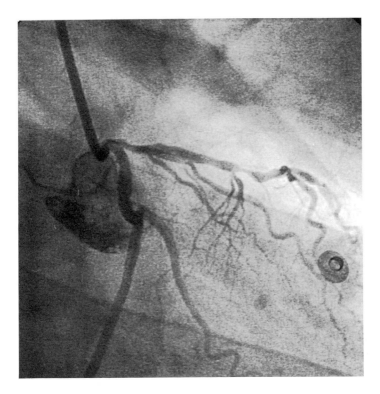

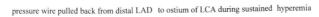

pressure wire pulled back from distal LAD to ostium of LCA during sustained hyperemia

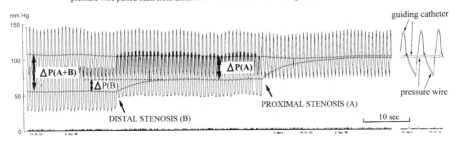

17.4 Identification of the culprit lesion.

Case 8:

Background: A 46-year-old man with stable angina pectoris (class II), treated medically, needed major abdominal surgery because of colonic cancer. An exercise test was performed to assess the cardiac risk and was positive at 60 W, whereafter coronary arteriography was performed. Three-vessel disease was present with anatomically significant lesions in the LAD, the obtuse marginal branch, and the right coronary artery (panel A and B).
Problem: Bypass surgery was contraindicated because of time constraints, the risk of dissemination of cancer, and the associated risk of gastro-intestinal bleeding. Can a culprit lesion be identified and dilated, in order to avoid bypass surgery but decrease the risk of major abdominal surgery ?
Solution: Myocardial fractional flow reserve of all lesions was determined, as shown in panel C to E. The LAD and LCX stenosis did not have a significant influence on the maximum achievable perfusion of the dependent myocardium (FFR_{myo} = 0.90 and 0.96, respectively). The RCA stenosis, however, was extremely severe from a functional point of view as indicated by a FFR_{myo} of 0.35. Therefore, this stenosis was subsequently dilated with a good anatomic and excellent functional result (panel F and G). The exercise test, performed 4 days later, reverted to negative and resection of a part of the large bowel was performed 6 days after PTCA. At present, 3 years later, the patient is free from cardiac complaints and free from cancer.
Comments: As FFR_{myo} is a lesion-specific index of epicardial coronary stenosis severity, it is extremely useful to identify one or more culprit lesions in case of multivessel disease. In a number of patients, bypass surgery can be avoided and PTCA of a culprit lesion performed. This is particularly beneficial if contra-indications for bypass surgery are present, as in this patient. In other patients, the choice for bypass surgery or minimal invasive surgery can be justified in that way. (see case 6 and 7)

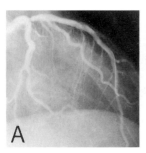
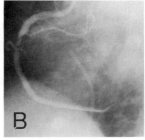
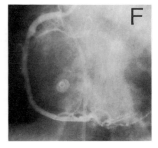

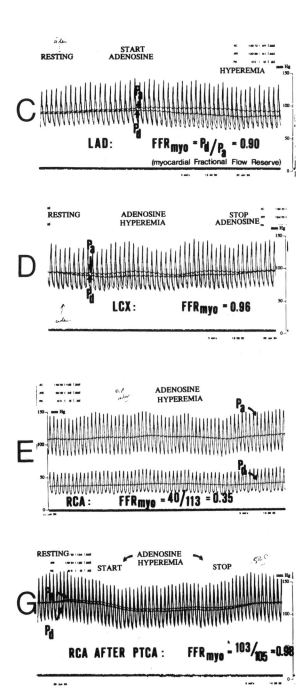

Case 9:

Case history: A 49-year-old man presented with typical, stable, exercise-induced angina. The exercise ECG performed without medication showed 2 mm horizontal ST-depressions in the anterior leads without chest pain and the MIBI spect scintigram at rest and during adenosine showed reversible flow maldistribution in the septal, inferior and anterior segments. At diagnostic catheterization global and regional left ventricular function was normal. On the coronary angiogram, a moderate left main stenosis was seen (diameter stenosis: 32%; minimal luminal diameter: 2.8 mm). Diffuse irregularities were present in the LAD, the LCx and the angular branch (panel A) and a tight stenosis was present in the mid-RCA (panel B). In some dynamic images of the coronary angiogram, there was a suspicion for a 'slit-like' stenoses in the very ostial LAD. This is not visible in the still frames as presented in panel A.

Problem (1): Discordance between the perfusion scan and the coronary angiogram: the flow maldistribution cannot be ascribed to the angiographically 'mild' stenosis in the left main.

Problem (2): Treatment strategy: a) if only the RCA is significant the patient's complaints could be attributed to this stenosis and an angioplasty of the RCA only could be proposed; b) if the left main stenosis is hemodynamically significant, a complete surgical revascularion should be proposed; c) if the hemodynamically significant stenoses are in the mid-RCA and the ostial LAD, a hybrid procedure could be proposed (angioplasty of the RCA and LIMA of the LAD)

Solution: The solution is given by the pressure tracings presented in panels C to F: In the LAD the FFR is 0.65, in the RCA 0.45, in the angular branch 0.92 and in the LCx 0.84. Only the RCA and the LAD should be revascularized as the left main stenosis cannot be considered significant.

Comments: Based on these multiple pressure measurements, it can be concluded that this patient could be treated by a so-called hybride procedure. Accordingly, a LIMA anastomosis was performed on the LAD by (minimal invasive) port access surgery and direct stenting of the RCA was performed. Six months later the patient was asymptomatic and the exercise ECG was normal. The control angiogram performed after 6 months is shown in panel G.

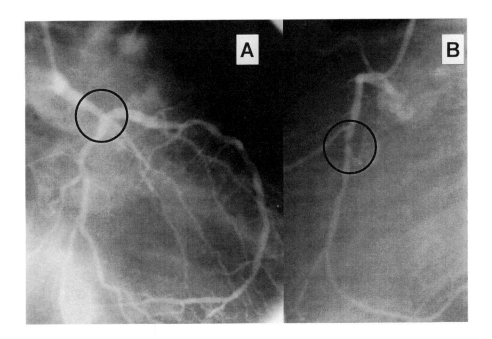

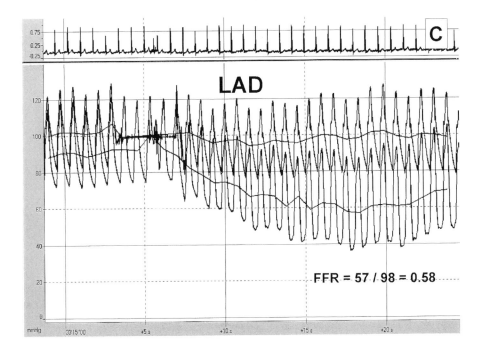

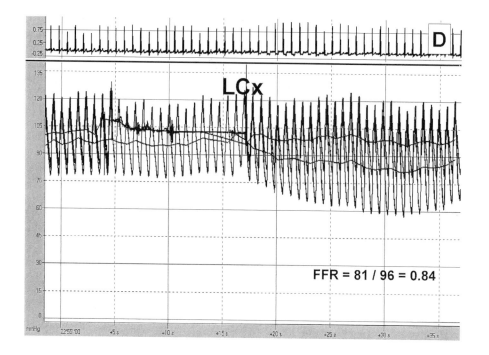

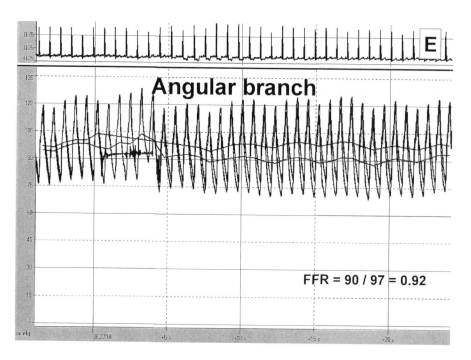

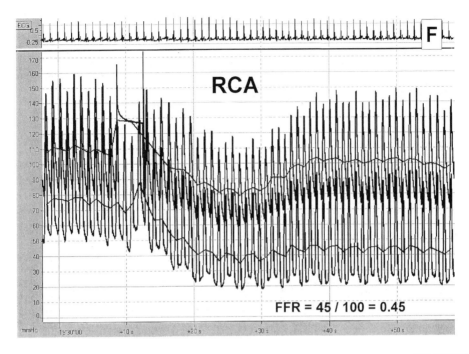

RCA

FFR = 45 / 100 = 0.45

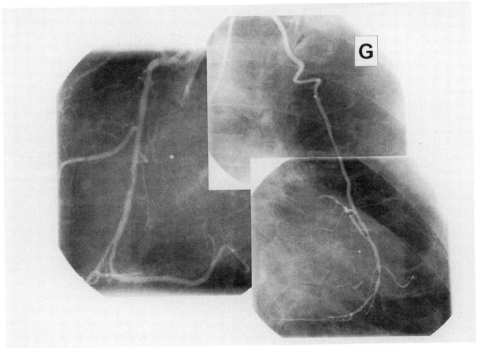

17.5 Left main disease.

Case 10:

Case history: A 36-year-old man was admitted because of recent onset typical chest pain with reversible ischemia on the ECG during episodes. At coronary angiography, a LM lesion of less than 50% was found (panel A and B). No other abnormalities were seen.

Problem: Does this lesion explain the ischemia on the ECG ? Could coronary spasm possibly play a role ?

Solution: When the pressure sensor is advanced across the left main stenosis into the LCX artery (panel D), a large resting gradient is present, which further increases at hyperemia and results in a FFR_{myo} of 0.45 (panel F). When the wire is placed in the LAD (panel C) and the sensor is moved across the LM stenosis and pulled back time and again during continuous hyperemia, a reproducible severe pressure drop is demonstrated (panel G). The patient had bypass surgery the next day with internal mammary grafts to both the LAD and LCX artery.

Comments: This case underlines the usefulness of coronary pressure measurements in intermediate stenosis. In particular, when the stenosis is

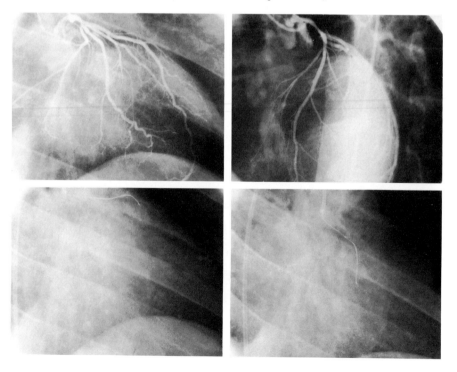

located in the left main coronary artery or the proximal part of a large branch, the consequences of demonstrating functional significance are important. In this patient, because of the ischemia on the ECG, surgery would probably have been performed anyhow. But often, when the anatomic severity is less than 50% and reversible ischemia less obvious, revascularization is deferred. In case of doubt, measurement of FFR_{myo} can either confirm the necessity of revascularization in some cases or avoid an unnecessary intervention in other cases.

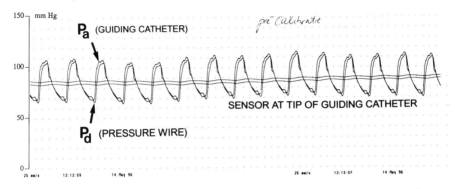

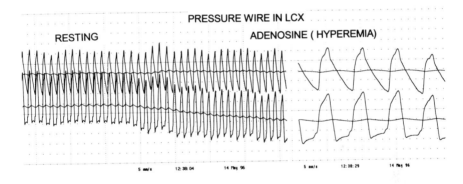

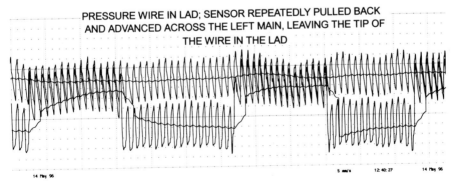

Case 11:

Case history: A 26-year-old man, with long-standing grade 2 aortic regurgitation and a mildly dilated and globally hypokinetic left ventricle, was admitted because of paroxysms of dyspnea and palpitations. He had never complained of chest pain. Aortic valve surgery was considered. At the pre-operative coronary angiogram, a stenosis of the left main stem was suspected (panel A and B, arrows). However, in no single projection this suspected ostial lesion appears really convincing.

Problem: Is there significant left main disease, which should also be treated and even may have contributed to the left ventricular dysfunction or to the paroxysmal complaints of this patient ?

Solution: Simultaneous pressure recordings are shown of the femoral pressure (through the side-arm of the femoral sheath), aortic pressure (through a 6F guiding catheter), and coronary pressure at the mid-LCX level (P_d, through a 0.014-in pressure guide wire). At rest, a gradient of 30 mmHg is already noticed, which increases to 54 mmHg after intracoronary adenosine injection. $FFR_{myo} = 54/117 = 0.46$ (panel C).

The gradient cannot be explained by the presence of the guiding catheter in the narrowed ostium since the femoral pressure and the pressure recorded through the guiding catheter, remain identical, even at hyperemia.

Comments: The presence of a tight left main stem stenosis was confirmed at surgery and the ostium of the left main stem was reconstructed.

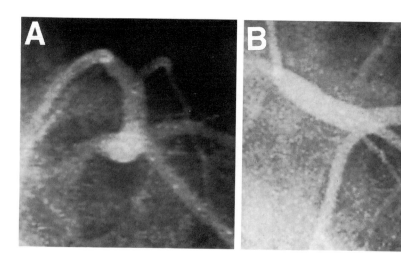

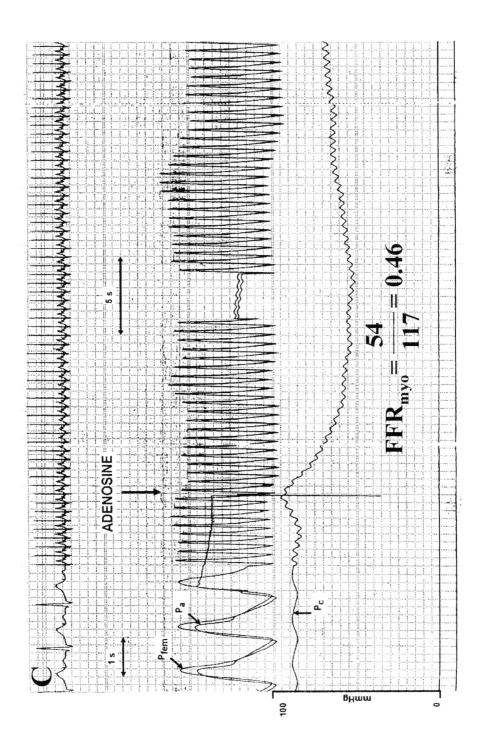

Case 12:

Case history: A 76-year-old man with non-insuline dependent diabetes and chronic renal insufficiency (creatinine: 3.7 mg%; ureum: 158 mg%) was admitted because of resting dyspnoe and thoracic complaints related to arterial hypertension (180/110 mm Hg at admission) with subacute pulmonary oedema. The resting ECG showed left axis deviation, high potentials and diffuse repolarisation abnormalities compatible with left ventricular hypertrophy. The echocardiogram, performed after disappearance of the pulmonary oedema showed a non dilated, mildly hypertrophic left ventricle with normal systolic function. At coronary angiography, diffuse coronary atherosclerosis was present without focal stenosis except at the level of the ostial left main where the angiographer described "a critical ostial stenosis with wedging of the pressure when intubating the main stem". The patient was referred for semi-urgent surgical revascularization.

Problem: Because of the operative risk in this old patient with diabetic nephropathy, it was decided to confirm the diagnosis of ostial left main stenosis by additional selective (panel A) and non-selective (panels B and C) contrast medium injections and intracoronary pressure measurements.

Solution: The non-selective injections in the left cusp showed a moderate ostial stenosis with a calculated minimal luminal diameter of 2.7 mm (panel C). The FFR across the stenosis was 0.94. Accordingly, the intervention was cancelled.

Case 11 and 12 illustrate the difficulties in evaluating left main stenosis especially when an ostial left main stenosis is suspected. The decision making process based on intracoronary pressure measurements had major prognostic implications in both cases and largely outweighted the minimal risk associated with the manipulation of a guide wire through a diseased left main. These examples also emphasize the need for a long-lasting hyperemic stimulus (papaverine or intravenous adenosine) as this is the only means to have a maximal vasodilation while disengaging the guiding catheter from the ostium.

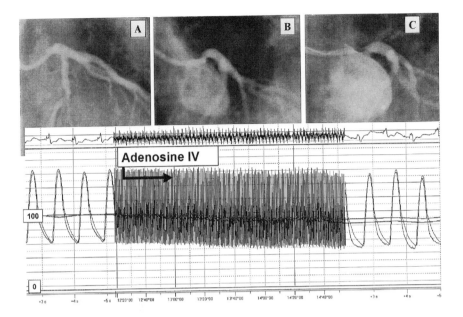

17.6   Epicardial versus microvascular disease.

Case 13:

Case history: A 68-year-old man was admitted for unstable angina with STdepression in the anterior leads. The coronary angiogram showed three-vessel disease with normal left ventricular function; chronic occlusion of the LCX (which had already been documented several years earlier), an angiographically tight stenosis in the proximal LAD (panel A) and a "moderate" stenosis in the mid-RCA (panel B). FFR associated with the stenosis in the proximal LAD was 0.42 (panel C); The latter stenosis was stented with good angiographic and functional result. The RCA stenosis was investigated by simultaneous Doppler flow velocity reserve (CFR) measurements and by pressure measurements (panel D).   CFR reached the too low value of 1.7.

Problem: Solely on the basis of this flow velocity assessment, it is impossible to determine whether the CFR is too low because of the presence of an epicardial stenosis or because of the presence of microvascular dysfunction.

Solution: FFR reached 0.86 suggesting that the contribution of the abnormal epicardial resistance to the decrease in CFR is probably small in the RCA.

Comments: This case illustrates the complementarity between CFR and FFR. More precisely, in this particular case the knowledge of both the CFR and the FFR enables us to predict that reestablishment of the epicardial conductance would lead to an increase in hyperemic perfusion pressure of 14 mmHg only and to an increase in CFR of (only) 14% (from 1.7 to 1.93).

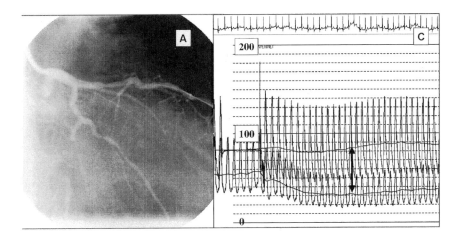

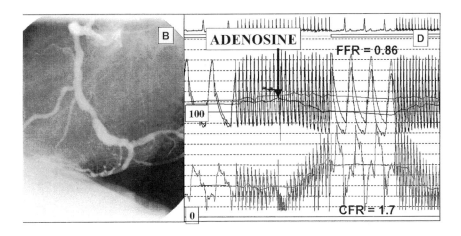

17.7 Previous myocardial infarction.

Case 14:

Case history: A 54-year-old man was admitted for "routine" coronary angiography after a transmural inferior wall infarction two weeks earlier. No non-invasive test had been performed. A subtotal stenosis in the dominant right coronary artery was seen. Coronary pressure measurement, however, showed a FFR of 0.78, apparently in contradiction with the severe stenosis.

Problem: How to proceed ? Should the lesion be dilated (as suggested by the angiogram) or does it make little sense to do PTCA (as suggested by the pressure measurement) ?

An additional measurement was performed by the Doppler wire and CFVR was as low as 1.2. The operator decided to perform PTCA, and a nice angiographic result was obtained (lower panels). However, despite this good angiographic result, CFVR did not increase at all and FFR only increased a little bit to 0.86.

Comments: Obviously, the reason for the low blood flow and CFVR in this patient was the simple fact that no or very little vital tissue was present anymore in the distribution area of the RCA. Therefore, PTCA was unnecessary and could have been avoided if one had relied upon the initial pressure measurement. If, across a severe lesion in an infarct-related artery, no significant pressure gradient can be provoked, this simply indicates transmural infarction with loss of vasodilatory response. The benefit of PTCA in such case is doubtful. In contrast, development of a significant pressure gradient at hyperemia not only indicates a significant stenosis but is also indicative of viable tissue (cf. case 15 in this chapter). At last, it is also important to realize that the functional significance of an epicardial coronary stenosis may change by decrease of the distribution area which can not be assessed by any anatomical method. These issues are extensively discussed in chapter 13.1.

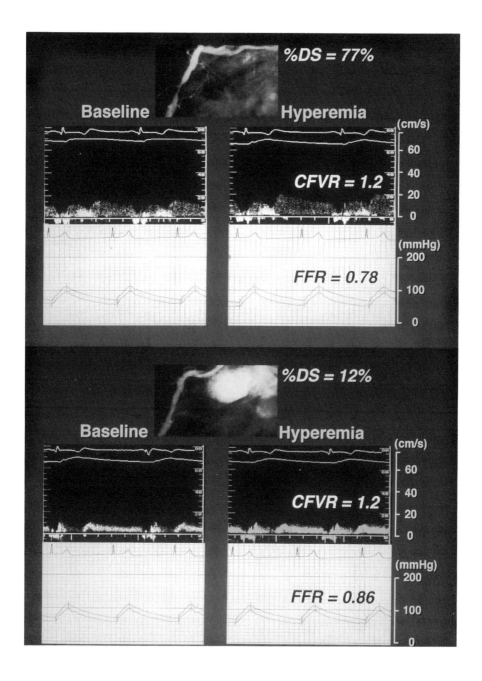

Case 15:

Case history: A 57-year-old male was admitted because of anterior wall infarction, successfully treated by r-tPA.

Five days later, coronary angiography was performed and a 67% stenosis was present in the proximal LAD-artery with a minimal luminal diameter of 1.34 mm (upper panel). Ventriculography showed akinesia of the complete anterior wall.

Problem: Is PTCA of the LAD-stenosis indicated ? Is there viable tissue in the anterior wall ?

Solution: Coronary pressure measurements were performed (middle panel) and a resting gradient was present of 10 mmHg which increased to 33 mmHg at i.v. adenosine induced hyperemia. This indicates viability of a significant amount of tissue in the anterior wall with preserved vasodilatory response, as well as functional significance of the LAD-stenosis (FFR 0.56), and justification of PTCA which was performed subsequently.

The lower panel shows the respective response to intracoronary injections of 20 μg of adenosine.

Echocardiography 6 weeks later showed only mild hypokinesia of the anterior wall and exercise testing was negative.

Comments: As extensively discussed in chapter 13.1, the response to vasodilatory stimuli and the ability to increase a transstenotic pressure gradient, is not only a measure for the residual significance of an infarct-related stenosis but also an indicator of myocardial viability. In contrast to the patient in case 14, an intervention was definitely indicated in this patient.

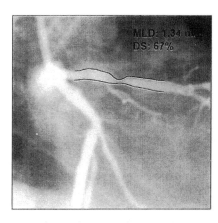
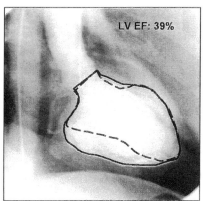
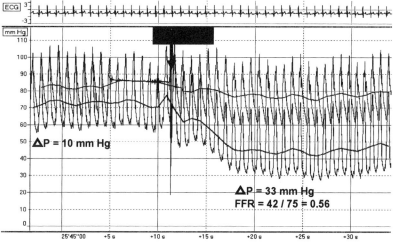
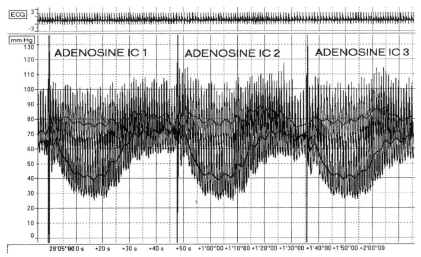

17.8 Diffuse disease.

Case 16:

Case history: A 54-year-old hyperlipemic male, heavy smoker, known for several years with typical exercise-induced angina and positive non-invasive tests, underwent coronary angiography. Diffuse disease was present in all 3 coronary arteries, but no significant anatomic stenosis was seen.

Problem: Can the diffuse disease or possibly small vessel disease explain the angina and the positive exercise test ?

Solution: After the pressure sensor has been placed in the very distal LAD, a significantly decreased FFR_{myo} of 0.72 is found. When the wire is pulled back during maximum hyperemia, however, no sudden pressure drop at a single location is seen, but a gradual decline of pressure along the complete course of the LAD. The same phenomenon was observed, to a somewhat lesser degree, in the LCX and RCA. Obviously, this patient cannot be helped by a coronary intervention. In this patient also Doppler derived CFVR was measured and equaled 1.52, 1.74, and 1.89 for the LAD, LCX, and RCA, respectively. This suggests that diffuse disease is not only present in the epicardial coronary arteries but also in the small vasculature.

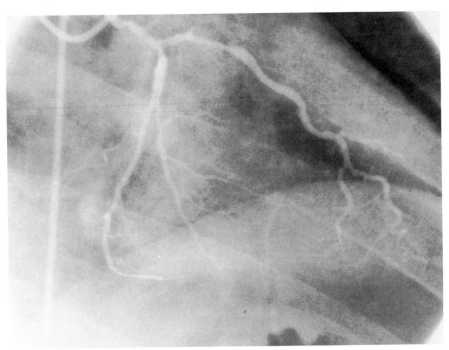

Comments: By proving that decline of pressure does not occur at one discrete site within the coronary artery, but is present diffusely along its entire course, potentially hazardous attempts to perform a coronary intervention, are avoided. Obviously, the treatment of choice must be medical (stopping of smoking, diet, statin therapy, and platelet-inhibitors).

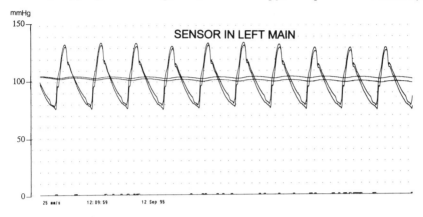

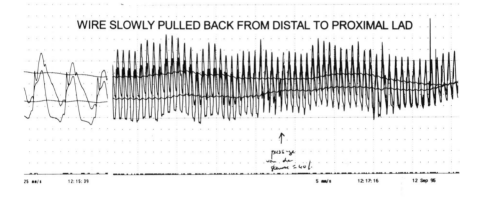

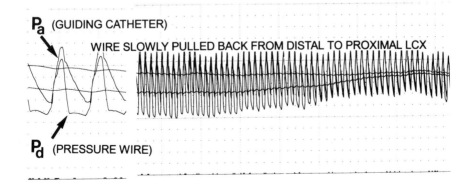

Case 17:

Case history: A 70-year-old lady with diabetes, hypertension, and a reversible perfusion defect in the inferior wall at MIBI-Spect imaging, was admitted for coronary angiography. Diffuse disease was present throughout the arterial tree, without any circumscript stenosis to which the complaints could be attributed (panel A).

Problem: Can this patient be helped by a coronary intervention or is medical treatment the best choice ?

Solution: Because the ischemia was located in the inferior wall, a pressure wire was advanced into the distal RCA, intravenous adenosine infusion was started, hyperemia induced (panel B), and a slow pull-back pressure recording was made under fluoroscopy during sustained maximum hyperemia (panel C). Although disease is diffusely present along the complete RCA, there was a sudden pressure drop at the mid-RCA and a stent was placed at that particular location. A good angiographic result was obtained (panel D) and when the pressure pull-back recording was repeated after stenting, only a minor pressure drop of a few mmHg was present across the stent, indicating good stent deployment (panel E). As also shown by the pressure pull-back curve in panel E, there is some gradient now in the more proximal part of the RCA, not visible before the intervention but unmasked now because of the increased blood flow through the vessel after stenting the most severe lesion. FFR after PTCA equals 70/81 = 0.88 which in this case can be considered as a satisfactory result.

Comments: Case 16 and 17 show the unique appropriateness of coronary pressure measurement to determine in patients with diffuse disease if adequate treatment and relieve of symptoms can be expected by a coronary intervention (local pressure drop) or that either medical or surgical treatment is indicated (diffuse decline of pressure along the artery).

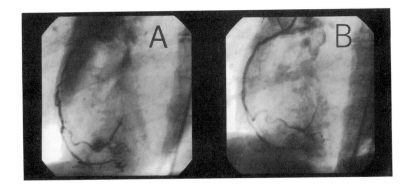

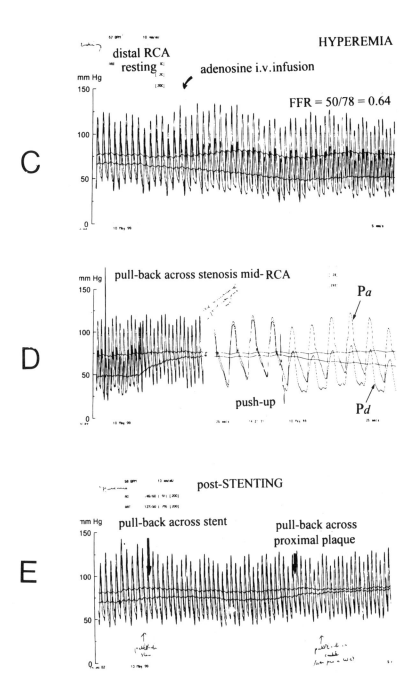

C — HYPEREMIA

distal RCA resting — adenosine i.v. infusion

FFR = 50/78 = 0.64

D — pull-back across stenosis mid-RCA

P*a*

push-up

P*d*

E — post-STENTING

pull-back across stent — pull-back across proximal plaque

17.9   Serial stenoses.

Case 18: Influence of the proximal lesion on FFR$_{myo}$ of the distal lesion.

Case history: A 71-year-old lady was admitted for PTCA of 2 sequential lesions in the proximal LAD-artery (left panel below). What is the influence of the presence of the proximal stenosis ("stenosis A") on the FFR$_{myo}$ of the distal stenosis ("stenosis B") ?

To answer this question, the pressure wire is positioned in the distal LAD and slowly pulled back to the ostium of the LAD artery during sustained hyperemia. The locations and respective pressure drops at the site of the stenosis are easily identified (arrows). Fractional flow reserve of the distal myocardium, called FFR (A+B), equals 52/80 = 0.65 (left hand side of the upper panel on the next page) and the apparent value of FFR (B) equals 51/63 = 0.81.

The value of FFR (B), predicted form the measured pressures by the equation in paragraph 13.4, equals 0.78 (P_a = 80; P_m = 63; P_d = 51; P_w = 24 mmHg, respectively).

After having stented the proximal stenosis, a similar pull-back curve is made (middle panel on the next page). The gradient across stenosis A has completely disappeared and, as a result, the gradient across stenosis B has increased from 12 to 17 mmHg. True FFR (B) equals 57/74 = 0.77. The lower panel on the next page shows the pull-back curve after having stented both lesions. Almost no hyperemic gradient is present anymore and FFR has increased to 0.98 (excellent result).

Comments: This case illustrates how serial lesions within one vessel can be separately assessed by coronary pressure measurements, and how the hemodynamic appearance and FFR$_{myo}$ of a distal lesion is influenced by the presence of a proximal lesion and can already be predicted by the equations in chapter 13.4.

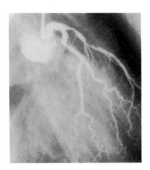 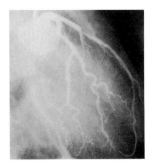 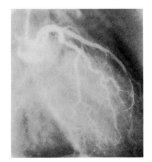

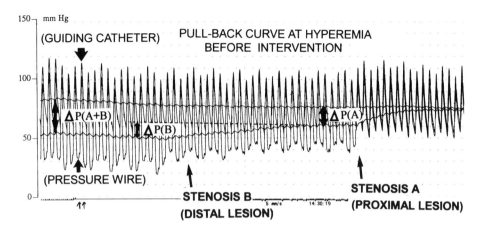

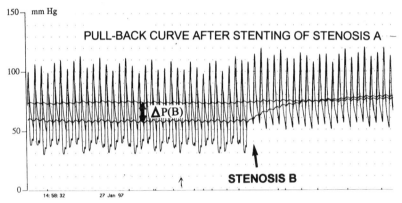

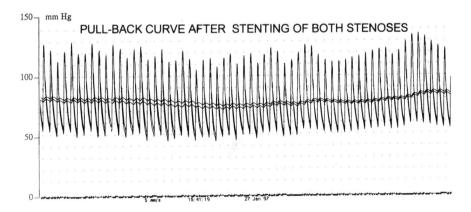

Case 19: Unmasking a proximal gradient by dilating a distal stenosis.

Case history: The left panel below shows the RCA of a 54-year-old male with several stenoses.
Problem: What is the contribution of each separate lesion to decreased blood flow and how do these lesions influence each other ?
Answer: In the *upper panel* on the next page the pressure wire is positioned distal to the distal stenosis (B), and pulled back slowly to the ostium of the RCA during sustained hyperemia. A large pressure drop, ΔP (B), is observed when the sensor crosses the distal stenosis, and a much smaller pressure drop, ΔP (A), is present across the mid-RCA stenosis (A), suggesting that stenosis A is not very severe from a functional point of view.
P_a, P_m and P_d in this tracing are 112, 98, and 51 mmHg, respectively and P_w equaled 21 mmHg. Therefore, the apparent value of the fractional flow reserve related to stenosis A, is 90/112 = 0.88, but the equation from chapter 13.4 predicts that its true value must be lower, i.e. 0.74 in this case.
Middle panel: After PTCA of the stenosis B, ΔP (B) has decreased from 46 to 15 mmHg and, as blood flow through the artery has increased, ΔP (A) has increased from 15 to 27 mmHg, unmasking the true severity of stenosis A. The value of FFR (A), derived from this tracing is 0.75 and very close to its predicted value. The *lower panel* shows the final pull-back curve after having stented both lesions. No residual gradient is present anymore across stenosis B and a residual gradient of 12 mmHg remains present across stenosis A. Final FFR of the myocardium supplied by the RCA has increased from 0.46 to 0.84 (moderate result).
Comments: Before the intervention, only a moderate pressure gradient was observed across the mid-RCA stenosis. After blood flow through the vessel had increased by stenting the distal stenosis, a large gradient developed across the proximal stenosis as predicted by the equation.

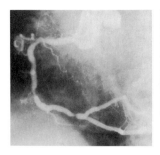
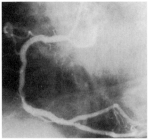
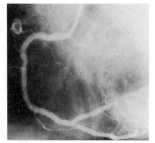

PULL-BACK CURVE AT MAXIMUM HYPEREMIA
BEFORE INTERVENTION

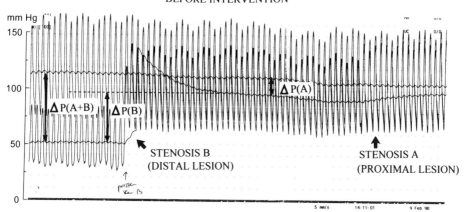

mm Hg
150
100
50
0

ΔP(A+B) ΔP(B) ΔP(A)

STENOSIS B
(DISTAL LESION)

STENOSIS A
(PROXIMAL LESION)

5 mm/s   14:11:01   9 Feb 98

PULL-BACK CURVE AFTER PTCA OF DISTAL LESION (STENOSIS B)

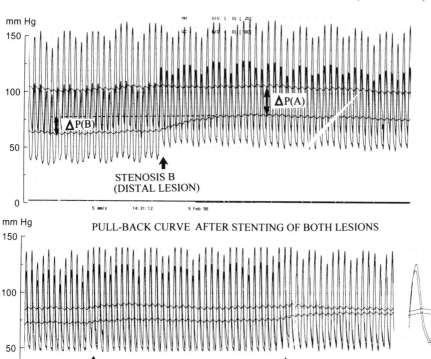

mm Hg
150
100
50
0

ΔP(B) ΔP(A)

STENOSIS B
(DISTAL LESION)

5 mm/s   14:31:12   9 Feb 98

mm Hg
150
100
50
0

PULL-BACK CURVE AFTER STENTING OF BOTH LESIONS

STENOSIS B
(DISTAL LESION)

STENOSIS A
(PROXIMAL LESION)

9 Feb 98   5 mm/s   15:09:11   25 mm/s

17.10 Collaterals.

Case 20: Protection by collaterals.

Case history: A 54-year-old man was referred for PTCA of a proximal LAD stenosis and 2 LCX stenoses (panel A). It is interesting to note that the LCX artery has 3 distal branches, 2 of which are filled by visible collaterals from the LAD and RCA, respectively (panel A and B). The third branch (the AV-groove branch) is not visually filled by collaterals.
Problems: 1.Should the LAD-stenosis be dilated ?
          2.How extensive is collateral flow to the different LCX branches.
Solution: At first, a pressure wire was advanced across the LAD lesion, which was not significant as indicated by a FFR_{myo} of 0.87. Therefore,

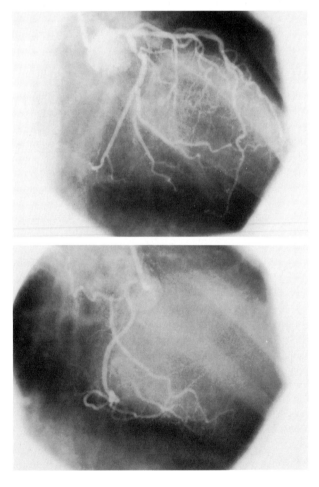

PTCA of the LAD was deferred. Second, a balloon was inflated in the proximal LCX lesion. Recruitable collateral blood flow was calculated by $(P_w - P_v)/(P_a - P_v)$ and equaled 0.24, which means that the recruitable collaterals can maintain at most 24% of normal maximum myocardial perfusion. No changes on the (already abnormal) ECG were seen at that 2-minute balloon occlusion. Next, the balloon was inflated in the more distal LCX-lesion, the pressure wire being positioned in the AV-groove branch. This time, recruitable fractional collateral flow to that part of the myocardium, was only 0.13, corresponding with 13% of normal maximum perfusion of that territory. As may be expected, severe ECG changes were seen at balloon occlusion.

Comments: The promising value of fractional collateral flow as a quantitative index of collateral development, and its value in predicting protection against ischemia, is demonstrated in this case.

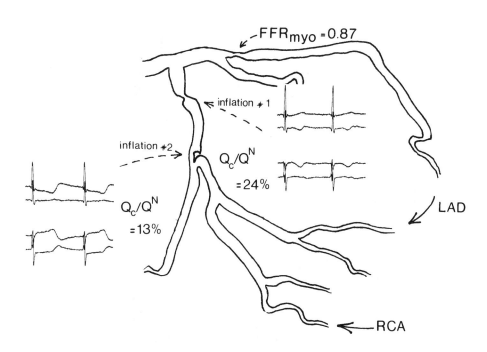

Case 21: Mild stenosis becoming significant by increase of the myocardial territory to be supplied.

Case history: A 52-year-old man presented with angina pectoris and a reversible perfusion defect at MIBI-Spect imaging in the inferior wall and apex. At coronary angiography, the RCA was completely occluded, and filled by collaterals from the LAD-artery which had a 50% stenosis in its proximal part.

Problem: Does this moderate lesion explain the perfusion defect ? What is the treatment of choice ?

Solution: Despite the only moderate stenosis in the LAD, coronary pressure measurement showed a significant gradient at hyperemia, resulting in a FFR of 0.68.

Comments: This large gradient and low FFR can be understood by realizing that the distribution area of the LAD has been largely increased beyond its normal size because also the inferior wall is supplied now by this artery. Therefore, a mild stenosis (which would probably not be significant by itself), becomes significant now and the patient underwent bypass surgery with 2 internal mammarian grafts to the LAD and RCA, respectively.

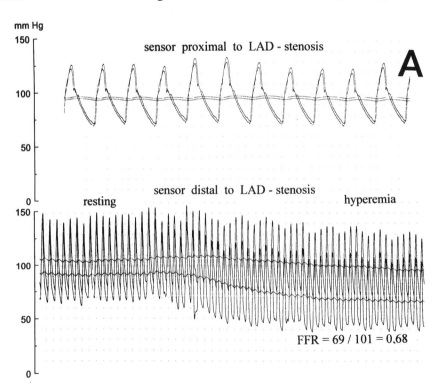

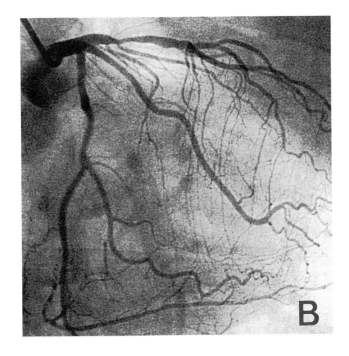

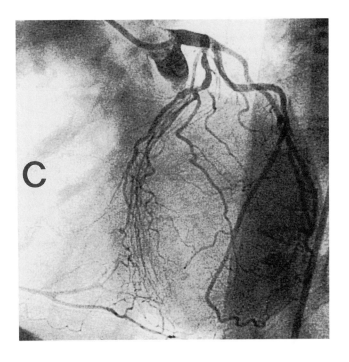

17.11 Evaluation of PTCA.

Case 22:

Case history: The angiograms of a 52-year-old male are shown before and after PTCA of a proximal LAD stenosis, monitored by intracoronary pressure recordings. The pressure wire was used as primary guide wire in this case. Therefore, all essential steps in monitoring an intervention are obtained and displayed on the next page. All pressures recorded at the different steps and the calculated values of FFR$_{myo}$, FFR$_{cor}$, and fractional collateral flow, are displayed in the matrix.

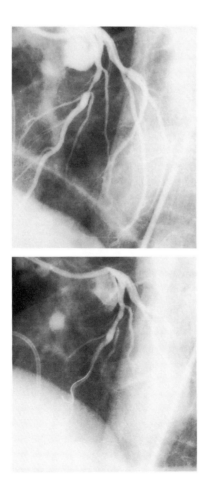

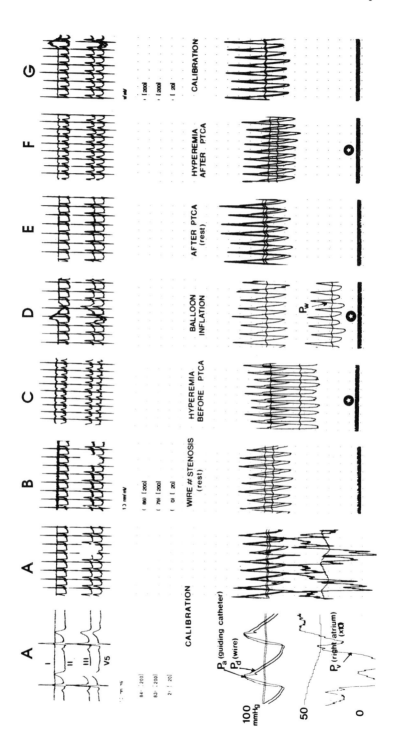

	Before PTCA	Balloon occlusion	After PTCA
P_a	81	85	83
P_d	53	-	76
P_v	4	5	6
P_w	(19)	21	(21)

	Before PTCA	Balloon occlusion	After PTCA
FFR_{myo}	0.64	0.20	0.91
FFR_{cor}	0.55	0.00	0.89
Q_c/Q^N	0.09	0.20	0.02

Comments: Such a matrix completely elucidates the functional effects of the stenosis and its influence on myocardial blood flow, both before and after PTCA. Moreover, as the post-PTCA angiogram is excellent, no significant dissection is present, and FFR_{myo} exceeds 0.90, no stent was placed. Follow-up after 2.5 years was excellent.

Case 23:

Case history: The angiograms (below) and all relevant pressure tracings (next page) are shown in a 74-year-old male before, during, and after PTCA of a RCA stenosis. Also in this patient, the pressure wire was used as primary guide wire. The matrix shows the relevant values of all fractional flow indexes.

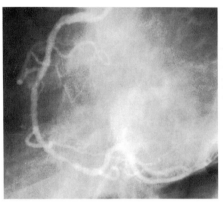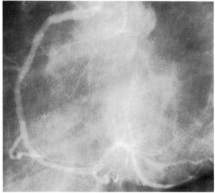

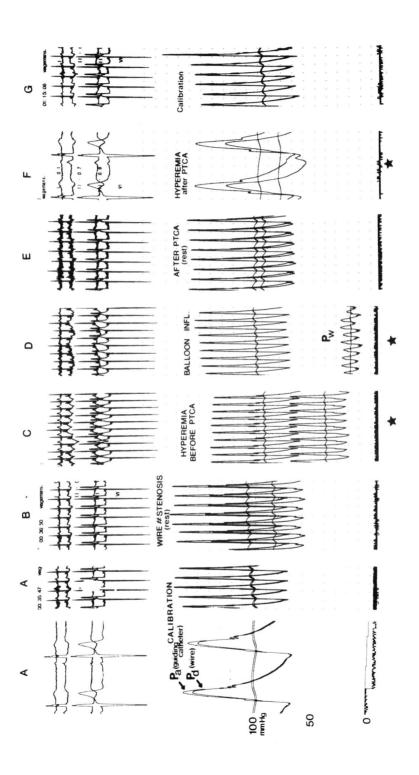

	Before PTCA	Balloon occlusion	After PTCA
P_a	90	101	98
P_d	42	-	82
P_v	2	5	2
P_w	(14)	18	(15)

	Before PTCA	Balloon occlusion	After PTCA
FFR_{myo}	0.45	0.14	0.83
FFR_{cor}	0.37	0.00	0.81
Q_c/Q^N	0.08	0.14	0.02

Comments: Post-PTCA FFR_{myo} equals 0.83, indicating a moderate functional result, despite the optimal angiogram. As this procedure was performed 4 years ago before the "stent-era" and at a time when we were not yet very well aware of the meaning and the interpretation of post-PTCA FFR_{myo}, no additional stent was implanted. Nevertheless, the clinical course was favorable and the patient is still in class I with minimal medication.

17.12 Evaluation of adequate stent deployment.

Note: A number of examples of FFR$_{myo}$ after stent implantation have been shown already in figure 14.7 and 14.11 and in case 18 and 19 of this chapter. Another example is given below.

Case 24:

Case history: A 38-year-old man was referred because of restenosis after regular PTCA of a proximal LAD stenosis 5 weeks earlier. It was decided to perform elective stenting, monitored by a pressure wire. The angiograms (below) and pressure recordings both before and after placement of a 3.0 Wiktor stent, are shown (next 2 pages). An inflation pressure of 12 atm was necessary to normalize the conductance of the stented segment, reflected by normalization of FFR$_{myo}$.

Note: If other disease is present in the stented vessel, to evaluate stent deployment, the ratio between the hyperemic pressure just distal to the stent and the hyperemic pressure just proximal to the stent, should be used.

Comments: If a pressure wire is used as first-line guide wire, all steps from initial diagnosis to final evaluation of the intervention can be made with one simple, relatively inexpensive, device.

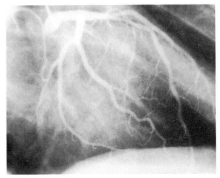
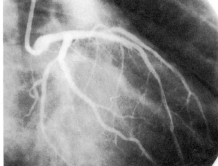

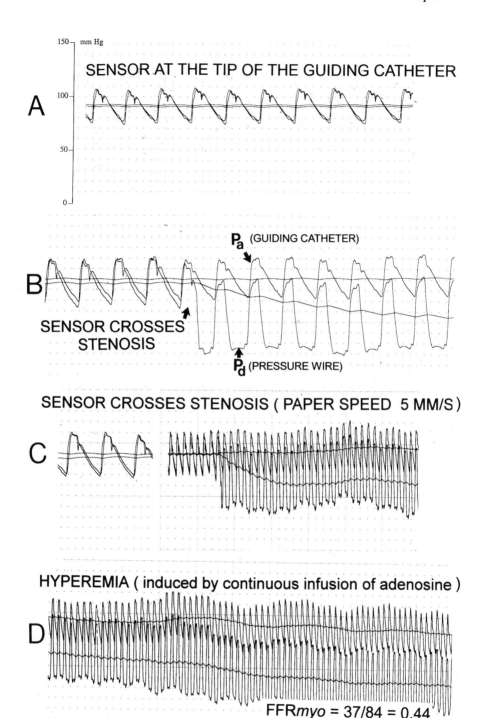

150 — mm Hg

SENSOR AT THE TIP OF THE GUIDING CATHETER

A 100 —

50 —

0 —

B

P$_a$ (GUIDING CATHETER)

SENSOR CROSSES STENOSIS

P$_d$ (PRESSURE WIRE)

SENSOR CROSSES STENOSIS (PAPER SPEED 5 MM/S)

C

HYPEREMIA (induced by continuous infusion of adenosine)

D

$FFRmyo = 37/84 = 0.44$

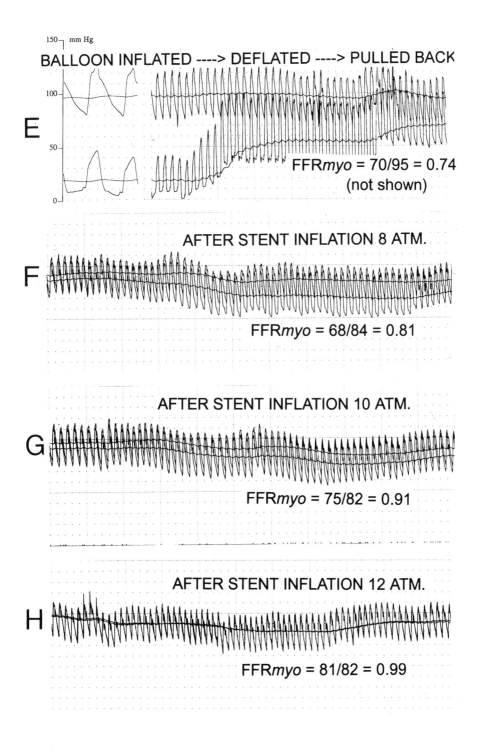

150 mm Hg

BALLOON INFLATED ----> DEFLATED ----> PULLED BACK

100

E

50

FFR*myo* = 70/95 = 0.74
(not shown)

0

AFTER STENT INFLATION 8 ATM.

F

FFR*myo* = 68/84 = 0.81

AFTER STENT INFLATION 10 ATM.

G

FFR*myo* = 75/82 = 0.91

AFTER STENT INFLATION 12 ATM.

H

FFR*myo* = 81/82 = 0.99

17.13 Unmasking of proximal gradient by PTCA or stenting a distal stenosis.

Case 25:

Case history: A 73-year-old man presented with typical crescendo anginal chest pain. No non-invasive stress testing was available before catheterization. The coronary angiogram (panel A and B) showed a 'critical' stenosis in the mid-RCA. Ad-hoc angioplasty (direct stenting) was performed. A pressure-monitoring guide wire was used to monitor the

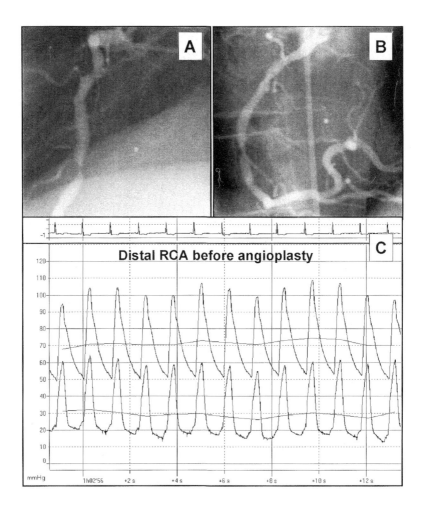

procedure. The pressure tracing during maximal hyperemia before angioplasty is shown in panel C. After stenting of the lesion in the mid-RCA (panel D and E), an unacceptable FFR of 0.62 (panel F) persisted in spite of a satisfactory angiographic result. Yet, when the sensor was pulled back

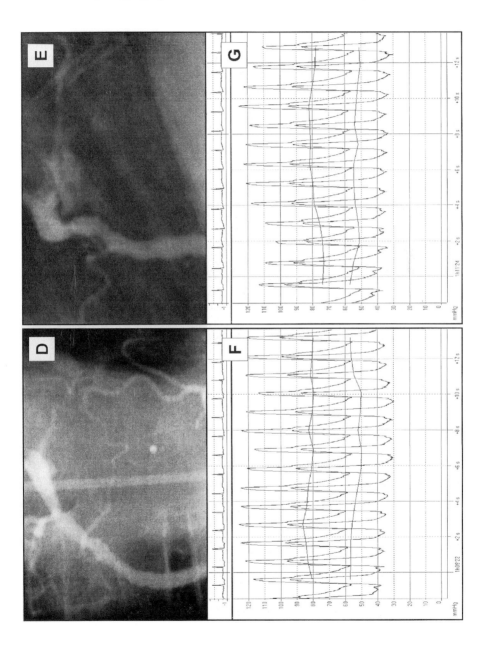

under hyperemia proximal to the stent, a similar value of FFR was observed (panel G). This indicated that the residual hyperemic pressure gradient was not due to the stented segment but to the segment proximal to the stent. Accordingly, a second stent was deployed in the proximal lesion with, this time, both a good angiographic (panel H and I) and functional result (panel J) with a FFR of 0.94.

Comments: This example illustrates that the hemodynamic significance of a stenosis, which is not immediately apparent at angiography, can be unmasked by reestablishment of the conductance of another stenosis (upstream or downstream). It is important to recognize that such gradient originating in the proximal part of the vessel, is not indicative for drift but a pathophysiologic phenomenon unmasked by the pressure measurement.

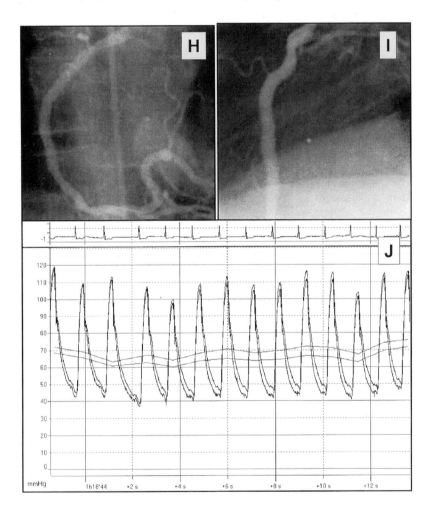

Chapter 18

CONCLUSIONS AND PERSPECTIVES FOR THE FUTURE

The usefulness of coronary pressure measurement has been recognized by the pioneers of balloon angioplasty, as testified by the presence of a fluid-filled lumen in the first generation of balloon catheters[1]. Since these early days, the interest in measuring distal coronary pressure has fluctuated between enthusiasm for having a simple index to assess coronary hemodynamics and disillusion due to the inconsistency of the results[2-6].

During the last years, the interest in coronary pressure measurement has revived because of two reasons, namely on one hand the technical progress in developing pressure-monitoring guide wires, and on the other hand a theoretical innovation, namely the concept of fractional flow reserve which closely relates distal coronary pressure to myocardial blood flow. Progress made in this field over the last 6 years is reported in this book and can be summarized as follows:

- Coronary pressure measurement can be performed easily, rapidly, and safely in patients with coronary artery disease and can be obtained in the setting of both diagnostic and interventional catheterization.

- As demonstrated theoretically and validated in-vitro, in animals, and in humans, pressure-derived fractional flow reserve (FFR_{myo}) represents the fraction of normal maximum myocardial flow which is preserved despite the presence of a coronary stenosis and can simply be derived from the ratio of two pressures recorded during maximal vasodilation.

- The contribution of collateral blood flow is taken into account by FFR_{myo}.

- The normal value of pressure-derived FFR_{myo} unequivocally equals 1.

- The values of pressure-derived FFR_{myo} are very reproducible irrespective of the prevailing systemic hemodynamic conditions and the contractility of the left ventricle.

- Pressure-derived FFR_{myo} can be used as a surrogate for a stress test for on-line clinical decision-making in the catheterization laboratory. Values lower than 0.75 are almost always associated with exercise-induced myocardial ischemia, while values higher than 0.75 most often exclude objective signs of ischemia during exercise. The accuracy of FFR_{myo} for that purpose is approximately 95% and higher than that of any single non-invasive test.

- The prognosis is favorable in patients in whom a planned angioplasty was deferred on the basis of coronary pressure measurements.

- After regular balloon angioplasty, the combination of a good angiographic result (residual diameter stenosis < 35% in the absence of a dissection type C to F) and a value of $FFR_{myo} \geq 0.90$, is associated with a very low cardiac event rate during a 2-year follow-up.

- After stent implantation, FFR_{myo} should normalize. If this is not the case, stent deployment was imperfect.

- FFR provides valuable information in many other and complex situations encountered in the catheterization laboratory, including multivessel and diffuse disease , previous myocardial infarction, serial stenoses, and intermediate left main disease.

- Fractional flow reserve is especially helpful in the selection of patients with multivessel disease who may be suitable candidates for either minimal invasive cardiac surgery or hybride revascularization.

Coronary pressure-measuring guide wires might play a dual role in the context of the diagnostic and therapeutic procedure: distal coronary pressure measurement may help in the decision whether or not to revascularize a coronary stenosis, and may also help in the assessment of the post-intervention result. A further expansion of coronary pressure measurement and the acceptance of coronary pressure-based clinical decision-making will depend on several factors:

(1) Further technical developments in pressure guide wires. At the time this book goes to press, the two pressure measuring guide wires which are commercially available now, are very close to regular angioplasty wires in terms of torquability, steerability, and trackability (Radi Pressure Wire and Endosonics Wavewire). With the latest version of these pressure measuring guide wires, progressive drift of the pressure recorded by the sensor is no longer a matter of concern. Some technical problems related the frequent disconnection and reconnection inherent to most interventional procedures still have to be solved.

Especially interesting is the development of sensors which combine pressure measurement and flow measurement, the latter based upon the thermodilution principle. By combining FFR and -independently measured- CFR within one sensor, complete insight will be obtained in the distribution of disease in both the epicardial coronary arteries and the microvasculature.

(2) The relationship between stenosis severity and prognosis. Coronary pressure and coronary flow reserve measurements determine whether or not the epicardial stenosis is "significant", i.e. flow-limiting or capable of causing reversible myocardial ischemia under conditions of increased demand. Like coronary angiography and most other diagnostic techniques, coronary pressure measurements provide an instantaneous picture of the severity of the coronary narrowing not taking into account its dynamic nature. Yet, whether the prognosis of patients with known coronary artery disease depends more on the propensity of a small plaque to rupture rather than on the presence of a "significant" stenosis, remains controversial. The prognosis of a patients with coronary artery disease being mainly determined by vessel occlusion, the classically accepted relationship between severity of the lesion and patient prognosis has recently been refuted. Myocardial infarctions have indeed been shown to result often from the occlusion of a previously mildly narrowed coronary segment assessed at angiography[7-10]. Even though these studies were small sized (less than 200 patients in total) this notion has rapidly been expanded in the believe that hemodynamically insignificant plaques bear a higher risk than flow-limiting stenoses. It should be reminded, however, that histopathological studies from patients with fatal coronary events have consistently shown that the stenosis underlying the site of plaque rupture was severe[11]. Data from the CASS study suggested that the individual risk of total coronary occlusion of a coronary stenosis after 5 years increased almost exponentially with its angiographic severity[12]. Furthermore, quantitative analysis of the angiogram

of these patients has demonstrated that besides left ventricular ejection fraction, the severity of coronary lesions as assessed by quantitative coronary angiography is a strong independent indicator of subsequent myocardial infarction over a long period of follow-up[13]. Recent data based on precise IVUS measure of stenosis severity demonstrated an almost exponential inverse relation between minimal cross sectional area and cardiac event rate after 13 months[14]. Finally, the powerful prognostic value of non-invasive stress testing in patients with coronary artery disease strongly supports the evidence that patients with lesions severe enough to induce reversible myocardial ischemia have markedly worse prognosis than patients with similar lesions but in whom stress testing is normal[15]. In particular, studies performed in large cohorts of patients have demonstrated a favorable prognosis in patients with documented coronary artery disease but a negative exercise-ECG[16-18]. Since we have demonstrated that pressure-derived fractional flow reserve can be used as a surrogate for a regular exercise-ECG in the clinical decision-making process during catheterization, it is likely that a high value of FFR_{myo} bears the same favorable prognostic information. If, in the next years, it would become apparent that there is no relationship between lesions severity and patients prognosis, coronary pressure (or any functional measure of coronary stenosis severity) would lose a lot of its value. In contrast, if it appears that functionally non-significant lesions are associated with a favorable prognosis without any mechanical treatment, coronary pressure measurements will be very useful for on-line clinical decision-making in such patients. The latter hypothesis is supported by preliminary results of the prospective, randomized DEFER trial reported in this book. The final results of that study are expected to be published soon.

(3) Decrease in restenosis rate after coronary stenting. The results of new methods aiming at reducing restenosis, particularly in-stent restenosis, will determine the usefulness of pressure-derived fractional flow reserve in the evaluation of coronary interventions. In the hypothetical (and unlikely) case where in-stent restenosis rate would be reduced to almost zero, no reason would persist for not stenting all lesions amenable to stenting. If, on the contrary, it appears that the restenosis rate after stenting of non-selected patients remains considerable, pressure-based provisional stenting could prove to be an elegant alternative to a "stent-them-all" policy. Similar considerations refer to brachytherapy.

(4) Cost of coronary stenting. In the present era of cost constraints, the price of coronary stenting will be important in distinguishing patients who would

and who would not benefit from coronary stenting after an angiographically successful balloon dilatation. In the hypothetical case where stents were free, stenting could be performed more liberally.

(5) The development of new techniques to investigate the coronary circulation. As long as coronary angioplasty and bypass surgery remain the main therapeutic options in coronary artery disease, coronary angiography will continue to serve as a road-map for the operator. The continuous improvement in quality of the radiographic images will facilitate further the introduction of guide wires into the coronary tree. It is therefore impossible to foresee to what extent emerging technologies like magnetic resonance imaging will replace the invasive assessment of the coronary circulation. To become a significant challenger to selective coronary catheterization in the diagnosis and treatment of coronary artery disease, these new technologies should be non-invasive and highly reproducible. Most importantly, new diagnostic techniques should provide information both on the lumen of the vessel and on the nature of the atherosclerotic plaque[19].

Whatever the future developments of interventional cardiology will be, it holds true that coronary pressure measurements and FFR_{myo} determine precisely to what extent a given epicardial stenosis limits hyperemic blood flow to the underlying myocardium. Given the fact that stenting is not possible in all coronary lesions, that the restenosis rate after a regular balloon angioplasty exceeds 30%, that in-stent restenosis is still a matter for concern, that angioplasty of a non-significant stenosis may transform the latter into a flow-limiting stenosis, and that coronary bypass surgery is not without morbidity and mortality, it seems desirable to demonstrate the hemodynamic significance of a lesion before embarking on any revascularization procedure. It is acknowledged, however, that the correlations between pressure measurement and signs of reversible myocardial ischemia were obtained only in stable patients. Therefore, these results should not be extended to patients with unstable ischemic syndromes. In the latter subset, clinical and electrocardiographic criteria must keep their prominent role in therapeutic decision-making.

With this caveat in mind, we believe that fractional flow reserve can be used for on-line clinical decision-making to justify ad-hoc angioplasty on one hand and to avoid unnecessary intervention in stable patients on the other hand[20]. This applies especially when the significance of the lesion is questionable and no non-invasive functional evaluation has been performed as is often the case[21], but also extends to many other complex diagnostic situations encountered in the catheterization laboratory. The role of fractional flow reserve for on-line evaluation of coronary interventions, is promising but its position has to be further established by some large prospective randomized studies.

References.

1. Gruentzig AR, Senning A, Siegenthaler WE. Non-operative dilatation of coronary artery stenosis. *New Engl J Med* 1979;301:61-68.
2. Rothman MT, Baim DS, Simpson JB, Harrison DC. Coronary hemodynamics during percutaneous transluminal coronary angioplasty. *Am J Cardiol* 1982;49:1615-1622.
3. Haraphongse M, Tymchak W, Burton JR, Rossal RE. Implication of transstenotic pressure gradient measurement during coronary artery angioplasty. *Cathet Cardiovasc Diagn* 1986;12:80-84.
4. Leimgruber PP, Roubin GS, Hollman J. Restenosis after successful coronary angioplasty in patients with single-vessel disease. *Circulation* 1986;73:710-717.
5. Anderson HV, Roubin GS, Leimgruber PP, Cox WR, Douglas JS, King III SB, Gruentzig AR. Measurement of transstenotic pressure gradients during percutaneous transluminal angioplasty. *Circulation* 1986;73:1223-1230.
6. Serruys PW, Wijns W, Reiber JHC. Values and limitations of transstenotic pressure gradients measured during percutaneous coronary angioplasty. *Herz* 1985;10:337-342
7. Ambrose JA, Tannenbaum MA, Alexopoulos D, Hjemdahl-Monsen CE, Leavy J, Weiss M, Borrico S, Gorlin R, Fuster V. Angiographic progression of coronary artery disease and the development of myocardial infarction. *J Am Coll Cardiol* 1988;12:56-62.
8. Little WC, Constantinescu M, Applegate RJ, Kutcher MA, Burrows MT, Kahl FR, Santamore WP. Can coronary angiography predict the site of a subsequent myocardial infarction in patients with mild-to-moderate coronary artery disease ? *Circulation* 1988;78:1157-1166.
9. Nobuyoshi M, Tanaka M, Nosaka H, Kimura T, Yokio H, Hamasaki N, Kim K, Shindo T, Kimura K. Progression of coronary atherosclerosis: is coronary spasm related to progression? *J Am Coll Cardiol* 1991;18:904-910.
10. Giroud D, Li JM, Urban P, Meier B, Rutishauser W. Relation of the site of acute myocardial infarction to the most severe coronary arterial stenosis at prior angiography. *Am J Cardiol* 1992;69:729-732.
11. Fishbein MC, Siegel RJ. How big are coronary atherosclerotic plaques that rupture? *Circulation* 1996;94:2662-2666.
12. Alderman EL, Corley SD, Fisher LD, Chaitman BR, Faxon DP, Foster ED, Killip T, Sosa JA, Bourassa MG. Five-year angiographic follow-up of factors associated with progression of coronary artery disease in the CASS-study. *JACC* 1993; 22: 1141-1154.
13. Mancini GBJ, Bourassa MG, Williamson PR, Leclerc G, DeBoe SF, Pitt B, Lesperance J. Prognostic importance of quantitative analysis of coronary cineangiograms. *Am J Cardiol* 1992;69:1022-1027.

14. Abizaid AS, Mintz GS, Mehran R, Abizaid A, Lansky A, Pichard AD, Satler LF, Hongsheng W, Pappas C. Kent K, Leon MB. Long-term follow-up after PTCA was not performed based on intravascular ultrasound findings. *Circulation* 1999; 100: 256-261.
15. Pavin D, Delonca J, Siegenthaler M, Doat M, Rutishauser W, Righetti A. Long-term (10 years) prognostic value of a normal thallium-201 myocardial exercise scintigraphy in patients with coronary artery disease documented by angiography. *Eur Heart J* 1997;18:69-77.
16. Weiner DA, Ryan TJ, McCabe CH, Chaitman BR, Sheffield LT, Fergusson JC, Fisher LD, Tristani F. Prognostic importance of a clinical profile and exercise test in medically treated patients with coronary artery disease. *J Am Coll Cardiol* 1984;3:772-779.
17. Wijns W, Musschaert-Beauthier E, van Domburg R, Lubsen J, Rousseau MF, Cosyns J, Detry JMR. Prognostic value of symptom limited exercise testing in men with a high prevalence of coronary artery disease. *Eur Heart J* 1985;6:939-945.
18. Mark DB, Hlatky MA, Harrell FE Jr, Lee KL, Califf RM, Pryor DB. Exercise treadmill score for predicting prognosis in coronary artery disease. *Ann Int Med* 1987;106:793-800.
19. Libby P. Lesion versus lumen. *Nature Med* 1995;1:17-18.
20. Meier B. Combining coronary angiography and angioplasty. *Heart* 1996;75:8-10.
21. Topol EJ, Ellis SE, Cosgrove DM, Bates ER, Muller DWM, Schork NJ, Schork MA, Loop FD. Analysis of coronary angioplasty practice in the United States with an insurance-claims data base. *Circulation* 1993;87:1489-1497.

Index